Get **more** out of libraries

Please return or renew this item by the last date shown.
You can renew online at www.hants.gov.uk/library
Or by phoning **0300 555 1387**

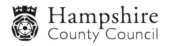

Hampshire
County Council

Oxford Handbook of
Expedition and Wilderness Medicine

Dr Chris Johnson
Consultant Anaesthetist, North Bristol NHS Trust
Southmead Hospital, Bristol, UK

Dr Sarah R. Anderson
Consultant in Communicable Disease Control
NorthWest London Health Protection Unit, London, UK

Dr Jon Dallimore
GP and Staff Grade Doctor,
Emergency Department, Bristol Royal Infirmary,
United Bristol Health Care Trust, Bristol, UK

Shane Winser
Geography Outdoors: the centre supporting field
research, exploration and outdoor learning,
Royal Geographical Society with IBG, London, UK

Professor David A. Warrell
Emeritus Professor of Tropical Medicine,
University of Oxford, Nuffield Department of Clinical
Medicine, John Radcliffe Hospital, Oxford, UK

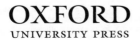

OXFORD
UNIVERSITY PRESS

Oxford is a registered trade mark of Oxford University Press
in the UK and in certain other countries

Published in the United States
by Oxford University Press Inc., New York

© Oxford University Press 2008

The moral rights of the authors have been asserted
Database right Oxford University Press (maker)

First published 2008
Reprinted in 2009

British Library Cataloguing in Publication Data
Data available

Library of Congress Cataloging in Publication Data
Data available

Typeset by Newgen Imaging Systems (P) Ltd., Chennai, India
Printed in China
on acid-free paper through
Asia Pacific Offset

ISBN 978–0–19–929661–3

10 9 8 7 6 5 4 3 2

Preface

Wilderness: 'a tract of solitude and savageness'
(A Dictionary of the English Language, Samuel Johnson, 1755)

Should the urge to explore, enjoy, and carry out research in wilderness environments be constrained in any way by considerations of health, safety, the environment, and the wellbeing of the local inhabitants? We think it should, but please read on.

Aims and scope of the speciality of expedition and wilderness medicine

Expedition medicine (known in North America as 'wilderness medicine') is concerned with maintaining physical and psychological health under the stresses and challenges of expeditions. Its aim is to encourage adventure but to attempt to minimize the risk of trauma and disease by proper planning, preventive measures such as vaccinations, sensible behaviour, and acquisition of relevant medical skills. Responsible attitudes towards the environment and the welfare of indigenous peoples in the area of travel are also of great importance.

Handbook of Expedition and Wilderness Medicine

This handbook is intended as a practical and portable guide to the prevention and treatment of those medical problems most likely to be encountered in extreme and remote environments. We hope that the book will be used in the planning and during the course of expeditions, by doctors, nurses, paramedics, and first-aiders, as well as by expedition members who are not medically qualified. The book is a product of the Royal Geographical Society (RGS) with the Institute of British Geographers' (IBG) Medical Cell, which was formed to provide medical advice to RGS-IBG expeditions. It has collected and summarized the enormous experience accumulated by UK-based explorers, expeditioners, researchers, and remote area travellers.

Are expeditions inherently dangerous?

Historically, exploration and wilderness travel have proved distinctly dangerous. In 1600, John Pory wrote of Leo Africanus, an early explorer:

'... I marvell much how he ever should have escaped so manie thousands of imminent dangers ... to have become captived ... his throte cut by the wilde Mores ... the Lyons greedie mouth, and the devouring jawes of the Crocodile ...'

Three centuries later, during Stanley's great trans-Africa expedition from Zanzibar to the Congo (1874–7), 114 of his original 228 expedition members died from battle, murder, smallpox, dysentery, drowning, crocodile attack, fever, execution, insanity, losing themselves and falling victim to cannibalism, opium, or starvation. This level of expedition mortality was unacceptable even in those days, and led to Stanley's being branded a ruthless and irresponsible leader.

Are expeditions safer in the modern era?

Only one historical expedition nightmare has disappeared from the face of the earth (smallpox). Many of the hazards facing Leo Africanus and Stanley still challenge expeditions in the 21st century, but we are now in a radically stronger position to minimize risk through careful planning based on a vast fund of medical knowledge and the development of drugs, vaccines, technology, and skills. The predominant aim of expeditions has shifted from discovery and sovereign possession in the 19th century to geographical and scientific discovery in the 20th century, and now to pleasure, personal development, and cultural exchange in the 21st century. The increasing popularity of 'gap year' adventure is acquainting school leavers and their anxious parents with some of the realities of wilderness travel.

Wilderness travel and exploration

We hope that this handbook will encourage many people to experience and enjoy expeditions and wilderness travel in a responsible way, and to identify and minimize avoidable risks without allowing these concerns to detract from the essential excitement and sense of achievement.

Chris Johnson
Sarah R. Anderson
Jon Dallimore
Shane Winser
David A. Warrell

August 2008

Foreword

If an expedition team in a remote region includes a key member who is prone to cardiac trouble, common sense would suggest that they take a portable defibrillator with them. But there are those who would scoff at this ... 'Why not take an X-ray machine and portable Intensive Care Unit, too?' This cynical point of view being that too much medical cover detracts from the very nature of a true wilderness expedition.

I once found myself, by myself, hauling a sledge towards the South Pole some 400 miles from the nearest human when the extreme pain of a kidney stone attack hit me without warning. Twenty years before I would have been in terminal panic for, in those days, I usually spurned any medical cover beyond a very basic First Aid pack. But Doctor Mike Stroud had, on this occasion, furnished me with an extensive array of painkillers, antibiotics and a mini handbook of instructions to cope with all likely and various less-likely ailments. So I was able to keep the agony of the stones at bay for the time it took to contact a ski-plane, and I was more than a little grateful for Mike's handbook and carefully thought out medical supplies.

Some years later, at 28,000 feet up the Tibetan side of Everest, the wire stitches that had held my chest-cage in position since a recent by-pass operation, suddenly felt as though they were tearing into and tightening my chest and lungs. Another heart attack, I realised, was imminent, and I grabbed for the Glycerine Tri Nitrate tablets which my wife had made me carry at all times on the climb. Thanks to their immediate 'dilating' effect, I survived the ensuing hasty midnight retreat back down to Base Camp, but a Scottish climber died of a heart attack at the same altitude the following night. He carried no GTN tablets, for he had no cardiac history.

If you can travel with a doctor, so much the better, but not everyone has that luxury. Full insurance cover is vital, and for Antarctica these days the Foreign Office Polar Department will, upfront, need to see proof that you have such cover.

The authors of this Handbook have all experienced travel in wild remote parts of the world and have learnt the hard way exactly what level of medical knowledge and supplies should be available to anyone or any group heading beyond the response reach of a 999 call.

Ranulph Fiennes
Expedition Leader
Exmoor, Somerset

January 2008

Dedication

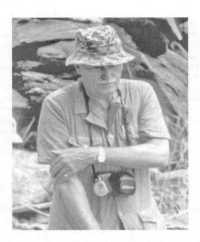

Dr Bent Einer Juel-Jensen (1922–2006)

MA, DM (Cand. Med. Copenhagen) FRCP, MRCGP, HonFRGS

This book is dedicated to the memory of our late very dear friend Bent Juel-Jensen who stimulated, encouraged and supported us together with generations of other young explorers and expeditioners at the Royal Geographical Society and the University of Oxford. He was the archetypal and model expedition medical officer.

Born in Odense, Denmark, Bent qualified in medicine in Copenhagen in 1949 but spent the rest of his life based in Oxford with his devoted wife Mary. At New College he studied physiology and Elizabethan literature and later became a loyal Fellow of St Cross College. His medical career began at the Radcliffe Infirmary with Dr Fred Hobson and Professor George Pickering, working on hypertension. In 1960, he became hospital Medical Officer and, from 1977 to 1990, University Medical Officer. Bent took charge of infectious diseases in Oxford and pioneered the treatment of *Herpes zoster* with antiviral drugs. Many of his protégés became consultants or professors of infectious diseases.

Bent's greatest enthusiasm was exploration and expeditions. He was passionately committed to the Oxford University Exploration Club, eventually becoming its Honorary President. Bent greatly improved the medical preparedness and training of its largely undergraduate members and was the inspiration, advisor and friend to many budding young explorers, including the editors of this Handbook. Pharmaceutical companies were pressurised into donating essential drugs for their medical kits. As founding medical advisor to the Royal Geographical Society he created a new awareness of the medical aspects of exploration. This contribution was recognised by his election to an Honorary Fellowship. The RGS-NMK Kora Research Project (Tana River, Kenya) in 1983 (Plate) had Bent as its energetic medical officer. He was friend and advisor to many famous explorers and travellers, the likes of Sir Wilfred Thesiger, Sir Vivian Fuchs and Bruce Chatwin.

After England and Denmark, Bent's favourite country was Ethiopia. Oxford expeditions to explore the rock hewn churches of Tigre in 1973 and 1974 resulted in his forming a close friendship with the local ruler, Prince Ras Mangashia. Bent's enthusiasm for Ethiopia stimulated him to learn Amharic and the priests' language Ge'ez, to embrace its history, literature, culture and food. He always carried his own supply of fiery berbera to ignite tame European dishes. His great physical courage, early displayed in his resistance to the Nazis in wartime Copenhagen, was again very much to the fore as he gave medical support across the Sudanese border to the Ethiopian Democratic Union's army battling the evil despot Mengistu Haile Mariam.

Bent Juel-Jensen, what an incredible man and a marvellous friend for all seasons!

Contents

Detailed contents

Reviewers

The Editors would like to thank the following people for their review comments.

Dr Mahreen Ameen

Dr Ian Davis

Dr Matthew Dryden

Dr Charles Easmon

Mr Paul Goodyer

Dr Sean Hudson

Dr Glynne Jones

Dr Caroline Knox

Dr David Lalloo

Dr James S Milledge

Dr Hugh Montgomery

Dr Edward Nicol

Dr Michael E Pelly

Mr Andrew Price

Professor John C Richardson

Dr Tim Rittman

Dr Stephan Sanders

Contributors

Dr Sarah R. Anderson
Consultant in Communicable
Disease Control, NW London
Health Protection Unit,
London, UK

Dr Kristina Birch
Consultant in Anaesthetics
and Intensive Care,
North Bristol NHS Trust, UK

Dr Julian Blackham
ST3 Emergency Medicine,
Severn Deanery and Air
Support Unit,
Great Western Ambulance
Service NHS Trust, UK

Dr Jim Bond
Freelance expedition leader,
doctor and ethnobotanist,
Renala Expeditions,
Edinburgh, UK

Mr Rupert Bourne
Consultant Ophthalmic
Surgeon, Hinchingbrooke
Hospital, Huntingdon and
Moorfields Eye Hospital,
London and
Professor of Ophthalmology,
Anglia Ruskin University,
Cambridge, UK

Dr Spike Briggs
Consultant in Intensive Care
Medicine and Anaesthesia,
Poole Hospital, Dorset, UK

Mr James Calder
Trauma and Orthopaedic
Consultant, North Hampshire
Hospital, and Clinical Senior
Lecturer, Imperial College,
London, UK

Mr Tim Campbell-Smith
Specialist Registrar in General Surgery,
South West Thames Rotation, UK

Dr Charles Clarke
Honorary Consultant Neurologist,
National Hospital for Neurology &
Neurosurgery, Queen Square,
London, UK and President of the
British Mountaineering Council

Dr Paul Cooper
Consultant Neurologist,
Hope Hospital, Salford
Greater Manchester, UK

Dr Jon Dallimore
GP and Staff Grade Doctor,
Emergency Department,
Bristol Royal Infirmary, United
Bristol Healthcare Trust, UK

Dr Richard Dawood
Specialist in Travel Medicine
& Medical Director, Fleet
Street Clinic, London, UK

Dr Sundeep Dhillon
Mountaineer and General
Practitioner,
Royal Army Medical Corps

Dr Andrew Drain
Specialist Registrar,
Cardiothoracic Surgery,
Papworth Hospital,
Cambridge, UK

Mr Jonathan Ferguson
Consultant Cardiothoracic
Surgeon, The James Cook
University Hospital,
Middlesbrough, UK

Prof. Karen Forbes
Consultant and Macmillan
Professorial Teaching Fellow
in Palliative Medicine,
United Bristol Healthcare Trust
and University of Bristol, UK

David Geddes
Dental Surgeon

Prof. Larry Goodyer
Head of the Leicester School of
Pharmacy, De Montfort
University, Leicester, UK
Paul Goodyer CEO
Nomad Travel and Pharmacy,
London, UK

Paul Goodyer
Food, water, and hygiene
Nomad Head Office
Unit 34, Redburn Industrial Estate
Woodall Road, Enfield,
Middlesex, UK

Mr Iain Grant
Senior Medical Officer,
British Antarctic Survey Medical
Unit, Derriford Hospital,
Plymouth, UK

Dr Mike Grocott
Senior Lecturer in Intensive
Care Medicine, Centre for
Altitude Space and Extreme
Environment Medicine, UCL
Institute of Human Health and
Performance, London, UK

Peter Harvey
Sentinel Consulting Ltd., Berkshire, UK

Dr Debbie Hawker
Consultant Clinical Psychologist
Interhealth

Dr Stephen Hearns
Consultant in Emergency Medicine,
Lead Consultant Emergency
Medical Retrieval Service,
Royal Alexandra Hospital
Paisley, UK

Mr Chris Imray
Consultant Surgeon UHCW
NHS Trust and Honorary
Reader in Surgery,
Warwick Medical School, UK

Dr Chris Johnson
Consultant Anaesthetist, North
Bristol NHS Trust, Southmead
Hospital, Bristol, UK

Dr Michael E Jones
Consultant Physician,
Regional Infectious Diseases Unit,
Western General Hospital,
Edinburgh, UK & HealthLink360
Edinburgh International Health
Centre Carberry,
Musselburgh, UK

Stephen Jones
Expedition Leader, UK

Dr Akbar Lalani
Royal Army Medical Corps.

Dr Christina Lalani
Trainee in Anaesthesia (ST1),
Frimley Park NHS
Foundation Trust, UK

Colonel Jonathan Leach
Director of General
Practice Education,
Defence Postgraduate
Deanery Edgbaston, UK

Nick Lewis
Environmental Consultant,
Poles Apart, Cambridge, UK.

David Lockey
Consultant Anaesthesia &
Intensive Care Medicine,
Frenchay Hospital, Bristol, UK

Dr Campbell J Mackenzie
Retired consultant nephrologist,
Bristol, UK

Carey McClellan
Extended Scope Physiotherapist,
Bristol Royal Infirmary,
United Bristol Health Care
NHS Trust, UK

Charlie McGrath
Travel Safety Specialist,
Objective Travel Safety Ltd,
Braunston, UK

James Moore
Charge Nurse, Emergency
Department, Royal Devon and
Exeter NHS Foundation Trust,
Exeter, UK

Professor Hugh Montgomery
Director, Institute for Human
Health & Performance,
University College London, UK

Mrs Clare Morgan
Sexual Health Advisor
Milne Centre for Sexual Health
Bristol Royal Infirmary, Bristol, UK

Dr Patrick Morgan
Anaesthetic Registrar,
Frenchay Hospital, Bristol, UK

Dr Daniel Morris
Specialist Registrar in Ophthalmology
Northern Rotation, UK

Dr Christopher Moxon
Research Associate,
Malawi- Liverpool- Wellcome
Clinical Research Programme,
Honorary Paediatric Registrar,
College of Medicine, Malawi

Dr Annabel Nickol
Clinical Lecturer in Respiratory &
General Medicine,
Oxford Centre for Respiratory
Medicine, UK

Dr Howard Oakley
Head of Survival & Thermal
Medicine, Institute of Naval
Medicine, UK

Prof Ian Palmer
Professor of Military Psychiatry,
Head of Medical Assessment
Programme, MoDUK,
St Thomas' Hospital,
London, UK

Alexander Phythian-Adams
Postgraduate student,
Institute of Immunology and
Infection Research,
University of Edinburgh, UK

Dr Andy Pitkin
Department of Anesthesiology,
University of Florida,
Gainesville, Florida, USA

Dr Andrew J Pollard
Reader in Paediatric
Infection and Immunity,
University of Oxford, UK

Dr Tariq Qureshi
Department of Emergency Medicine,
John Radcliffe Hospital,
Oxford Radcliffe Hospitals,
NHS Trust, UK

Dr Paul Richards
General Medical Practitioner,
South Essex Teaching PCT,
Director Medical
Expeditions, UK

Barry Roberts
Commercial Director,
Wilderness Medical Training,
UK

Dr George Rodway
Research Fellow,
Center for Sleep and
Respiratory Neurobiology,
University of Pennsylvania,
Philadelphia, USA

Assoc Prof. Marc Shaw
Specialist Travel and
Geographical Medicine,
Worldwise Travellers Health
Centres, New Zealand

Dr Joe Silsby
Consultant in Anaesthesia and
ICM Taunton and
Somerset NHS Foundation
Trust, UK

Dr Charlie Siderfin
General Practitioner,
Heilendi Family Medical Practice,
Kirkwall, Orkney, UK

Dr Julian Thompson
Specialty Registrar in
Anaesthesia Royal Berkshire,
Hospital, Reading, UK

Andrew Thurgood
Consultant Nurse and Immediate
Care Practitioner,Birmingham, UK

Prof. David A. Warrell
Emeritus Professor of Tropical
Medicine, University of Oxford,
Nuffield Department of Clinical
Medicine, John Radcliffe Hospital,
Oxford, UK

James Watson
Physiotherapy Officer,
Medical Support Unit, Headquarters,
Hereford Garrison, UK

Dr Andy Watt
Consultant Physician/Geriatrician,
Biggart Hospital, Prestwick, Ayrshire, UK

Dr Jane Wilson-Howarth
GP Partner, Petersfield Medical
Practice and Medical Director of the
Travel Clinic Cambridge, UK and
advisor to Engineers without Borders

Dr Jeremy Windsor
Specialist Registrar in
Anaesthetics and Intensive Care,
University College London
Hospitals, UCLH Foundation
Trust, London, UK

Mrs Shane Winser
Geography Outdoors: the centre
supporting field research exploration
and outdoor learning
Royal Geographical Society with IBG
London, UK

Symbols and abbreviations

ABC	Airway, Breathing, Circulation
ACE	Angiotensin converting enzyme
ACL	Anterior cruciate ligament (knee)
ADL	Activities of daily living (disability)
AED	Automated external defibrillator
AIDS	Acquired Immune Deficiency Syndrome
AMS	Acute mountain sickness
AMTS	Abbreviated mental test score
ARDS	Acute respiratory distress syndrome
ARI	Acute lower respiratory infection
ART	Atraumatic restorative technique (dental)
ASAP	As soon as possible!
ATLS	Advanced trauma life support
AVPU	Scale to evaluate conscious level (Awake/Verbal/Pain/Unresponsive)
BAS	Broad arm sling
BLS	Basic life support
BM	Blood glucose measurement
BMI	Body mass index
BNF	British National Formulary
BP	Blood pressure
BS	British Standard
BTS	British Thoracic Society
CAGE	Cerebral arterial gas embolism
CMV	cytomegalovirus
CNS	Central nervous system
CO2	Carbon dioxide
COPD	Chronic obstructive pulmonary disease
CPP	Cerebral perfusion pressure
CPR	Cardiopulmonary resuscitation
CRT	Capillary refill time
CSF	Cerebrospinal fluid
CVA	Cerebral vascular accident (stroke)
DCI	Decompression illness
DCS	Decompression sickness
DEET	Diethyl toluamide insect repellent

DKA	Diabetic ketoacidosis
DSH	Deliberate self-harm
DTI	Department of Trade & Industry
DVT	Deep venous thrombosis
EAV	Expired air ventilation
EBV	Epstein-Barr virus
ECG	Electrocardiogram
ELISA	Enzyme-linked Immunosorbent assay
ELT	Emergency locator transmitters (aircraft)
ENT	Ear, nose, throat
EPA	Environmental Protection Agency (US)
EPIRB	Emergency position indicating rescue beacon
ERP	Emergency response plan
ETT	Endotracheal tube
FCO	Foreign and Commonwealth Office (UK)
GCS	Glasgow coma scale
GI	Gastrointestinal
GMC	General Medical Council (UK)
GORD	Gastro-oesophageal reflux disease
GP	General Practitioner
GPS	Global positioning system
GSM	Global system for mobile communications
GTN	Glyceryl trinitrate
HAART	Highly active anti-retroviral therapy
HACE	High altitude cerebral oedema
HAPE	High altitude pulmonary oedema
HAR	High altitude retinopathy
HAS	High arm sling
HELP	Heat escape lessening position
HiB	Haemophilus influenzae b
HIV	Human immunodeficiency virus
HPV	Human papilloma virus
HPVR	Hypoxic pulmonary vasoconstrictive response
HRT	Hormone replacement therapy
HSV	Herpes simplex virus
HVR	Hypoxic ventilatory response
IBRD	International beacon registration database
ICP	Intracranial pressure
IHD	Ischaemic heart disease
IM	Intramuscular (drug administration)
IPJ	Inter phalangeal joints (digits)

IRM	Intermediate restorative material (dental)
IUCD	Intrauterine contraceptive device
IV	Intravenous
JME	Juvenile myoclonic epilepsy
LA	Local anaesthetic (eg. lidocaine)
LCL	Lateral collateral ligament
LIF/RIF	Left/Right iliac fossa of abdomen
LMA	Laryngeal mask airway
LUQ/RUQ	Left/Right upper quadrant of abdomen
LZ	Landing zone (aircraft)
MAP	Mean arterial pressure
MCA	Marine & Coastguard Agency
MCL	Medial collateral ligament (knee)
MCPJ	Metacarpophalangeal joints (digits)
mg	milligram
MI	Myocardial infarction
ml	millilitre
MMR	Mumps, Measles, Rubella
MO	Medical officer
MRI	Magnetic resonance imaging
NFCI	Non-freezing cold injury
NGO	Non-Governmental organisation
NHS	National Health Service (UK)
NICE	National Institute for Health & Clinical Excellence (UK)
NPA	Naso-pharyngeal airway
NSAID	Non-steroidal anti inflammatory drug (eg. ibuprofen)
O2	Oxygen
OCP	Oral contraceptive pill
OPA	Oro-pharyngeal airway
ORS	Oral rehydration solution
P	Pulse
PASP	Pulmonary artery systolic pressure
PCL	Posterior cruciate ligament (knee)
PCR	Polymerase chain reaction
PE	Pulmonary embolism
PEFR	Peak expiratory flow rate
PEPSE	Post-exposure prophylaxis following sexual exposure
PF	Peak flow (asthma)
pH	Acid/base scale

P-I	Pressure immobilization
PID	Pelvic inflammatory disease
PLB	Personal locator beacons (ground personnel)
PO	Oral (drug administration)
PPE	Personal protective equipment
PPI	Proton-pump inhibitor drug
PR	Rectal (drug administration)
PTSD	Post-traumatic stress disorder
RGS	Royal Geographical Society
RICE	Rest, Ice, Compression. Elevation
RR	Respiratory rate
RSI	Repetitive strain injury
RSV	Respiratory syncitial virus
RTC	Road traffic collision
SAR	Search and Rescue
SARS	Severe acute respiratory syndrome
SC	Subcutaneous (drug administration)
SCUBA	Self-contained underwater breathing apparatus
SPF	Skin protection factor (sunscreen)
STI	Sexually transmitted infection
TB	Tuberculosis
TDS	Three times daily (drug administration)
TMJ	Temperomandibular joint
TPR	Temperature, Pulse, Respiration (Chart)
UC	Ulcerative colitis
UK	United Kingdom
URTI	Upper respiratory tract infection
USA	United States of America
UTI	Urinary tract infection
UV	Ultraviolet (radiation)
UVA, UVB, UVR	Ultraviolet radiation
VEGF	Vascular endothelial growth factor
VHF	Very High Frequency (radio waveband)
WBGT	Wet bulb globe temperature

Chapter 1

Expedition medicine

Sarah Anderson, Chris Johnson, David Warrell,
and Shane Winser

The nature of expeditions

This book is about the physical and mental wellbeing and healthcare of travellers to remote areas. Remote areas are defined as places where access to sophisticated medical services is difficult or impossible and the responsibility for dealing with medical problems falls on expedition members. In the UK this branch of medicine is usually called 'expedition medicine'.

An expedition is an organized journey with a purpose. Early expeditions sought new lands to claim, develop, and exploit. In the 20th century, as gaps on maps shrank, geologists, naturalists, and ecologists added detail to the knowledge, while physiologists explored human responses to extreme environments. Today, new scientific knowledge requires a highly technological approach and considerable funding, so personal development, cultural exchange, and fundraising have become an increasingly important justification for travel.

Exploration and adventure travel organizations, some commercial, others charitable, now send thousands of people overseas each year, and the distinction between an expedition and a leisure trip is becoming blurred. North Americans recognize this and call what we are describing in this book 'wilderness medicine'.

Groups travelling to remote areas now include:
• Well organized and funded expeditions
• Small groups of independent travellers
• Commercial trips to remote destinations
• Charity fundraising treks to exotic destinations
• Participants in adventure holidays
• Competitors in extreme sporting events
• Gap year travellers.

Expeditions travel to all parts of the world but, for British expeditions, mountain ranges and tropical jungles are the most popular destinations (Fig. 1.1). Inevitably, expeditions involve greater exposure to environmental extremes and novel hazards than other forms of travel. Participants in groups that organize their own journey should anticipate, understand, and prepare to deal with at least the obvious hazards that they will encounter on their journey.

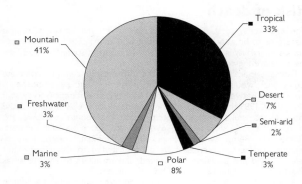

Fig. 1.1 Expedition destinations.
Source: Royal Geographical Society Medical Database.

Risk of death

The explorer's worst nightmare may be to catch a dreaded tropical disease or to be attacked by a ferocious wild animal, but for most expeditions the reality is more mundane. Stomach upsets, sprains, bruises, and insomnia are the common problems.

Expeditions are becoming safer. In the 18th and 19th centuries complete expeditions would disappear into the wilderness and never be heard from again. Between 1943 and 1985, 1% of British Antarctic Survey staff died; since 1985 there has been only one death. In the 20th century, the ratio of successful summit attempts to deaths on Mount Everest was 1:7; in 2007 the ratio improved to 6 deaths for 500 successful summits[1] (Table 1.1). Better weather forecasting, equipment, communications, training, and rescue services have all contributed to this change, but safety should not be taken for granted, and travellers to remote areas should strive to minimize risk and be self-sufficient.

A death during an expedition is rare and tragic but should be kept in perspective (Tables 1.2 and 1.3). The media love dramatic stories but ignore the hazards of daily life. With the exception of extreme sporting activities, the risk for participants in a well-planned expedition is not that different from the risks faced during an active life at home[2]. Fatal road accidents, drowning, or falls can occur anywhere; effective advanced planning can reduce their incidence. Unfamiliar environmental hazards cause both deaths and injuries. In some countries, insect-borne diseases such as malaria and dengue are a significant hazard. Proper briefing of travellers, together with good risk management, can reduce harm. Sadly, the risk of violent death overseas from crime or terrorism has climbed from a low point in the mid-20th century.

> Expeditions are getting safer. . . . .
>   BUT Society is less tolerant of risk.
> Deaths occur on expeditions . . . . .
>   BUT deaths also occur in the UK and receive less publicity.
> All deaths are a tragedy . . . . .
>   BUT—by **not** travelling do you reduce the number of deaths?
>
> *Only join a trip if you know, understand and accept the risks.*

---

1 http://www.everestnews.com/history/everestsummits/summitsbyyear.htm
2 Anderson S.R, Johnson C.J.H. Expedition health and safety: a risk assessment. *Journal of the Royal Society of Medicine* 2000; **93**: 557–62.

Table 1.1 Relative risk of death in remote areas

Everest summit ratio (to 1999)	1 in 7
Himalayan mountaineering	1 in 34
Everest summit ratio (2007)	1 in 83
Antarctica over-wintering (1943–83)	1 in 100
All cause risk of death after major surgery	1 in 250
Royal Geographical Society Survey (1995–2000)	1 in 1500
Himalayan trekking	1 in 7000
Gap year travel	1 in 7500
Low altitude jogging	1 in 7700

Table 1.2 Deaths in UK travellers during 2002

Deaths from natural causes	1111
Non-natural causes	316
Total deaths	1427
Journeys made:	59,200,000
One death per 41 500 journeys	
(Typically between one and three deaths a year are linked to expedition travel.)	

Table 1.3 Non-natural deaths in UK travellers 2002

Road accident	158
Suicide	57
Drowned	21
Air accident	14
Murder (non-terrorist)	10
Terrorism (Bali bombs 26)	29
Balcony accidents	14
Skiing and mountaineering	12
Rail death	1
Total deaths	316

Expedition morbidity

Several studies have looked at the type of medical problems encountered during expeditions. Fig. 1.2 shows a summary.

Gastrointestinal upsets (30%)

Diarrhoea and vomiting are an inevitable hazard of travel and are usually self-limiting. However, serious cases lead to dehydration and hospitalization. Dysentery, cholera, and giardiasis can infect the unwary. Simple hygiene measures can reduce the incidence of problems, but all travellers need to carry basic remedies for days when travel is unavoidable, and larger expeditions ought to have the facilities to rehydrate a seriously affected member.

Medical problems (21%)

Simple medical problems such as respiratory infections and headache are very common, and are usually easily treated. Insect-borne diseases such as malaria and dengue fever can be incapacitating and sometimes fatal. Appropriate precautions should be taken.

Orthopaedic problems (19%)

Sprains and back strain are common; rest and simple painkillers help. Fractures and serious trauma will require evacuation.

Environmental problems (14%)

Environmental extremes may cause problems for the unprepared. Altitude sickness affects many travellers ascending rapidly to altitude; heat exhaustion and heatstroke can be a serious problem, while at the other extreme frostbite and non-freezing cold injury can cause long-term disability. When environmental problems occur they can be serious, and require urgent treatment and evacuation, often in difficult circumstances.

Fauna (8%)

Unfamiliarity with local animal life can lead to injury. Scorpions and sea urchins commonly cause problems. Wherever rabies is endemic, dogs should be treated with caution. Although it is very unusual to be eaten or sat upon, large animals throughout the world present a hazard.

Feet (4%)

Good footcare is always essential. Blisters cause misery and can become infected on a long expedition. Regular cleansing and use of foot powder reduces fungal infections and sores.

Surgical problems (1%)

Acute abdominal crises, gynaecological pain, and renal stones are very alarming and generally require evacuation of the patient, but are fortunately rare.

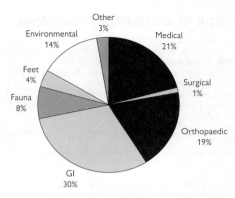

Fig. 1.2 Categories of 1263 medical problems recorded by Royal Geographical Society Survey 1995 to 2000.

The scope of expedition medicine

Expedition medicine is about:
- Preparing for an expedition—to minimize ill health and maximize expedition achievements
- Working during the expedition—in a professional capacity to diagnose, treat, and manage disease
- Managing expedition emergencies and potential evacuations
- Finally, advising on health issues once the expedition has returned home.

Organizing the medical care of an expedition takes time and includes tasks such as:
- The assessment of risk and processes to manage this
- Team selection
- First aid training
- Preventive medicine both before departure and in the field
- Organization of a suitable medical kit
- Knowledge of special health problems
- Provision of medical skills in the field
- Arrangements for medical back-up and evacuation
- Organization of medical insurance.

Each of these aspects will be covered later in this book.

Expedition medicine is not just about the treatment of disease; it should permeate all facets of the expedition. Health criteria must be considered when the location of the base camp is decided and the activities of the trip planned. Food, sanitation, and psychology are part of the medical officer's work. The medical officer will fulfil many roles and will certainly be expected to be nurse as well as doctor. At times this may involve listening to and encouraging those who are finding the expedition stressful. The need to accompany a casualty during evacuation may mean that certain personal goals are not attained.

Correctly practised, expedition medicine should not constrain the enthusiasms and ambitions of an expedition but, by anticipating preventable medical problems, facilitate the achievements and enjoyment of all participants.

Preparations

Section editor
Sarah Anderson

Contributors
Sarah Anderson, Jim Bond, Jon Dallimore,
Richard Dawood, Peter Harvey, Tariq Qureshi,
Barry Roberts, Jane Wilson-Howarth, David Warrell
and Shane Winser

Joining an expedition

The Royal Geographical Society estimates that more than 1,000 overseas expeditions leave the UK annually. These will range from solo travellers or teams of two up to expeditions involving 100 or more participants. Expeditions typically last for as little as 1–2 weeks to many months, if not years in the case of continuing research programmes. The shear volume of expedition traffic represents great scope for joining an expedition, assuming one is not inclined to organize a journey independently. Expeditions occur throughout the year but are usually timed for a variety of reasons; for example, to coincide with a certain event (summer holidays, animal migration patterns), climatic conditions (avoiding monsoons or other 'rains') and the seasons (avoiding the Himalaya or north polar areas in the northern hemisphere winter).

Potentially there is a huge choice of where to go and what to do. Think first about your motivation:
- Science
- Adventure
- Personal challenge
- Community involvement.

Think second about your personal circumstances:
- Relevant skills and experience
- The level of responsibility you desire
- Time available
- Financial commitments/resources
- Personal interests.

Unless you fully appreciate the demands of expedition travel, as opposed to independent travel, it is worth initially considering joining a short expedition before committing yourself to a prolonged and arduous journey in a very remote area, with little chance of repatriation if you find you cannot cope or hate the experience.

Expeditions are costly enterprises and normally each participant has to pay their way. At best you might get your costs covered by the expedition but it is unrealistic to expect a wage, unless you have a special skill and/or are vastly experienced. There is also the opportunity cost to consider while on an expedition when mortgages, pensions, and other bills have to be paid, and there is no corresponding income. In addition there are 'hidden' costs which might include upgrading clothing, camera equipment, special insurance, etc. It all adds up.

Types of expedition

Institutional expeditions

Universities, research groups, and public institutions (such as the Natural History Museum and Royal Botanic Gardens, Kew and Edinburgh) are examples in this class.

Commercial expeditions

Commercial operators charge a fee to join their expeditions and aim to make a profit. They range from 'one-off' projects to 'adventure travel' companies who offer land-based expeditions and ocean sailing opportunities. Such businesses may be run by sole traders, as partnerships, or as limited companies. The Department for Trade and Industry (DTI) regulates 'package' holidays. These regulations can apply to not-for-profit organizations as well, such as charities. A travel package is offered when at least two of the following three components are included: transport, accommodation, or other tourist service accounting for a significant proportion of the package. Anyone offering a 'travel package' is legally required to be 'bonded' so that any fees paid are protected if the company folds prior to travel. For the current regulations see:
http://www.dti.gov.uk/consumers/buying-selling/holidays-travel/
package-holidays/index.html

Charity organizations

The Charity Commission is the regulator and registrar of charities in England and Wales. There is great variety in the expedition activities of such bodies. For example, they range from medical research expeditions, aid and relief work, youth expeditions, conservation and science projects to expeditions for medically disadvantaged people and 'charity challenges' (such as treks, cycle rides, and climbs) in aid of a specific cause. See http://www.charity-commission.gov.uk for the register of organisations. Remember that companies that run 'charity treks' on behalf of registered charities are *not* charities and may be profit-driven businesses.

Private expeditions

Anyone can set up an expedition and recruit team members to join it. This is not regulated and no qualifications are necessary to do so. A one-off expedition is outside the scope of the 'travel package' DTI rules discussed above.

Film/TV projects

There is great public interest in the adventures, suffering, landscapes, and human dramas associated with expeditions. These adventures are made more accessible by low cost filming and production techniques, and are another route by which aspiring medical officers (MO) might get an opportunity to join an expedition. This offer is not without risk, both professional and psychological.

Assessing an expedition opportunity

While you might be grateful to any expedition that accepts you, you are also about to invest time and finances to get involved, so do some research to satisfy yourself that the organization is capable of achieving the expedition aims and meeting your expectations.
- How long has the company/organization been trading and what is its financial structure and bonding system?
- Are they aligned to a standard, e.g. BS8848 (see box) or screened via an external organization such as the RGS or Young Explorers Trust?
- What are the credentials of the expedition leader(s)?
- How much do you have to pay and what does it include/exclude?
- How are participants selected and medically screened?
- What pre-expedition meeting/training plan is in place?
- What medical kit is provided?
- What insurance, risk assessment, and emergency back-up arrangements are in place?
- Will your medical defence organization cover you if there are Americans/Canadians or other nationals on the team?
- Don't ignore your instinct or 'gut feeling'; sloppy administration might be a tell-tale sign of poor field organization.

Information sources on expedition opportunities
- The internet
- Word of mouth
- Contacts through companies that offer expedition medical training
- The Royal Geographical Society maintains a:
  - Register of personnel available for expeditions, which is used to help expeditions to recruit an MO (http://www.rgs.org/medicalcell)
  - Bulletin of expedition vacancies
  - List of organizations that recruit expedition members http://www.rgs.org/je

Keep a logbook

It will become increasingly common for organizations to ask for an applicant's logbook of experience, which should detail your outdoor and travel-related experience, expedition experience, and qualifications. An example is available to download at http://www.rgs.org/JE

BS 8848: a specification for visits, fieldwork, expeditions, and adventurous activities outside the UK

This new British Standard aims to reduce the risk of injury or illness on overseas ventures by specifying the safety requirements that have to be met by providers of these activities. Intended for expedition organizers, universities, and other organizers of field research, gap year travel companies and providers of adventurous holidays, BS 8848 provides organizations that comply with the specified requirements with a way of being able to demonstrate to participants and other interested parties that their venture provider is following good practice to manage the venture safely. BS 8848 can also be used to identify areas for improvement in existing safety management procedures.

See http://www.bsi-global.com/BS8848 for further details.

Human dynamics on expeditions

Expeditions create their own unique (social context) atmosphere, perhaps akin to being in a theatre of war. There can be enormous strain on individuals and the team, brought about by the intensity of living in a group, which is amplified by physical hardship, deprivation of normal western comforts, climatic and cultural demands, and the stress of striving to achieve the expedition's objectives. This is one of the great attractions of expedition life; to put oneself to the test and willingly forego the relative safety and security of home in exchange for the deep satisfaction, elevated self-esteem, and close human bonds that can be one of the greatest benefits of the expedition experience.

To optimize the expedition experience for all participants, particular attention must be paid to appropriate team selection, team building, effective leadership, and an understanding of the dynamics of groups in the field.

Team selection

There is great variation in how individuals come to join (or be selected for) an expedition. This is related to the myriad expedition styles, be they scientific, exploratory, adventure-related, for personal and social development, other reasons or some combination thereof, and whether the expedition is institutional, charitable, commercial, or private. At one end of the spectrum there are arguably no selection criteria save for the applicant's bank balance. In contrast, one can draw on a number of tools with which to vet and select potential team members.

Any comprehensive, formal selection process involves
- Resources and cost
- Ethical issues
- Data protection issues
- An assessment of the attitude and aptitude of the applicant
- A wise investment in assembling a compatible team with the skills and motivation required to achieve the expedition objectives.

Any selection process less than comprehensive relies on
- The 'old boy's network'
- Wishful thinking
- Criteria irrelevant to the demands of the expedition
- A 'face fits' mentality.

Selection tools
- Verifiable previous experience:
  - Relevant country experience
  - Similar conditions/season
  - Role to be fulfilled
- Verifiable specific skills/qualifications to fit a particular role:
  - Ask for bona fide documentation
- Application forms:
  - Is penmanship or the ability to compose an essay relevant?
  - Is it appropriate to request a photo?
  - Are the questions relevant, unambiguous, and non-discriminatory?

- References:
  - A weak tool, even if submitted in confidence
- Selection events to observe applicant's behaviour directly:
  - Use tasks/projects that simulate the demands of the expedition
  - Beware the 'horns and halo' effect, when observers only pay attention to behaviour that supports their 'first impression', whether this is favourable or unfavourable
  - Inform candidates about the selection criteria
- Interviews:
  - Some people do not interview well despite being highly suitable
  - Most interviewers are poorly trained
- Ability and personality tests:
  - Potentially expensive; requires professional administration
  - Beware of pseudo-psychometric 'team role' tests
  - Ethical issues related to appropriate test use and debriefing of applicant
  - Don't use in isolation of other data
- Fitness tests:
  - Must be appropriate to the demands of the expedition
- Technical skill tests (e.g. mechanical skills, driving).

Arguably, it is simpler to de-select candidates, despite the negative connotations this has. Some de-selection criteria include:

- Medical/psychiatric history
- Lack of physical fitness
- Incompatibility with other team members
- Lack of experience
- Lack of relevant skills.

Self-selection

The number of applicants can be reduced by providing sufficient information about the *objectives* of the expedition and the *selection criteria* to help applicants gauge their own suitability before applying.

Debriefing of results

If the selection criteria are public, clear, and unambiguous, and the selection process is fair and unbiased then it should be straightforward to inform failed applicants about their shortcomings and reasons for not being selected. There is no legal requirement to provide reasons for not selecting someone but it is obviously polite to do so. Conversely, it is in the direct interests of the expedition to take the opportunity to inform successful applicants that they have been selected on certain merits but may have shortcomings that they should address.

Personality characteristics

Technical skills, experience, and physical fitness aside, expedition members should possess an abundance of the following personality traits and abilities:

- Tolerance
- Resilience
- Adaptability/flexibility
- The ability to work well with others
- A sense of humour
- Emotional maturity
- Communication skills
- Problem-solving skills
- A reasonable degree of autonomy
- Self-insight—someone who knows their own strengths and weaknesses.

In corporate recruitment circles it is accepted that *'Past performance predicts future behaviour'*. This is equally true when applied to expeditions. Finally, all other factors aside, consider whether the applicant would pass the 'blizzard test'—that is, would you be happy to spend long periods of time with this person confined to a tent in a blizzard?

Team building

Time is well invested prior to the expedition in building the expedition members into an effective team so that the team is ready to handle the demands of the expedition. The time devoted to this should be proportional to the size of the team and the complexity and longevity of the expedition. For large multinational expeditions it is impracticable to get the team together before the expedition; in these circumstances a period of time should be devoted in-country to team building, skill development, and briefings, before the party is deployed to the field.

Team building is focused on developing

- Friendship and relationships—a support network
- Open communication processes
- Decision-making processes
- Conflict resolution processes
- Clarity of the expedition objectives and priorities, and building confidence in these being achievable
- Faith in the team leader(s)
- Clarity of roles and responsibilities
- Trust, mutual respect, and cohesion
- The skills required for the expedition
- An appreciation of personality differences
- An appreciation of each member's aspirations, fears, and concerns.

Normal expedition preparation and planning activities are effective vehicles for team building and include

- Menu planning
- Logistical planning
- Making, sourcing, and buying equipment and supplies
- Testing equipment

- Press and public relations
- Financial planning and fundraising
- Skill training
- Fitness training
- First aid training and simulations.

Thought should be given to
- Assigning specific responsibility/accountability for tasks
- Ensuring that all team members have a chance to work together on a variety of tasks to prevent cliques forming
- Holding formal review sessions to report on progress and outstanding challenges
- Informing the team of normal group dynamics and the phases a group typically passes through 'forming, storming, norming, and performing'.

Leadership

Leadership is a kind of behaviour that guides others to reach a desired objective or outcome. All teams require leadership. A small private expedition of friends may not have a formal leader and therefore be 'leaderless' but there is no such thing as a 'leadershipless' team. Leadership manifests itself in a number of ways. A leader may be formally appointed (or self-appointed). Otherwise leadership is transient and is exerted by individual team members from the position of an assigned role or responsibility, personal expertise, or personality.

By definition, a leader would be deemed effective if the team achieves the expedition objectives, but in practice it is not so simple. Therefore consider two questions: What should leaders <u>do</u>?

What should leaders <u>be?</u>

Leaders should <u>do</u> the following
- Lead by example
- Set achievable goals and communicate priorities to the team
- Ensure that resources are available to achieve those goals, including appropriate training
- Give the team permission to make decisions within defined limits
- Give honest, direct, and timely feedback about performance
- Encourage effective team processes—planning, problem-solving, and decision-making
- Work to promote harmony and group cohesion
- Protect the team from outside interferences.

Leaders should <u>be</u>
- Organized
- Decisive but flexible
- Effective communicators
- Emotionally stable and physically robust
- Good problem-solvers
- Good listeners—to the team's concerns and views.

Leaders will engender discontent and will be criticized for
- Unfairness (real or perceived)
- Inconsistency
- Withholding information
- Favouritism
- Not doing what they ask others to do
- Lack of supervision and guidance
- Oversupervision
- Being dogmatic/inflexible
- Being indecisive
- Putting their own needs ahead of the team's
- Lacking the courage to make unpopular decisions.

A leader's checklist
- Does the team know what's expected of them?
- Do they have the resources to do the job?
- Does each individual have an accurate perception of what they are contributing?
- Is the team on track to achieve the expedition's goals based on current performance?
- Does each team member feel appreciated, motivated, and committed to the team and its purpose?

Being a leader is a challenging role, for which most people are not trained. Individuals have unique needs and this is perhaps the greatest leadership challenge—to connect equally with all team members and steer their energy and efforts towards achieving the expedition's goals. Often several individuals evolve to produce a leadership team to fulfil the diverse leadership roles.

Group dynamics

A cohesive team is more likely to achieve the expedition aims than a fragmented group so it is desirable to promote this through pre-expedition team building and effective leadership. A cohesive team will be happier and more confident than a less cohesive group.

Morale and cohesion can be adversely affected under the following conditions
- Communication breakdowns
- Illness and inability to cope with the physical demands of an expedition
- Bad weather
- Boredom—lack of structure and purpose
- Splinter groups—cliques
- Exclusive relationships in the group
- Poor food
- Unfairness and inequalities in food, assignments, accommodation, etc.
- Failure to achieve expedition objectives
- Exhaustion, lack of recovery time, and recreation opportunities.

The performance of individual team members can also be adversely affected by

- Culture shock
- Homesickness
- Breakdown of close relationships within the team
- Lack of fitness, poor health, and hygiene
- Mental/psychological illness.

It is unrealistic to expect all team members to become great friends with each other. Team cohesion relies on trust, fairness, tolerance, and acceptance of different personalities, opinions, and habits within the framework of a workable team structure, an appropriate resource base, effective leadership, and a mutually agreed purpose that the team is motivated to achieve.

Role of the expedition medical officer

The expedition MO is key to the success of an expedition. Success is achieved by preventing expedition members becoming ill and treating, quickly and appropriately, those who become unwell or have an accident. This does not mean that, as MO, you must treat everything that is presented to you, but rather you must use your knowledge to advise on the best course of action. As MO you are unlikely to be busy with medical problems but, if someone is ill or injured, you may be the only person who can deal with the situation. These can be stressful times, with no advice available from seniors and no one to relieve you for a break. Good communication between you, your patient, and other expedition members is essential, as is strong decision-making, based on the knowledge and facilities available to you.

To prepare for the role of expedition MO

- Carefully research the geographical area where you are traveling
- Improve your knowledge of local medical problems
- Attend relevant courses in expedition medicine, first aid, advanced life support, basic dental skills or a Diploma in Tropical Medicine and Hygiene
- Prepare physically.

Pre-expedition roles

- Advise and brief the team on medical issues (general and specific to the expedition environment)
- Undertake medical screening of all expedition members (📖 p. 58)
- Encourage all participants to have a pre-expedition dental check-up
- Document the blood group of each expedition member (obtained free by donating blood at a local blood donor centre)
- Consider subscribing to the Blood Care Foundation to ensure access to safe blood abroad http://www.bloodcare.org.uk
- Provide advice on immunizations and malaria prophylaxis (📖 p. 32)
- Organize appropriate first aid training for all expedition members (📖 p. 54)
- Educate the team on health and hygiene issues (📖 Chapter 3)
- Obtain, pack, and transport medical supplies and kits (📖 p. 46)
- Undertake a risk assessment and prepare associated documents (📖 p. 74)
- Review local health services and medical facilities
- Anticipate and plan evacuation of a severely ill or injured person
- Prepare a communication network to support your medical diagnosis and decision-making and in case of evacuation (📖 p. 136)
- Prepare an emergency response plan (📖 p. 132)
- Organize medical insurance with full emergency evacuation cover (📖 p. 82)
- Confirm professional indemnity insurance will cover expedition MO role.

Medical screening of expedition members is essential to ensure tailored pre-travel advice and to expand the expedition first aid kit. Ask each member to complete a personal medical questionnaire and emphasize the need for full disclosure due to insurance cover. Make three copies of the questionnaire: leave one in the UK with a nominated contact and take two on the expedition, in case an emergency evacuation is needed.

Pre-expedition Medical Questionnaire

NAME:

DATE OF BIRTH:

ADDRESS:

NEXT OF KIN:
  Name
  Address
  Tel./contact details
  Relationship

GP DETAILS:

CURRENT MEDICAL PROBLEMS:

PAST MEDICAL HISTORY (including past psychiatric history):

CURRENT MEDICATION:

ALLERGIES:

LAST DENTAL CHECK-UP:

IMMUNIZATIONS: DATES:
  Polio
  Tetanus/Diphtheria
  Pertussis
  Hib (*Haemophilus influenzae* b)
  MMR (Mumps, Measles, Rubella)
  Meningococcal Meningitis ACWY
  Pneumoccal
  BCG
  Cholera
  Hepatitis A/B
  Japanese B encephalitis
  Rabies
  Tick-borne encephalitis
  Typhoid
  Yellow fever

BLOOD GROUP:

Roles during the expedition
- Reiterate rules of camp and personal hygiene (📖 Chapter 3, p. 89)
- Continue to reinforce these at regular intervals during the expedition
- Ensure a safe, copious water supply
- Undertake brief medical review of expedition members on arrival
- Revise basic first aid and management of minor injuries with all expedition members
- Place expedition medical kits in a designated place and inform all expedition members
- Organize a routine for patient consultations
- Oversee the safety of expedition members
- Reassess the risks posed by the natural environment, instruct the team on prevention and early suspicion (e.g. heat illness, altitude sickness), and alter emergency plans as appropriate
- Review evacuation plans
- Consider visiting the local hospital early to introduce yourself
- Practice a mock evacuation
- Write up accident reports as necessary
- Enjoy being part of the expedition.

Camp health and hygiene
As MO you are responsible for base camp health and hygiene. Contribute to the designs of the camp layout to ensure water supplies and waste disposal are correct. Undertake regular checks of latrine and kitchen hygiene, food storage, and rubbish disposal (📖 Chapter 3, p. 89). If anything is substandard bring it to the attention of all expedition members and rectify. Strict adherence to the rules of camp and personal hygiene is essential to minimize gastroenteritis, the most common complaint of all expeditions.

Consultations
A consultation service for non-urgent problems is one of the main roles of an MO; how you do this will depend on the size and structure of your expedition. Allocate a regular time each day when you are exclusively available for consultation; consider before or after meals. It is important to try to ensure complete privacy (not always easy). Briefly record consultations and any treatment given.

Treatment
Most expedition MOs are simply equipped owing to the size and mobility of their expedition. This can mean that few diagnostic aids are available. MOs should ensure that they have medical supplies sufficient for treating minor illnesses and are able to provide emergency care for more serious conditions until a patient can be evacuated.

Most problems are straightforward and can be dealt with on the spot. The role of the MO is therefore uncomplicated: to make a diagnosis and treat. In urban settings, help is available to confirm intuitive feelings or doubts; however, in the field it is not, and as expedition MO you therefore have to assume the worst case scenario. This may mean causing a lot of inconvenience and concern, for example, by sending someone with stomach ache to hospital with possible appendicitis, or making someone with a headache descend 1000 m. You will provoke grumbling and hostility if the person recovers without intervention, but you really have no choice other than to take the safest course of action.

MOs are also there to offer reassurance. People come with genuine symptoms, whether major or minor, and the significance may not always be apparent to the sufferer. You will not know what the situation is until you have made a serious attempt at a diagnosis, so *never fail to take this step*. If you think nothing is wrong, friendly reassurance is very important. Remember that psychological or psychiatric problems, fears, and tensions may manifest themselves as physical symptoms. Expeditioners tend to be self-sufficient people, and the circumstances of an expedition often reinforce this. There is a tendency for MOs to overdo the self-sufficiency; this can lead them to try and solve all problems single-handedly. Always ask yourself whether extra advice is available and if it would be useful.

Confidentiality

All patients rightly expect that medical information will be confidential. People also have a right to refuse treatment, even if, in the MO's view, this will not be in their best interest. However, the General Medical Council has made it clear that doctors also have a duty to the public at large. On expeditions circumstances can arise where confidentiality may need to be broken so that the health and safety of other expedition members is not jeopardized. The expedition leader may need to be informed that an individual is concealing an illness or refusing treatment.

Consent

Without consent, treatment is assault. Consent to emergency life-saving treatment is usually presumed by the law if the patient is unconscious or too ill to consent. The law presumes that a reasonable person would wish his/her life to be saved. In the case of a healthcare professional acting within his/her sphere of clinical competence, consent is usually implied, i.e. the patient does not resist the treatment and therefore is presumed to consent. In other situations where treatment carries considerable risk, or is controversial, informed expressed consent should be obtained. For consent to be informed the individual must understand the proposed treatment and the risks involved in accepting or refusing that treatment. This means that the patient should be made aware of material risks and common or serious side effects, as well as the likely consequences should treatment be withheld. Verbal consent, especially in an expedition setting, is usually adequate.

For an individual over 16 years of age, only that individual is able to give consent. Remember, patients have the right to refuse treatment. Children under 16 can consent to medical treatment themselves if, in the opinion of the doctor, they are capable of understanding the nature and consequences of that treatment (Gillick Competence). The child should, however, be given information that is relevant to his/her age and understanding. When taking under-16s on an expedition it is wise to gain written permission from the parent or guardian that medical care can be given if it is thought to be in the child's best interest.

Incident reports

Incidents may happen. One of the roles of the expedition MO is to write up an incident report if necessary. Information should be collected on:
- The site and time of the incident/accident
- The people involved
- Who else was present (witnesses)
- What happened
- What action was taken
- The outcome.

Assessing risk

Medical risk management should form part of overall risk assessment (📖 p. 74). The assessment of risk is made just as well by people who commonly encounter the hazard, such as climbers, cavers, and divers, as by MOs. In these activities, participants are usually well informed and are trained to advise beginners. Risks can be minimized by the use of sensible precautions such as safety belts in vehicles and wearing helmets while climbing.

Once in the field, it is important to *reassess* the risks, particularly local flora and fauna, and the climate—both heat and humidity—in addition to the risks posed by the physical environment. Situations may arise in the field where the MO will either have to give an opinion about a proposed activity, or give unsolicited warnings when activities have already started. Once in the field, assessment of risk by the MO is essential and a crisis management strategy should be prepared (📖 p. 130).

Evacuation

An essential role of the MO is the ability to make a decision on evacuation. Consider the following:
- The need to choose the safest option when diagnosis cannot be confirmed by colleagues or tests
- The often conflicting needs of the other expedition members
- The lack of privacy and confidentiality, all part of expedition life.

Plans should be prepared on communication and transportation methods in case an emergency or evacuation occurs. (See 📖 p. 136 for further details on evacuation.) If the evacuation is to be funded by an insurance company it will be critical to liaise with the insurance company's medical assistance agent. This individual will hold the approval for financing evacuations. Failure to do this has and will result in the insurance company's not paying for evacuation costs.

Treating people not on the expedition

In many parts of the world expeditions are perceived by local people to be rich and endowed with clinical skills and drugs. The apparently universal human desire to take medication may be stimulated by the arrival of the expedition, and the slightest hint that you will treat people in the local community may produce a flood of 'ill' people. It is tempting to try to 'help' and to establish goodwill by offering medicines to all but, before you do, consider the potential harm:

- You may not understand local people's health problems and therefore misdiagnose
- You may endanger your own expedition members by using drugs intended for them
- You may be blamed unreasonably for adverse outcomes
- You may offend local healers (and health services)
- Treatment may be incomplete and thus ineffective or harmful
- You might be exploited for your novelty value
- You may not be in a position to follow up treatment
- You may encourage expectations among local people that the local medical services cannot meet.

Nevertheless, you cannot avoid doing what you can to help other people. Local people, particularly children, who are severely ill or injured, should be treated, but not necessarily by you; evacuate these patients if possible. Your authority may help to achieve this. As the expedition MO, you should not treat chronic disease. You will not have the resources or the time, and it would be better for everyone if patients are treated by the local health service. (📖 p. 122).

Post-expedition

- Repeat advice on continuing malaria prophylaxis for the full prescribed period if appropriate
- Provide health and medical advice and support as necessary
- Warn team members about non-healing skin lesions (leishmaniasis) and the need to seek medical help if a fever develops within the first few weeks after return (malaria), etc.

If participants have no symptoms post-expedition, it is probably unnecessary to recommend a post-expedition medical review. For participants with symptoms, the MO should recommend urgent review by a doctor, to examine, investigate, and treat as appropriate. The most helpful tests post-expedition are:

- Full blood count with white cell differential to detect an increase in eosinophils (an eosinophilia is seen with parasitic disease)
- Urine dipstick for blood, protein, or sugar
- Stool specimen for ova, cysts, and parasites
- Urine specimen and serology for schistosomiasis (>6 weeks after expedition) if exposed to fresh water in endemic areas (📖 p. 490).

Do not forget that tropical diseases such as malaria and schistosomiasis may present weeks, months, or even years after the expedition has ended. A single case in your expedition team should alert you to suggest the screening of other members since they are likely to have shared the same risk of exposure. In general, the role of the MO post-expedition will be to direct individuals to the best local UK health provider to treat the problem.

Ethics of expeditions

The importance of ethical considerations and behaviour on an expedition cannot be overstated. Whatever adventurous goals or scientific outcomes are achieved, it is often how the expedition is approached or conducted which leaves the most lasting impression. This is particularly true among people of the host country.

The study of ethics is as complex or as simple as you make it. We each have a conscience and a sense of social responsibility to guide us. However, on an expedition, there are (at least) four other sets of ethical standards also operating:

• Personal ethics of other individuals
• Group ethics that the team adopts, deliberately or subconsciously
• The religious beliefs, values, and cultural mores of the people in whose territory you are journeying
• Universal human rights.

Below is a recognized framework to help make some of these standards explicit—and defendable.

Principles

The 'four principles plus scope' model of biomedical ethics[1] should be familiar to most recent medical graduates. It can, if thought through, be applied to almost any situation.

The 'four principles' of ethical debate and behaviour

1. Respect for **A**utonomy: the right to individual self-determination
2. **B**eneficence: the doing of good
3. **N**on-maleficence: the avoidance of doing harm
4. Respect for **J**ustice: equity, fairness.
(Mnemonic: **A B**eautiful **N**ose **J**ob)

There is no hierarchy to the 'four principles'; they simply form a 'checklist' for assessing the ethical dimensions of a decision or dilemma.

The task of the responsible person is to consider a question from each perspective, and then make a judgement on balance.

What do the four principles mean in practice (and plain English)?

A.   *Autonomy* involves respecting an individual's right to choose treatment or refuse it. Respect for the autonomy of others carries with it the moral obligation to maintain (appropriate) confidentiality, to keep one's promises, not to deceive one another, and by extension, to communicate well at all times.

B, N.   *Beneficence* ('doing good') and *non-maleficence* ('not doing harm') are complimentary obligations. Examples include ensuring that all team members, including the expedition doctor, have adequate training for what they would reasonably be expected to do, and

1 Beauchamp TL, Childress JF (1989). *Principles of biomedical ethics*, 3rd edn. OUP, New York, Oxford.

providing clear information about the risks that people will be undertaking.

Empowerment, whether of individuals or local communities (see Scope, below), can be seen as an overlap of the first three principles (A, B, and N). It is arguably a core function of any expedition.

J. Respect for *justice* is the moral obligation to act on the basis of fair adjudication between competing claims. This can be to do with:
- The fair distribution of scarce resources (distributive justice)
- Respect for different peoples' rights (rights-based justice)
- Respect for morally acceptable laws (legal justice).

Scope
When applying the four principles, you need to determine the boundaries within which your ethical question lies.[2]

One rule of thumb for expeditions is to consider all people directly affected by the expedition's presence (See 📖 p. 30: Care of local staff). For environmental effects, your scope may be much wider.

Examples
There are often no easy or absolutely right answers for what constitutes ethical practice. Part of the fun of an expedition is the new and unexpected challenges that make you think about, or re-think, your position.

Acknowledge your mistakes, apologize if you have got it wrong and learn from them. The following sections are peppered with a few examples, the ethical principles involved being indicated by the A, B, N, or J annotation used above.

Cultural clashes
Definition
When cultural differences come to the surface, or are no longer tolerated.

Incidence
Cultural clashes occur surprisingly commonly on expeditions, even more so than with tourists, who are often seen as passing through, or 'doing their own thing'.

Underlying causes
Cultural miscommunication → loss of mutual respect/trust.

NB. Any situation where a mixed group of people is working together under arduous conditions for some time has some potential for a clash. The difference in cultures may merely be a focus of attention.

Risk factors
- History of colonialism in either the host or guest peoples
- Apartness (or apartheid), in eating, sleeping, travelling arrangements.

---

2 Gillon R (1994). Medical ethics: four principles plus attention to scope. *BMJ* **309**: 184.

Symptoms and signs
- Paternalism (real or perceived)
- An obvious disagreement
- Silence ...

Prevention
Attention to appropriate:
- Communication:
  - Translation skills—e.g. making implicit meanings explicit
  - Listening skills, including body language
  - Serious effort to understand socially and culturally determined references and attitudes
  - Awareness that you are operating in a different cultural norm
  - Openness, honesty, good humour, and inclusiveness at all times.

- Behaviour, e.g. drugs, alcohol, sexual licentiousness.
- Values, e.g. humility, respect for differing beliefs, taboos, and work ethic.

At the very least, a cultural clash has the potential to cause upset. In extremes, it can wreck the whole expedition.

Personal/professional clashes
Background
People do not always get on well with each other, even with the best intentions and a shared, common purpose. The hardships, close working conditions, and interdependency of the expedition environment can turn minor irritations into resentments.

If everyone on the team has a clear role to play, it may be easier to respect each other's contribution while accepting joint responsibility for helping out in any way possible when things go wrong.

Causes
- Poor communication—both expressive and receptive
- Unrealistic expectations—which may in themselves be a result of poor communication.

NB. Personal clashes sometimes masquerade as professional clashes and vice versa.

Risk factors
Certain roles on an expedition may inevitably pull in different directions at certain times, e.g. leader vs MO, logistician vs health and safety person.

Prevention
- *Before setting off:* choose your team carefully. Consider team building exercises, e.g. imaginary worst-case scenarios.
- *At the start:* establish ground rules, e.g. no criticism of people behind their backs; respect for personal space. Acknowledge the potential for falling(s) out and work out clear ways in advance to air grievances and resolve disputes early.

- *During:* aim to build on shared group values and develop a sense of group responsibility. Communicate with each other—no one should be expected to carry all the weight of their particular role alone.
- *In a crisis:* depending on the particular hazards of the expedition, you may ultimately need to have a formal chain of command.
- *After:* be self-critical and prepared to learn from your mistakes for next time.

Management of disputes

Although this should ideally be a group responsibility, it often falls on the leader or the expedition doctor (in his confidential capacity) to sort these conflicts out. Allowing each person to have his/her say is important; however 'time-out' may need to be called first before a resolution is attempted.

Care of local staff

Duty of care

An expedition's duty of care extends to all participants (J). A participant could be defined as anyone who would not be in a given situation if it were not for the expedition, e.g. local drivers, porters, guides, cooks (N).

Potential areas to consider, with examples

- Bare essentials of life
  - Are your porters adequately fed, watered, clothed, shod, and sheltered at night for the conditions you are asking of them? (N, J)
- Health and safety
  - Are there enough life jackets/helmets to go round, and does everyone know how to use one? (N, J)
  - Are some participants expected to take greater risks than others, e.g. local people riding in the back of a pick-up? (N, J)
- The right to be consulted and to say no
- Access to (appropriate) medical attention
  - Standards of medical care on the expedition should be no different for local participants
  - This does not necessarily mean expatriation for treatment of serious injury or illness, but could well entail having to arrange casualty evacuation to appropriate in-country medical facilities
- Fair recompense for any work carried out, or extra risks taken
  - This should be commensurate with local wages, costs, etc., so as not to distort the local economy completely (B, N, J)
- Respect for home/family life
  - Setting off at a certain time may mean a man can't milk his goats and he has to arrange someone else to do it for him (A, J)
- Respect for feast days, time to pray, etc.
- Long-term consequences for local participants
  - Are you empowering them?
  - Is anything you're asking them to do (e.g. to translate) likely to compromise their social standing in the community? (N)

Good practice

Duty of care, whether moral or legal, is only a minimal requirement. Good practice, enabling you and your team to get the most out of the expedition, demands a lot more.

Scope

NB. The boundaries between expedition participants, their dependents, and the rest of the local population may be rather blurred at times (📖 see Indigenous people p. 122).

Immunizations

Introduction

Vaccines offer reliable protection against an increasing range of important disease hazards abroad. Where travellers sometimes go wrong is to assume that when they have had the injections, there's nothing more to be done. Unfortunately, this is not the case, and careful attention to the other health precautions covered in this book remains of paramount importance, before, during, and after every successful expedition. An important benefit of going to be vaccinated is the opportunity to discuss a wider range of health concerns and precautions that may be even more beneficial than the vaccines themselves, an opportunity that should always be used to the full.

Timing

Immunizations should be obtained at least 6 weeks before departure, to allow time to give vaccines requiring more than one dose, and to avoid having to travel with a sore arm or other side effects. Vaccine supply problems do occur from time to time, and this can be a further reason for seeking protection well in advance.

Background

Everyone attending for immunization should bring with them any available records of previous vaccines received, to avoid unnecessary repeated doses.

Immunization schedules are becoming more complicated and more crowded, and, especially where groups of young people are concerned, 'catch-up' protection may be necessary for any missed doses, notably MMR and diphtheria, tetanus, and polio (Table 2.1). Recent outbreaks of mumps and measles have occurred in young people in whom MMR vaccine has been omitted. HIV-positive and other immunosuppressed people require special advice about immunizations. See http://www.bhiva.org/files/file1001634.pdf

Table 2.1 UK childhood immunization schedule

At 2 months old:
- Diphtheria, tetanus, acellular pertussis, inactivated polio vaccine, and Hib (DTaP/IPV/Hib)
- Pneumococcal (PCV)

At 3 months old:
- Diphtheria, tetanus, acellular pertussis, inactivated polio vaccine, and Hib (DTaP/IPV/Hib)
- Meningitis C (Men C)

At 4 months old:
- Diphtheria, tetanus, acellular pertussis, inactivated polio vaccine, and Hib (DTaP/IPV/Hib)
- Meningitis C (Men C)
- Pneumococcal (PCV)

At around 12 months:
- Hib
- Men C

At around 13 months:
- Measles, mumps, and rubella (German measles) (MMR)
- PCV

3–5 years (pre-school):
- Diphtheria, tetanus, acellular pertussis, inactivated polio vaccine (DTaP/IPV) or (dTaP/IVP)
- Measles, mumps, and rubella (German measles) (MMR)

13–18 years:
- Diphtheria, tetanus, and inactivated polio vaccine (Td/IPV)

BCG is no longer routinely given to children aged 10–14 years.

Source: UK Department of Health, Sept 2006.

Certificates and regulations

Yellow fever remains the only disease for which international, WHO-approved vaccination certificates still apply as a condition of entry to some countries. Travellers to Saudi Arabia during the Haj (pilgrimage to Mecca) may be asked to show a vaccination certificate for meningitis; long-term travellers to certain countries may very occasionally also be asked to show a so-called 'AIDS-free' certificate or HIV test result.

Choosing which vaccines to have

Beyond compliance with international health regulations, travel vaccines are not required formally as a condition of entry. They are 'optional' and are based on recommendations that take account of the likely health risks such as: locally prevalent diseases, the precise details of a trip or expedition, including its duration, conditions of accommodation, the likely level of contact with local people, and the environment.

In the UK, the Department of Health issues general guidelines[3], and the WHO also issues information. Many GPs, travel clinics, and other sources also formulate their own policies.

On an expedition, participants inevitably compare the vaccines and medication they have received; inconsistencies tend to be the rule rather than the exception, which can lead to unnecessary anxiety and can undermine confidence in the advice that has been given.

The best option is for an expedition's MO to draw up some general guidelines or a formal policy, seeking specialist advice if this is needed. The best care comes when one clinic or practice takes responsibility for the entire group. If this is not possible, the MO should circulate guidelines to all expedition members to give to the individual clinics or practices that will carry out immunization.

In the UK, only a small number of travel vaccines can be provided free of charge on the NHS, and travel vaccines are becoming increasingly costly—a factor that needs to be considered in the context of an expedition's overall budget.

Table 2.2 Vaccine guide

Vaccine	No. of doses	Initial course		Duration (years)	Lead time for protection (single dose vaccines)
		Interval between first and second doses	Interval between second and third doses		
Polio booster (injected)	3*	6 weeks*	6 months*	10	
Diphtheria/tetanus booster				10	
Cholera, travellers diarrhoea (Dukoral)	2	1 week		2	2 weeks from start
Diphtheria/tetanus/polio				10	
Typhoid injected (Typhim Vi)	1			3	10 days
Typhoid oral (Ty 21a)—capsules	3	2 days	2 days	1	10 days
Hepatitis A vaccine—adult	2	6–12 months		>10	2 weeks
Hepatitis A vaccine—child under 16 years	2	6–12 months		>10	2 weeks
Typhoid/hepatitis A (combined)	2	6–12 months		Typhoid: 3 years; hepatitis A: 1 year then >10 years	2 weeks
Hepatitis B—standard schedule (adult & child)	3	1 month	5 months	5	
Hepatitis B—rapid schedule	4	7 days	14 days	1, then 5	

Table 2.2 (Contd.)

Vaccine	Initial Course			Duration (years)	Lead time for protection (single dose vaccines)
	No. of doses	Interval between first and second doses	Interval between second and third doses		
Twinrix hepatitis A/hepatitis B	3	1 month	5 months	10/5	
Yellow fever	1			10	10 days
Rabies	3	7 days	21 days	3	
Pneumonia (Pneumovax)	1			5+	
Meningitis A/C/Y/W	1			5	2 weeks
Japanese B encephalitis	3	7 days	7–23 days	2+	
TB: BCG (must have skin test first)	1				
Tickborne encephalitis	2–3	28–42 days		3+	
MMR (mumps/measles/rubella)—adults	1				
Varicella	2	4 weeks			

Live vaccines: to be given on same day or 3 weeks apart.
* These courses are usually completed during childhood.

Individual vaccines for travel

Bacterial meningitis (📖 p. 468)

Most travel clinics are able to provide up-to-date information about areas of risk. Travellers who have had their spleen removed may be more vulnerable to this condition.

A new vaccine is available that protects against the A, C W, and Y strains of the disease. This is highly effective, and provides protection for 5 years. Other vaccines are in development, including vaccines against the problematic B strain.

Vaccination is important for travellers at high risk (e.g. those who have had a splenectomy), and for travellers to high-risk destinations (see Fig. 2.1), especially if they will be in close contact with local populations.

Cholera

The old injected cholera vaccine provided no useful protection, and is no longer available. A cholera vaccination certificate is no longer necessary as a condition of entry for any destination.

A new, oral vaccine is now available (since May 2004). This vaccine uses killed cholera bacteria and a modified form of the cholera toxin to generate localized antibody protection on the surface lining of the intestine. Other diarrhoea-causing organisms produce a very similar toxin, which is why this vaccine also has a protective effect against some types of traveller's diarrhoea (notably enterotoxigenic *E. coli*—ETEC—which accounts for as many as 40% of cases).

Cholera remains endemic in many parts of the world, but outbreaks tend now to be limited to settings with severe overcrowding, such as in refugee camps, or under conditions of extreme poverty. Improved ability to treat cholera with simple fluid replacement means that the consequences of infection are no longer as severe, though they can still sometimes be devastating. Cholera vaccine may be a sensible precaution for situations involving close contact with local communities in developing countries, though many people additionally use the vaccine for protection from ETEC.

- Cholera causes catastrophic, watery diarrhoea
- It is a disease of poor hygiene, transmitted via the faecal/oral route, usually by water
- It can therefore also be prevented by water purification, hygiene, and food and water precautions
- The oral cholera vaccine available in the UK is Dukoral™
- Dukoral™ is a suspension given in the form of a drink, in two doses, 1 week apart; protection is simple and safe
- The course should be completed 1 week before departure
- Protection lasts approximately 2 years.

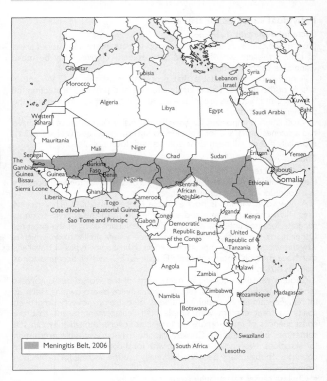

Fig. 2.1 Distribution of annual epidemics of meningococcal meningitis in Africa: the "meningitis belt".

Table 2.3 Live and inactivated vaccines

Live vaccines	Killed/inactivated vaccines
Measles/MMR	Cholera (Dukoral™)
Oral polio (no longer given)	Diphtheria
Tuberculosis (BCG)	Hepatitis A
Typhoid (Ty 21a)	Hepatitis B
Yellow fever	Japanese B encephalitis
	Meningitis ACWY
	Polio (injected)
	Rabies
	Tetanus
	Tick-borne encephalitis
	Typhoid (Vi antigen)

Live vaccines should be avoided during pregnancy and in people suffering from
reduced immunity—specialist advice may be needed.

Hepatitis A (📖 p. 456)

Hepatitis A is common in hot countries and countries with poor hygiene
(Fig. 2.2). Modern hepatitis A vaccines are given in a two-dose regimen
that provides reliable, longlasting protection.

Hepatitis A vaccines were originally predicted to protect for 10 years.
However, the latest vaccine product licences have been extended to
25 years. Growing experience with these vaccines suggests that their
protection may in fact be lifelong, in the same way that hepatitis A infection
confers lasting immunity.

- The risk of a serious infection increases with age: during early childhood,
  complications are rare, but by the age of 40, there is a 2% risk of
  severe liver failure.
- Hepatitis A is one of the commonest vaccine-preventable diseases.
- Hepatitis A vaccine is safe, highly effective, and longlasting.

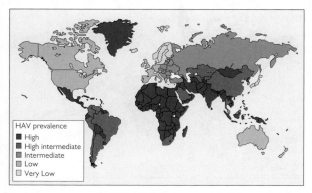

Fig. 2.2 Geographical distribution of hepatitis A prevalence.

Hepatitis B (📖 p. 456)

Hepatitis B is spread by sexual exposure, and by blood and blood products, including non-sterile medical instruments; it is a hazard in all developing countries (Fig. 2.3). It is a sensible precaution for anyone planning to spend a prolonged period abroad, particularly if they will be sexually active, in close contact with local communities, or at increased risk of needing medical treatment.

In addition to the standard methods of giving the vaccine, accelerated schedules can be used when less time is available prior to departure (for example, doses on days 0, 7, 21–28 with a booster dose at 1 year).

- Hepatitis B vaccination has already become part of the standard childhood vaccination schedule in many countries, and there is much pressure for it to be added to the UK schedule.
- Many consider it to be a sensible precaution for all sexually active young people.
- It should also be considered for anyone at increased risk of accident or injury abroad, who might need medical attention in circumstances where sterile medical instruments and screened blood transfusions might not be readily available.

Influenza (📖 p. 492)

Some people regard seasonal influenza (flu) as the world's most highly prevalent vaccine-preventable disease; it is certainly a disease of travel.

Although it occurs seasonally during the winter months in the northern and southern hemispheres, it is a year-round problem in the tropics.

Expeditions, by their very nature, tend to involve groups of people spending much time together. It would seem sensible to protect members against this common, troublesome problem.

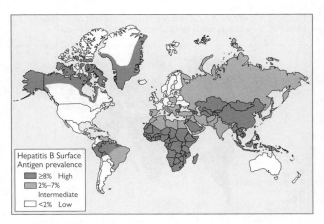

Hepatitis B Surface
Antigen prevalence
■ ≥8% High
■ 2%–7%
   Intermediate
□ <2% Low

Fig. 2.3 Geographical distribution of hepatitis B prevalence.

Japanese encephalitis

Japanese encephalitis is a viral disease transmitted by mosquito bites. Although rare, it carries a high risk (around 30%) of serious neurological side effects. It occurs throughout Asia (Fig. 2.4; there were 1800 fatal cases in India in 2005), with greatest risk between the months of April and October. It occurs mostly in rural areas—farm animals are the source of the infection (baby pigs and ducks).

The vaccine should certainly be considered by anyone likely to spend much time in rural and some urban parts of Asia.

- Historically associated with a moderate risk of allergic-type side effects, the current vaccine is safe and effective
- Three doses of vaccine are required for protection, usually given at days 1, 7, and 28
- New vaccines are in development
- Vaccination should be considered by anyone planning to spend time in rural parts of Asia.

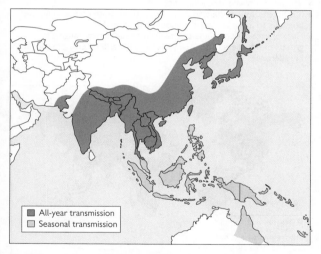

Fig. 2.4 Geographical distribution of Japanese encephalitis. Reproduced with permission from Tsai TR, Chang GW, Yu YX (1999). Japanese encephalitis vaccines. In: Plotkin SA and Orenstein WA (eds) *Vaccines*, 3rd edn. WB Saunders, Philadelphia, PA, 672–710.

Rabies (📖 p. 458)

Good quality vaccine may not be available in a high proportion of the places where rabies is a problem. Rabies immune globulin can be even more difficult to obtain, and can be extremely expensive (approximately £1000–£2000 per person). Obtaining correct treatment may require a trip to be curtailed or abandoned (Fig. 2.5).

Pre-exposure vaccination simplifies the treatment necessary after a bite: fewer vaccine doses, and no need for immune globulin injections. It is increasingly recommended for travellers likely to be exposed, particularly for travel to India, Burma (Myanmar), and Thailand, and parts of Africa and South America.

The new rabies vaccines are safe and cause little or no reaction; three doses of vaccine are necessary (days 0, 7, and 21), so some advance planning is required.

- Pre-exposure vaccination is strongly recommended, particularly for long stays in countries with a high prevalence of animal rabies, or when taking part in activities that involve close contact with animals
- Vaccination is safe and highly effective
- It is best to follow the standard vaccine three-dose course whenever possible, to avoid any doubts about protection
- Cost of vaccination can be substantially reduced by arranging for groups of travellers to share a vial of vaccine and receive the injections intradermally.

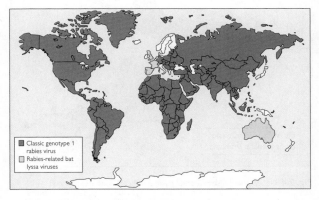

Fig. 2.5 Rabies-endemic areas of the world.

Tick-borne encephalitis (📖 p. 458)
A safe vaccine is available, and medical experts in the affected regions strongly advise visitors to be vaccinated if they will be exposed to possible risk (Fig. 2.6). (In Austria, the entire population is vaccinated as a matter of routine!) The vaccine requires two, or preferably three, doses for protection, starting at least 3 weeks prior to travel. A common approach is to give two doses 28 days apart, or three doses at days 0, 7, and 21.
- Vaccination is strongly advised for people at risk, particularly those visiting forested areas in late spring. For short-term travellers many advise tick avoidance measures only.

Tuberculosis (📖 p. 470)
Immunization with BCG is now no longer routinely offered to school-children in the UK, though it is offered at birth to targeted risk groups.
  Expeditions involving travel to parts of the world that are highly endemic for TB—especially if there will also be a close degree of contact with local people—should consider the need for BCG protection.

Typhoid (📖 p. 471)
Typhoid remains common in all developing countries, and in most hot countries with poor hygiene conditions. Vaccination is advisable for travel to Africa, Asia (especially the Indian subcontinent), and Latin America, and should also be considered for travel to Mexico and the Caribbean.
  Two vaccines are available: an oral vaccine (Ty 21a), consisting of three capsules to be swallowed on alternate days, that only provide full protection for about 1 year; and an (Vi antigen) injected vaccine, that provides 3-year protection after a single dose.
- The oral vaccine contains live, modified bacteria, so should not be taken at the same time as antibiotics
- Previous generations of typhoid vaccines caused unpleasant reactions (local pain, fever, illness), so travellers may be concerned about side effects
- Current oral and injected vaccines are extremely safe and do not cause these effects
- Vaccine protection is approximately 80% effective.

Yellow fever (📖 p. 460)
Worldwide, the risk of yellow fever is growing (Fig. 2.7). Vaccination against yellow fever is necessary for travel to many parts of Africa and South America, either as a certificate requirement or for personal protection. It is also a certificate requirement in Asia for travellers arriving from affected regions of Africa and South America. The certificate lasts 10 years, but does not become valid until 10 days after vaccination: anyone likely to need to travel at short notice should have the vaccine in advance.
- International regulations are aimed at protecting countries from importation of the virus rather than at protecting travellers
- The vaccine is live, so must be avoided in pregnancy and people with reduced immunity
- The vaccine is extremely safe, though a tiny number of serious reactions in elderly people has led to increased caution in its use
- Only a single dose is necessary.

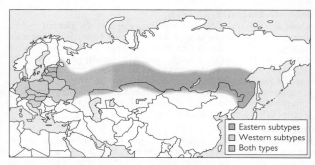

Fig. 2.6 Geographical distribution of tick-borne encephalitis.

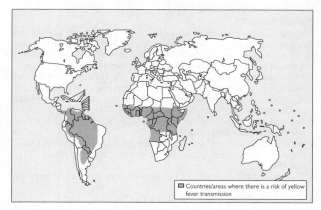

Fig. 2.7 Geographical distribution of yellow fever.

Resources and further advice
http://www.dh.gov.uk
http://www.fitfortravel.scot.nhs.uk/
http://www.nathnac.com
http://www.who.int/ith
http://www.cdc.gov
http://www.fleetstreetclinic.com

Dr Richard Dawood (ed.) *Travellers' Health: How to stay healthy abroad.* (OUP)
Dr Richard Dawood
info@fleetstreetclinic.com
http://www.fleetstreetclinic.com
The Fleet Street Travel Clinic
29 Fleet Street, London EC4Y 1AA
Tel: +(0)20 7353 5678
Fax: +(0)20 7353 5500

Medical kits and supplies

It is never possible to deal with every possible accident or illness—even with a large amount of medical equipment. Items from medical kits are used most frequently for blisters, headaches, minor cuts and sprains, sunburn, diarrhoea, and insect bites. Similar illnesses and accidents occur on all expeditions, but clearly extra drugs and equipment may be needed to deal with problems in particular environments.

It is often difficult to judge how much medical equipment to take and this will depend on:

- The size of the party, the duration of the trip, and its remoteness
- The number of outlying camps
- The likelihood of having to treat local staff and villagers
- Local medical facilities
- The medical knowledge of the team members/medic
- Communications with other camps and remote medical help.

Obtaining supplies

Buying medical supplies from a retailer can be costly, and acquiring, packing, and labelling a medical kit can be time-consuming. UK drug companies may provide samples or donate medication, particularly if there is some formal recognition of the company's sponsorship. Local pharmacists and NHS hospital trusts may be able to help by providing drugs at cost. Technically, GPs should not give NHS prescriptions for illnesses which may be acquired outside the UK, but many do.

In some parts of the world, prescription drugs are available over the counter but they may be counterfeit and the quality cannot be guaranteed.

Drug export

Expeditions carrying reasonable quantities of drugs are unlikely to encounter problems at customs when entering a country. However, it may be useful to have a doctor's letter stating that the drugs are for the personal use of the expedition team members and are not the subject of any commercial transaction.

Controlled drugs

Wherever possible, avoid taking 'controlled' drugs. A Home Office licence is required (Tel: 020 7273 4085 for more details) and must be returned within 28 days of return to the UK. Tramadol is a suitable alternative for most conditions. Any controlled drugs dispensed should be recorded in a controlled drugs register.

Storage and transport
- Where possible, avoid liquid medicines
- Obtain tablets in blister packs—loose-packed tablets can disintegrate during the rigours of an expedition
- Avoid splitting the medical kit between several team members—a vital piece of equipment may be 2 hours' walk away!
- Wrap the whole kit in waterproof/dustproof packaging (e.g. re-sealable polythene bags, old film canisters, and Tupperware boxes)
- Try to pack items which are used together in the same box, e.g. cotton buds, fluorescein strips, tetracaine, and chloramphenicol ointment for eye problems
- Label each box with a laminated, waterproof list of its contents on the lid. If the kit is marked with a large red cross it may attract attention and be a target for thieves—medical supplies are very valuable in many parts of the world
- Full instructions should be provided with each medical kit.
- A small personal medical kit should be carried by each expedition member at all times

Personal medical kit

Each team member should carry a small supply of first aid equipment for their own personal use.
- Paracetamol or preferred painkiller
- Adhesive plasters
- Antiseptic wipes
- Blister kit
- Piriton or similar antihistamine
- Insect repellent
- Sunblock cream
- Iodine for water purification
- Rehydration sachets (e.g. Dioralyte®)

In addition, team members should carry sufficient personal medication for the duration of the trip, including antimalarials.

Recommended medical kit

Quantities are for a group of 20 people on a 6-week high-altitude mountaineering expedition. The list may be useful as a checklist when preparing kits for other types of expeditions (see notes below for other environments).

Antimicrobials	Amounts
Ceftriaxone for injection 1 g	5 ampoules
Chloramphenicol (eye) ointment 1%	3×4 g
Clarithromycin or erythromycin 250 mg	40 tablets
Ciprofloxacin 500 mg	50 tablets
Co-amoxiclav 375 mg	84 tablets
Doxycycline 100 mg	80 capsules
Flucloxacillin 500 mg	100 capsules
Fluconazole 150 mg tablets	4 tablets
Gentisone HC® (ear drops)	10 ml × 4
Mebendazole 100 mg	20 tablets
Metronidazole 400 mg	100 tablets
Metronidazole suppositories 1 g	10
Penicillin V 250 mg	56 tablets
Valaciclovir 500 mg	10 tablets
Riamet®	48 tablets
Painkillers, local anaesthetics/sedatives	
Aspirin 300 mg	32 tablets
Co-codamol 30/500	80 tablets
Diclofenac 50 mg	100 tablets
Ibuprofen 400 mg	80 tablets
Ketamine for injection (500 mg/10 ml)	2
Lidocaine 1% for injection	5 ml × 10
Lidocaine gel	2
Lorazepam for injection 1 mg	5 ampoules
Midazolam for injection (10 mg/5 ml)	5 ampoules
Paracetamol 500 mg	100 tablets
Tetracaine (amethocaine) eye drops	6 minims
Tramadol for injection 100 mg	5 ampoules
Tramadol 50 mg	50 tablets
Zopiclone 7.5 mg or temazepam 10 mg	20 tablets

Gastrointestinal

Bisacodyl laxative	20 tablets
Gaviscon® (antacid)	100 tablets
Dioralyte® sachets	40
GlucoGel®	2 ampoules
Loperamide	50 capsules
Prochlorperazine 5 mg	56 tablets
Ranitidine (Zantac) 150 mg	60 tablets
Stemetil® for injection 12.5 mg	5 ampoules
Stemetil® suppositories 25 mg	10

Cardiovascular

Bisoprolol 5 mg	20 tablets
Atropine for injection 600 mcg	5 ampoules
Furosemide 40 mg	10 tablets
Glyceryl trinitrate spray	1

Respiratory/allergy

Adrenaline 1:1000	10×1 ml
Beclomethasone inhaler 100 mcg	2
Chlorphenamine 4 mg	60 tablets
Chlorphenamine injection 10 mg	5 ampoules
Cetirizine 10 mg	20 tablets
EpiPen®	1
Hydrocortisone injection 100 mg	5 ampoules
Otrivine-Antistin® (eye drops)	2
Prednisolone EC 5 mg	100 tablets
Salbutamol inhaler (Ventolin®)	2

Altitude

Acetazolamide 250 mg	100 tablets
Dexamethasone 2 mg	40 tablets
Nifedipine MR caps 20 mg	20 capsules

Creams and ointments

Aciclovir cream (Zovirax®)	$2 \text{ g} \times 6$
Anusol-HC® cream	$15 \text{ g} \times 1$
Mupirocin cream	$15 \text{ g} \times 6$
Betadine	$500 \text{ ml} \times 1$
Clotrimazole cream	$20 \text{ g} \times 6$

Crotamiton (Eurax®)—anti-pruritic	30 g × 2
Cyanoacrylate tisssue glue	1
E45 cream	50 g tube
Flamazine® cream	50 g tube
Hydrocortisone cream 1%	15 g × 6
Magnesium sulphate paste	50 g × 1
Savlon® concentrate	100 ml
Silver nitrate cautery sticks	5
Tisept® sachets (chlorhexidine and cetrimide)	25 ml × 15
Tropicamide 1%	3 ampoules
Sunblock SPF 25+	1

Hardware

Blood glucose monitoring equipment	
BNF—British National Formulary (most recent edition)	1
Head torch, pen torch	1
Dental first aid kit	1
Disposable scalpels, scissors, forceps, wooden spatulas	2
Fluorescein eye test strips	10
Kendrick traction device	1
Gloves sterile (medium)	10 pairs
Isolaide resuscitation aid	2
Latex gloves (non-sterile)	100
Safety pins	12
Sam splint	2
Sterile supplies kit	1
Stifnek™ select neck immobilizer	2
Thermometer (digital)	1
Tuff Cut® scissors	1

Dressings

Adhesive plasters	50 assorted
Alcohol swabs	100 × 2
Crepe bandages 7.5 and 10 cm	4
Dressing No. 15	2
Eye dressing No. 16	4
Gallipot	5

Gauze swabs 5 × 5 cm^2	100
Inadine dressings	10
Melolin dressing 10 cm^2	5
Melolin dressing 5 cm^2	5
Micropore tape 2.5 cm	2 rolls
Nasal tampons	5
Steri-Strips™, assorted	4 packets
Sutures 3/0, 4/0, 5/0	4 of each
Triangular bandages	8
Tubigrip (knee/ankle)	10 m of each
Tubinette (size 01)	5 m
Tubinette finger applicator	1
Vaseline gauze 10cm^2	10
Zinc oxide roll plaster	2 rolls
Injection equipment and intravenous fluids	
2 ml, 5 ml, 10 ml syringes	20 of each
Blue, green, orange needles	20 of each
iv cannulae 14G, 18G	10 of each
Giving sets	5
Normal saline 1 l	6
Gelofusine	500 ml × 8
Dextrose 5%	500 ml × 4

In addition
An up-to-date *BNF* should be carried at all times. It should be referred to to check drug doses, side effects and contraindications. Also see: http://www.bnf.org/bnf/index.htm

Other equipment to consider
The use of these items requires special training and so will depend on the medical skills in the group:
• Stethoscope
• Anaeroid sphygmomanometer
• Auriscope/ophthalmoscope
• Oropharyngeal/nasopharyngeal airways
• Nasogastric tube
• Urinary catheter
• Chest drains and Heimlich valves for pneumothorax
• Suturing equipment
• Dental forceps, if skilled
• Snake (or other) antivenom.

Extra drugs and equipment for specific environments

Malarious areas (📖 p. 474)

Take spare prophylactic antimalarials if the expedition is going to a region where malaria is endemic—someone always loses their tablets! Also take a different and appropriate drug for standby (prospective) treatment of a fever that could be malaria (e.g. Riamet®/coartemether). Rapid diagnostic tests for malaria can be very useful (📖 p. 475). Mosquito nets should be re-treated with permethrin every 3–6 months (depending on the amount of rain and UV exposure); always carry spare permethrin together with protective gloves.

Sailing, boating, or canoeing (📖 p. 633)

Participants develop chapped hands, salt water boils, and sunburn. Lanolin-based hand cream is useful and Dramamine® or cinnarizine are recommended for seasickness.

Tropical areas (📖 p. 675)

Wound infections are common, and small individual iodine tincture bottles are recommended to clean wounds plus additional topical antibiotics. Antivenoms for snakes, scorpions, etc. may be considered for high-risk areas and occupations plus several long 10 cm-wide crepe bandages for pressure immobilisation (📖 p. 531).

Diving expeditions (📖 p. 658)

Otitis externa (diver's ear) is common; take extra antibacterial eardrops (e.g. Gentisone HC®) and consider aluminium acetate or distilled water after each dive. Oxygen, chest drains, and ventilation equipment may be needed. Find out where decompression facilities exist before you need them! Consider additional antibiotics for marine wound infections.

Mountain expeditions (📖 p. 607)

Oxygen is bulky and heavy but is essential for any trip above 6000 m. Acetazolamide, nifedipine, and dexamethasone should certainly be carried. Consider the excellent Kendrick traction device for thigh fractures as these can be life-saving in remote areas—they are lightweight (around 500 g) and are very popular with mountain rescue teams.

Desert environments (📖 p. 675)

Dehydration and heat-related illnesses are of major concern. Strongly consider iv fluids and plenty of cannulae and giving sets. Total block suncream and goggles to keep sand out of eyes are recommended. (A hand-held global positioning system is very reassuring when wells or wadis are few and far between.)

Caving (📖 p. 665)

Histoplasmosis, a fungal infection of the lungs, may be contracted while caving. Symptoms of severe pneumonia which are unresponsive to antibiotics would merit evacuation for a chest X-ray and investigation (treatment is with iv amphotericin B). Rabies was once contracted by some cave explorers in Texas, but since many caves are bat-infested and bats of all kinds may carry rabies, pre-exposure rabies prophylaxis should be considered. A number of other infections, bacterial, viral, fungal, and protozoal, have been contracted in caves; some are bat- or bird-related. See http://www.latech.edu/tech/education/cavedis/cave-disease-table2_1.html. Siopel® silicone cream is recommended for macerated skin produced by prolonged contact with wetsuits. Foul air can cause lethal carbon dioxide poisoning, and carbon monoxide monitors and oxygen may be required.

Useful addresses

Home Office Drugs Branch, 50 Queen Anne's Gate, London SW1H 9AT (0207 273 4085).

Medical Export Services Ltd, PO Box 179, London SW5 9DS (0207 404 5011).

Medicines Control Agency, Market Towers, 1 Nine Elms Lane, London SW8 5NQ.

Nomad Medical Ltd, 3–4 Turnpike Lane, London N8 0PX (0208 889 7014).

Further reading

A'Court CHD, Stables RH, Travis S (1995). Doctor on a mountaineering expedition. BMJ **310**: 1248–52.

Auerbach PS, Donner HJ, Weiss EA (2003). *Field Guide to Wilderness Medicine*. St Louis, Mosby.

Du Pont HL, Steffen R (1997). *Textbook of Travel Medicine and Health*. Hamilton, Ontario, BC Decker.

Medical and first aid training

Managing sudden illness or injury on an expedition is very different from giving conventional first aid in a developed country where there is rapid recourse to definitive care. It may be necessary to render first aid in difficult environmental conditions—desert heat, Siberian cold, at high altitude, in darkness, rain, or snow. Evacuating a patient to definitive medical care may take days because of a remote location, poor weather conditions, or lack of communications and suitable transport. This means that expedition team members need to be prepared to give first and second aid while on an expedition. Some medical conditions encountered on expeditions will be very unusual in the UK and are not covered in standard first aid texts, e.g. malaria, altitude illness, and venomous bites and stings. Learning advanced first aid techniques such as straightening broken limbs or using antibiotics to treat infections will be essential and the use of any special medical equipment or drugs will require careful training.

Ideally, all expedition team members should have a basic first aid qualification. Basic first aid training should cover:
- Scene assessment and safe approach to the injured casualty
- Basic life support
- Control of bleeding and the management of shock
- Simple fracture treatment
- Care of the unconscious patient
- Safe movement of the injured patient.

If it is not possible to train all team members, then a trained first-aider should be available at each expedition project site.

First aid courses
Basic first aid
This is best learnt by attending one of the many standard courses run by the St John Ambulance or the British Red Cross. In addition, many other providers run courses aimed at those wanting to work in an outdoor environment.
See http://www.sja.org.uk and http://www.redcrossfirstaidtraining.co.uk

Aims of first aid

- To preserve life
- To limit worsening of the condition
- To promote recovery

Principles of first aid

- Assess the situation
- Make the area safe
- Assess all casualties
- Start with the ABC of resuscitation
- Identify the injury or illness
- Prioritize giving appropriate and adequate treatment
- Organize appropriate removal of casualties to secondary care
- Make and pass on a report

Specialist courses on expedition medicine

Expedition Medicine—http://www.expeditionmedicine.co.uk/
Expemed—http://voyageconcepts.co.uk
Medical Expertise—http://www.medical-expertise.co.uk/
Wilderness Medical Society—http://www.wms.org/
Wilderness Medical Training:
http://www.wildernessmedicaltraining.co.uk/
MEDEX—for specialist courses in mountain medicine—
http://www.medex.org.uk/courses_mountain_medicine_2005.htm
Wilderness Emergency Medical Service Institute—
http://www.wemsi.org/
See also RGS website—http://www.rgs.org/GOseminars

Expedition medical skills for the medical officer

The expedition MO (and as many of the expedition team as possible) should have basic first aid skills, be able to measure vital signs, and be able to diagnose and treat important, common illnesses and injuries. For an expedition MO the bare minimum of skills needed is listed in Table 2.4.

More detailed information on how to diagnose and manage each of the conditions listed in Table 2.4 can be found within this book. To gain the necessary experience to deal with such conditions, it is advisable to attend a specialist course on expedition medicine (☐ p. 55).

Table 2.4 Essential expedition medical skills

Knowledge and management of:

1. Common expedition complaints:
- Blisters
- Bruises
- Sprains and strains
- Cuts/grazes
- Splinters
- Burns/scalds
- Bleeding

2. Common medical conditions:
- Infections, such as diarrhoea, URTI, and urinary infections
- Asthma
- Fits
- Headaches

3. Serious medical problems:
- Anaphylaxis
- Chest and abdominal pain
- Dyspnoea and cough

4. Important injuries:
- Head and spinal injuries
- Fracture and dislocation reduction and splinting

5. Environmental injuries:
- Altitude-related illness—AMS, HAPE, HACE (☐ p. 620)
- Heat illnesses—heat exhaustion and heatstroke
- Cold injuries—frost bite, hypothermia
- Diving injuries
- Venomous bites and stings (☐ p. 517)

6. Patient handling:
- Moving, lifting, and straightening of injured casualties
- Patient transportation, including improvised stretchers

7. Ability to provide remote advice and coach first-aiders through treatment.

Medical screening

Selection vs inclusiveness

Some potential expedition team members, including leaders, have pre-existing health problems or disabilities. The majority of these people can still enjoy safe, successful trips with careful planning.

There are several issues:
- Team leaders and group members may be concerned that some disabilities or chronic illnesses may prevent individuals from participating fully in the physical and emotional challenges of an expedition
- It is possible that the rigours of expedition life may worsen the underlying condition (and possibly compromise others)
- If the underlying condition does deteriorate, adequate facilities may not be available.

It is therefore essential to weigh up the possible risks to an expeditioner's health against the potential benefits of travel for any individual who has significant pre-existing health problems. It would be nice to include all applicants, but for some the risk of serious illness, even death, may be unacceptable.

Minimizing the risks—things to consider

- Ensure all participants complete a health questionnaire—preferably at least 6 months before planned departure (Table 2.5).
- Follow up any significant issues with the patient or request a GP report or report from a specialist
- How stable is the condition, and how severe?
- Exclude those with:
  - Unstable, severe mental illness, e.g. schizophrenia, bipolar disorder, hypomania, depression
  - Any current untreated psychological disorder
- Consider carefully whether to take or exclude those with:
  - Repeat episodes of anxiety or depression
  - Recent loss events
  - Eating disorders
  - Deliberate self-harm and previous suicide attempts
- Ask for any previous remote travel experience and how they coped
- Ask about travel environment, expedition duration, medical back-up, communications in the field, and evacuation logistics
- Make a decision—will this individual be travelling at unacceptable risk?
- Sometimes acceptance on a trip is provisional pending performance on training exercises or a full medical examination and review
- Occasionally, significant pre-existing illness is not declared until the expedition is in the field. This can be a very risky situation where there is inadequate information about the condition, additional medication is not available, and the expedition is very remote from expert medical help. If the applicant is uninsured because the insurers will not cover this particular condition, it may be necessary to repatriate that person.

Table 2.5 A health questionnaire for pre-existing conditions

1. Do you suffer from asthma, epilepsy, or diabetes?

2. Are you allergic to anything?

3. Have you ever had any heart problems?

4. Do you suffer from recurring back or joint problems?

5. Have you ever had psychological or psychiatric illness, including eating disorders, deliberate self-harm, overdoses, depression, anxiety, or psychosis?

6. Do you have any objections to any form of treatment, including blood transfusions or immunizations?

7. Do you have any current medical problems?

Uninsured psychiatric problem—case history

A 19-year-old gap year student had a previous history of bipolar affective disorder. He told the company organizing the placement in Ecuador and they requested information from the treating psychiatrist. The psychiatrist provided a letter stating that she was confident that the student would be able to cope with the rigours of a 6-month trip to Ecuador, that he was stable on medication, and she had no concerns that he would not be supervised during the placement. Two weeks after arrival in-country the student stopped taking medication and became violent and deluded. It was clear he would need to be repatriated for inpatient treatment and the company started to arrange this via the insurers. At this stage it emerged that the student had not declared the psychiatric illness to his insurance company, and the insurers declined to meet the cost of the claim. After 2 weeks' inpatient treatment in Ecuador the student was flown home accompanied by his father and a consultant psychiatrist from Quito. The parents had to pay £7500 to cover these costs.

Generic pre-expedition advice
- Staff and other team members should have a working knowledge of any disability or illness and immediate treatment that may be necessary, such as management of hypoglycaemia, anaphylaxis, or convulsions in fellow expeditioners
- Review the group medical kit—will any extra items be required?
- What are the medical skills of the expedition MO?
- How long will the group be remote from definitive medical care?
- What local medical facilities exist?
- Look at evacuation logistics before they are needed
- Remember adverse weather conditions will affect air evacuation plans, and in many parts of the world night-time flying is not possible, even in an emergency
- Plan escape routes so that a journey can be curtailed if necessary
- Anticipate what means of communication will be needed—telephone, email, satellite phones, radios, EPIRB (emergency position indicating radio beacon), mobile phones
- Ensure that the expedition insurers are fully informed—some pre-existing medical conditions attract a higher insurance premium, and insurers may not meet a claim if they have not been informed of all material facts.

Pre-expedition advice for the participants
- The individual should be able to demonstrate a good level of fitness appropriate to expedition activities to be undertaken. Short, low-intensity trips to a similar environment with different activity levels will be particularly useful for people with conditions such as diabetes where the individual needs to learn to manage their illness in varied conditions
- Optimize the illness and monitor with a diary of blood sugars, blood pressure, peak flow rates, etc.
- Each individual should have a self-management plan after discussion with the GP, specialist nurse, or consultant. This can be summarized in a letter from the treating doctor together with any significant past illnesses and medications
- Individuals need to carry their own medication with some in reserve
- Discuss the risks openly, and ensure participants are prepared to accept them.

During the journey
- Flying west results in a long day, flying east a short day
- People who take regular medication should stay on home time and then adjust timings on arrival
- All travellers need to keep hydrated and mobile, particularly while flying
- Pro-thrombotic conditions may benefit from aspirin, compression stockings, even low molecular weight heparin injections.

During the expedition
- Advice and support should be available—from group leaders/medical team or local medical staff
- Where good communications exist it may be possible to obtain advice from the home country and treating doctors
- Encourage the 'buddy system', particularly for younger groups, so that all individuals are looking out for any problems.

After the expedition
- Encourage reassessment of the medical condition with the expeditioner's GP/specialist
- Send a report of any significant problems to the GP
- Consider contributing to the RGS Expedition Health and Safety Survey—medical problems and 'near misses', available at: http://www.rgs.org/medicalcell

Advising those with pre-existing conditions

Notes on common problems

Asthma (📖 p. 362)

15–20% of young people have asthma
- Optimize control before departure to enable a good level of fitness.
- Consider carrying a peak flow meter and spacer (probably not a nebulizer as this is bulky and heavy, but consider if on-board ship or on a larger expedition)
- Carry a supply of oral and injectable steroids
- Consider antibiotics
- Follow the British Thoracic Society (BTS) guidelines for management.
- Each individual should discuss a treatment plan with GP, asthma nurse, or respiratory specialist before departure
- May need to exclude those with very severe, brittle asthma.
- High-altitude travel is not a provoking factor for asthma, but an asthma exacerbation at high altitude will be more serious because of the hypoxic environment.

The management of acute asthma is discussed in Chapter 11.

Diabetes (📖 p. 238)

Diabetes need not be a contraindication to travel; however, a person with diabetes needs to be confident monitoring their blood sugars and adjusting their diabetes control. Those who have recently been diagnosed with diabetes should consider deferring a trip to a very remote area until they are completely confident that they can manage the disease safely without outside support.

The main concerns regarding travel with diabetes are:
- The risk of hypoglycaemia because of changes in time zones, food intake, and energy output. Some blood sugar monitors are less reliable in extreme conditions such as sub-zero temperatures
- Infections are more likely and may be more serious, especially gastro-enteritis
- In those who have had diabetes for many years there is an increased risk of heart attack or stroke. Reduced kidney function, disturbances in skin sensation (particularly the feet), and ulceration should be considered.

Before the expedition

Antimalarials and immunizations should be advised as for other travellers.

It is useful to have the following information from the GP, diabetes nurse, or specialist
- Date of diagnosis
- How well controlled is the patient's diabetes (HbA1c level)?
- Do they follow medical advice?
- Insulin type, dosage, frequency?

- Have there been admissions to hospital with hypoglycaemia/hyperglycaemia?
- Any complications—neuropathy, ulceration, insulin resistance?
- Has treatment varied over last year?

This information can be written in a letter and given to the patient. If appropriate, it can also usefully mention the need for carrying needles and syringes. Those who are insulin-dependent should consider switching to soluble insulin four times daily with very frequent blood sugar measurements.

Even if not eating, people with diabetes continue to need regular insulin, and frequent blood sugar testing becomes even more important. Intravenous fluids and injectable antiemetics may be needed if vomiting occurs, and the use of these items may need special training or the presence of a suitably qualified healthcare professional.

Other group members should be trained in recognizing the symptoms of hypoglycaemia and the treatment needed—GlucoGel®, Glucagon, or, rarely, intravenous glucose 10%.

During the expedition
It is important to consider:
- Will there be medical/nursing staff available to supervise/advise treatment?
- The expedition organizers need to consider the dietary needs of those with diabetes. Snacks should be readily available in case of delays or low blood sugar levels
- 'Ideal' blood sugar levels may not be possible because of varying diet and activity levels. The main concern is preventing hypoglycaemia, so a little latitude is reasonable for a few weeks during the trip
- People with diabetes are more susceptible to infections and should report any symptoms at an early stage before blood sugar levels become erratic. Foot infections may be particularly serious in those who do not have normal sensation—wounds must be treated promptly to prevent ulceration and other complications.

Checklist for the individual
- Should have usual immunizations and antimalarials
- Ensure adequate supplies of insulin, lancets, sugar testing sticks, syringes/pens, needles, sharps disposal, glucometer, Hypostop, and glucagon
- A talisman such as a MedicAlert® bracelet should be worn
- Are the insurers aware, as diabetes is a significant pre-existing condition?
- If the individual suffers from travel sickness, consider an antiemetic to prevent vomiting/dehydration
- Insulin storage (see box)
- Oral rehydration solutions and an antiemetic should be available.

Insulin

Ideally insulin should be stored at 4–8°C. At these temperatures it will remain active for up to 2 years. At 30°C it will remain effective for about 2 months.

Frio® insulin storage pouches keep insulin vials cool in hot climates for up to 45 h (http://www.friouk.com).

Insulin should be carried in hand luggage, although a medical letter of authorization may be required. X-rays do not affect insulin.

Vacuum flasks can be used to protect insulin from climatic extremes.

If insulin is 'clumped' or turbid it should not be used.

Other resources:
http://www.diabetes.org.uk
http://www.diabetes-exercise.org

Hypertension

Isolated, well-controlled hypertension is not a problem for most people travelling to remote areas. However, if there is evidence that organs have been damaged secondary to hypertension (heart failure, renal failure) the risks of stroke or heart attack will be much higher. Consider:
• Blood pressure should be stable before travel
• Consider an ECG and an exercise tolerance test if there are risk factors
• Check renal function before travel
• Ensure that there is a good level of fitness and that individuals can cope with activity levels similar to those likely to be encountered on the trip
• Blood pressure may improve with weight loss and increased exercise during an expedition. Consider whether measuring blood pressure during the trip will be feasible or even sensible
• Antihypertensive medication:
  • May affect exercise tolerance
  • Beta-blockers can cause lethargy and limit maximum heart rate response. They also reduce the blood flow to the extremities, which may become important when travelling to cold areas
  • Diuretics increase urine output and can lead to hypotension if an individual is already dehydrated
  • Angiotensin-converting enzyme (ACE) inhibitors can also cause hypotension after exercising
  • Calcium channel blockers affect heart rate during exercise and side effects include ankle swelling and flushing which may be worse in hot climates
  • Consider carrying aspirin 300 mg for angina or heart attacks, GTN spray for angina, and blood pressure monitoring equipment
• After return, people with hypertension should be medically reassessed to check current blood pressures and renal function.

Cardiovascular disease (📖 p. 351)

A history of angina, previous MI, diabetes, hypercholesterolaemia, family history of ischaemic heart disease or claudication will all be worrying. Stresses of expedition life may provoke symptoms of chest pain (📖 p. 351) or breathlessness on exertion.

Six months after heart attack or coronary artery bypass graft/ angioplasty or stenting it is possible to undertake remote foreign travel provided there are no symptoms of chest pain or breathlessness while exercising to the level required on the expedition.

There always remains the risk of recurrence and this must be accepted by the individual and team members. Formal exercise tolerance testing prior to travel is essential. Ask the question: can the individual undertake vigorous activity at the same level as expected on the expedition (i.e. can they spend long days walking in the British hills)?

Epilepsy (📖 p. 296)

The consequences of a seizure during an expedition activity could be very serious; for instance, falling from the back of an open vehicle, being tossed overboard during white water rafting, collapsing on steep ground. Dehydration, alcohol, stress, and lack of sleep may all provoke convulsions. Gastroenteritis may affect antiepileptic levels and result in fitting.

Before the trip more information will be required regarding the frequency, severity, preventive medication, and treatment of convulsions. Other team members need to be aware and know what to do in the event of a fit (📖 p. 236). Antiepileptic medication may interact with other drugs, particularly antimalarials (chloroquine and mefloquine) and quinolones such as ciprofloxacin.

Treatment of status epilepticus (a seizure lasting longer than 30 min) is very difficult in a remote environment and the condition can be life-threatening. Those with epilepsy should follow guidance regarding swimming, driving, operating machinery, and dangerous activities such as diving and rock climbing as they would at home. Epilepsy is a significant pre-existing health problem and insurers must be aware of the diagnosis in the event of a claim. Consider taking rectal and iv diazepam together with an oropharyngeal airway and a hand-held suction device.

People with epilepsy are definitely travelling at increased risk but this can be minimized with preparation—some activities such as SCUBA diving may be unacceptably risky and this should be understood before departure.

Allergy and anaphylaxis

Anaphylaxis is a severe form of allergic reaction (📖 p. 220). It may be provoked by food, drugs, or insect bites and stings. Knowledge of the allergy is essential for cooks, expedition staff, and other group members.

All expedition members need to be aware of the symptoms and signs of severe allergic reactions and should know how to give adrenaline (epinephrine), if required. A MedicAlert®/MediTag bracelet or similar talisman should be worn at all times.

Adrenaline (epinephrine) in the form of an EpiPen® (simpler to use than Anapen), if recommended by the GP or specialist, needs to be carried at all times and must be kept in hand luggage during air travel. It is useless unless the person at risk knows how to use it, without delay, in an emergency. Consider taking extra drugs for anaphylaxis—epinephrine, chlorphenamine, hydrocortisone, ranitidine, and a salbutamol inhaler.

In those with severe allergies, consider oral antihistamine for the duration of the trip (beware of interactions with older antihistamines such as terfenadine). This should be discussed with the GP or specialist. Remember that severe allergy can be induced by aspirin in some people, and that aspirin and widely used non-steroidal anti-inflammatory agents, such as ibuprofen (Nurofen®) and diclofenac (Voltarol®), can cause or aggravate urticaria and angioedema.

Useful addresses
http://www.anaphylaxis.com
http://www.allergyfoundation.com

Suggested questions for those with allergies

1. What are you allergic to?
2. How do you react to this substance and how often?
3. When did you last have an allergic reaction?
4. What treatment is necessary when you have an allergic reaction?
5. When, if ever, have you required hospital treatment for an allergic reaction?

Inflammatory bowel disease

Inflammatory bowel disease such as Crohn's disease or ulcerative colitis (UC) may predispose individuals to severe, possibly life-threatening diarrhoea and gastrointestinal haemorrhage. Other complications such as anaemia, dehydration, and generalized infection may also occur. The drugs used to treat inflammatory bowel disease may, depending on the dose, have an effect on the immune system so that infections may be easier to acquire.

Individuals with inflammatory bowel disease should be fully aware of the potential risks. Severe, bloody diarrhoea, particularly if associated with a fever or abdominal pain, require prompt medical attention.

For those with inflammatory bowel disease:
• Avoid traveller's diarrhoea if at all possible
• Inform the MO immediately if there is any flare-up of disease—particularly bloody stools and fever
• The group should carry oral rehydration solutions, iv fluids, antibiotics, and steroids
• A casualty evacuation plan should be in place.

Further information may be found at http://www.crohns.org.uk

Psychiatric illness (📖 p. 495)

Depression, anxiety, DSH (deliberate self harm), and eating disorders are all common, but there is often non-disclosure and this may affect insurance cover (see case history).

A carefully worded pre-expedition questionnaire is needed to ensure that psychiatric and psychological illness is not overlooked.

Some expedition companies will not accept those still taking antidepressant medication because of the difficulty of managing an exacerbation and for arranging regular supervision.

Involve the GP and/or psychiatrist in making the decision regarding fitness to travel—an expedition is not the place to convalesce from a serious mental health problem.

If there is a history of psychotic illness some psychiatrists recommend that the individual has been stable for 2 years, is off medication and can show evidence of coping with stressful situations, including foreign travel.

Disabilities

Remarkable achievements on expeditions have been made by those with significant disabilities. Appropriate challenges can be identified which help to maintain independence and dignity by the use of special adaptations. A multidisciplinary team (occupational therapists, physiotherapists, nurses, rehabilitation physicians, and prosthetists) can all contribute to identifying these challenges and advising on safe travel.

The needs of those with disabilities may be considered under the following headings:

• Mobility (prostheses, wheelchair, ability to transfer)
• Seating (are specialized cushions required?)
• ADLs (activities of daily living)—what help is needed for activities of daily living—washing, feeding, shaving, toileting?
• Communication—consider the safety aspects for those with hearing or visual impairment
• Bladder/bowel control—self-catheterization, use of suppositories, changing ileostomy bags are all possible issues which will need sensitive management
• Skin—prolonged walking, immersion in sea water, and the effects of heat may affect the skin under a prosthetic limb or the prosthesis itself. Those with paraplegia may quickly develop pressure sores or blisters without realizing so skin care in this group is very important
• Cognitive and behavioural—are there any difficulties with thinking, understanding, behaviour, or psychological issues?

HIV and immunosuppression

Expedition members who are HIV positive or immunosuppressed for other reasons need special advice about immunizations and prophylaxis against opportunistic infections.

See http://www.bhiva.org/files/file1001634.pdf
http://www.cdc.gov/mmwr/preview/mmwrhtml/rr5315a1.htm

Child health in remote areas

Exploring with children and adolescents broadens everyone's horizons and facilitates introductions to people who might otherwise have been passed by. It does, however, often mean adapting the style and pace of travel. Goal-driven trips where the targets have been set by adults without consulting younger members can be disastrous. Involve everyone in the planning and allow time for everyone to indulge their interests. The trip will be most successful if the adults are performing well within their levels of competence. Children are often more adaptable and resourceful than the adults with whom they travel.

Immunization

Parents will need to ensure their child is up to date with the routine childhood vaccines (📖 p. 33) because, in less well resourced regions, levels of local immunization will be low and thus 'herd' immunity is poor. Travellers are therefore at increased risk of measles, pertussis, diphtheria, etc. For other immunizations the family should probably consult a travel health expert. Intrepid children are more likely to get bitten by dogs and monkeys; rabies immunization is therefore especially relevant for any child capable of independent propulsion.

Yellow fever immunization is not given to infants under the age of 9 months so this might preclude family travel to regions where yellow fever is common.

Typhoid immunization has poor efficacy in children under the age of 18 months and gives no cover at all against paratyphoid. Parents must therefore be especially aware of the means of reducing the risk of these and other faecal–oral infections (📖 p. 382).

Antimalarials

Both Lariam (mefloquine) and Malarone (atovaquone + proguanil) can be given to children. Mefloquine does not seem to cause the problems with mood that adults sometimes experience; the tablets crack easily into quarters for children's doses. It should be noted, however, that travel into highly malarious regions with small children or in pregnancy may be unwise and expert advice should be sought before travel.

Unfamiliar environments

Odd and unexpected things can faze children and adolescents, including weird food, unfamiliar lavatorial arrangements (toddlers can't squat over long drops), and issues surrounding personal space. Small children prefer to be down at a level where they too can explore; they get bored if carried all day, and it is sobering to realize that every year in the Alps children die from hypothermia while being carried in backpacks by skiing or mountaineering parents. A thermometer is not necessary to assess if a baby or toddler is chilling dangerously. Compare his skin temperature on the limbs with trunk temperature; if the limbs feel colder then the child needs to be warmed in a place of shelter.

Sunshine

Sunburn in childhood is associated with an increased risk of skin cancer in adulthood. It also makes the whole family miserable. Severe sunburn can lead to hypothermia, disastrous loss of fluids, and secondary infection. It is crucial, therefore, that children are protected with long clothes, hats, sun-protective swimsuits, umbrellas (if carried in a backpack), sunscreens, and avoidance of exposure at the very hottest times of the day. So-called sunblocks reduce exposure to the wavelengths that cause sunburn without necessarily giving adequate protection to cancer-causing wavelengths. SPFs of 15 to 30 are therefore recommended; sunscreens need to be reapplied frequently (see also Skin 🕮 p. 246).

A fine pimply, very itchy rash is probably *prickly heat*. Unlike many of the other causes of itching in children, this is not a histamine-mediated response and so it doesn't respond to antihistamines. The treatment is getting the child cool—either by immersing or splashing with cold water, dabbing (not rubbing) with damp a cloth, and/or retreating to a room with a fan or air conditioning. Calamine lotion is soothing. Dressing the child in loose fitting, 100% cotton clothes will help avoid the problem, and so will a rest during the hottest part of the day.

Bite prevention (🕮 see p. 264)

It is wise to embrace precautions that avoid insect and tick bites, not least because an itching bitten child is miserable but, in hot climates, scratched bites often lead to skin infections. Hydrocortisone 1% or Betnovate® RD ointments are the best treatment for bites and stings, although could promote infection if the skin is broken. Skin infections (🕮 p. 272–280) cause spreading redness, oozing, sometimes red tracking on the affected limb, and, later, fever.

In addition to the discomfort of insect bites, there is—of course—also the possibility of acquiring a serious vector-borne disease (including malaria) from a bite. As children grow older and more adventurous they are probably more prone to picking up ticks, which puts them at risk of further significant infections—even in the UK. Choosing the right clothes and footwear helps keep biters away, as does spraying these clothes with permethrin. At dusk, any remaining exposed skin can be covered in a repellent based on up to 30% DEET, or Merck 3535. Repellents that are based on citronella or lemon eucalyptus are less effective alternatives and are not suitable for malarious regions. Children find applications of repellent to the face very unpleasant and it is easily rubbed into the eyes. Fortunately, plastering the face with repellents is seldom necessary. If the child is small then he can be protected under a cot net (preferably also proofed with permethrin), and older children are partially protected by the fact that malaria mosquitoes tend to hunt at ankle level; thus applying repellent to the clothes usually discourages mosquitoes from searching up and biting the face. Further information on bite avoidance, bed nets, etc., is on 🕮 p. 477.

Ill or bored?

When children become unwell, they can become precipitously ill within hours, and diagnosis can very difficult, especially if the patient isn't yet capable of explaining where it hurts. A toddler with tonsillitis, for example, will often point to his tummy when asked where the pain is. Many cautious paediatricians advise against intrepid travel with children who cannot yet talk because:

• It is difficult to distinguish boredom from disease
• Small children are fearless and fall off things, or drown
• Children explore and swallow things they shouldn't
• If they get bacillary dysentery they can become dangerously ill rapidly
• Dehydration becomes an issue sooner and can be difficult to manage
• Malaria is a huge risk and bite precautions are difficult to enforce.

Once a child has reached the age of 4 years they become fun to travel with and they'll enjoy sharing your adventures. They can also be bribed to put on long clothes at dusk and apply repellent. They are also better able to communicate about any symptoms that they have. Illness with fever can initially be treated with both paracetamol and ibuprofen. In a non-malarial region it is probably safe to delay consulting a doctor if the child perks up, although meningitis or typhoid are always possible. In areas where malaria is a risk, a child with a fever over 38°C must be evacuated to a clinic or hospital.

Diagnostic aids

Diagnosis in an ill child is challenging whoever you are and travel makes this task even more difficult. The designated adult responsible for children would be well advised to travel with *urine dipsticks*, a *thermometer* and a *child health book*. The *Baby Check* scoring system is invaluable for grading the severity of illness in babies under 6 months (see Further reading). The responsible adult should also know the location of the nearest competent medical facility.

Common causes of high fever in children

• Tonsillitis (toddlers usually refuse food)
• Middle ear infection (with ear ache on one side only)
• Pneumonia/lung infection (>40 breaths/min)
• Bacillary dysentery (fever can start before the diarrhoea; blood is sometimes visible in the stools)
• Sepsis arising from wound infections
• Malaria (has the child been in a malarious region for >1 week?)
• Meningitis and meningococcal septicaemia
• Dengue fever (children raised in temperate zones often avoid the severe 'breakbone' illness of adults).

Common causes of drowsiness in children

• Fatigue
• Dehydration, especially secondary to diarrhoea
• Malaria
• Significant infection, including typhoid, meningitis, UTI, etc.
• The child has swallowed something noxious (e.g. someone's sleeping pills or paraffin in a coke bottle).

Diarrhoea

In diarrhoea, fluids are lost through increased bowel actions and from sweating (especially if there is also fever), yet the appetite will be wanting and often it is difficult to get the child to drink. Standard oral rehydration salts and even fruit-flavoured oral rehydration solutions taste unpleasant because of the potassium content, and many children—even if somewhat dehydrated—will refuse them. In most situations all that the child needs is water with some kind of solute in it. Sugars and/or salts enhance fluid transport into the body, so that water is absorbed more efficiently than if pure water is drunk.

Examples of rehydration solutions include:
- Young coconut
- Crackers and water
- Thin soups
- Colas (but not Diet Coke); add a pinch of salt
- Banana and water
- Toast, jam, and fluids
- Water or dilute squashes with honey or sugar added
- Weak herb teas with sugar added
- Blackcurrant juice
- Sweet drinks that you can see through
- Drinks made with Bovril, Marmite, or Oxo
- Plain carbohydrate foods such as boiled rice and noodles also enhance fluid absorption.

Dehydration

Paediatricians make meticulous calculations of what is required to rehydrate an ill child, but a child who is controlling fluid intake through drinking is most unlikely to overhydrate. An early sign of dehydration is to look at the lips and inside the mouth; if these areas look dry then the child needs more fluids. A child who is continuing to pass urine is not significantly dehydrated. Comparing the child's current weight with a recent reliable weight is a useful method of assessing whether there is dehydration. If the child becomes too drowsy to drink then intravenous or nasogastric fluids will be required.

Some causes of abdominal pain in children

- Diarrhoea/gastroenteritis (pain often relieved by passing wind or stool)
- Constipation (give more to drink, and lots of fruit; increasing pain often heralds stool passage)
- Tonsillitis (in the under-3s, antibiotics are recommended)
- Urinary tract ('bladder') infection (serious in the under-5s—treat with antibiotics and arrange further investigation by a doctor at home).
- Fatigue (equivalent to a grown-up's migraine)
- Appendicitis (usually in children >5 years; pain starts around navel and moves to right lower abdomen; a child with an appetite does not have appendicitis, nor does one who can jump around, or sit up from lying without pain). Suspected appendicitis needs evacuation to a hospital
- Meningitis 📖 p. 468 (an emergency—evacuate)
- Malaria 📖 p. 474 (an emergency—evacuate)

- Lower lobe pneumonia (respiratory rate is usually increased >40/min); antibiotics by mouth may cure. Hospital assessment is recommended
- Typhoid or paratyphoid (note that paratyphoid is not covered by current vaccines); this is a serious condition that needs expert treatment
- Hepatitis A or E (often mild in small children) and some other viral infections
- Intussusception (in child 3 months to 2 years; needs surgical treatment)
- Threadworm (there will also be anal itching); treat with oral mebendazole and repeat after 1 week
- Twisted testicle (some children are too shy to mention where it hurts); needs an urgent operation

Generally the further away the pain is from the navel the more likely it is to have a significant or serious cause. Pain that wakes a child at night suggests real illness and is seldom benign.

Breathing problems

Respiratory problems are common in travelling children. Perhaps a fifth will have asthmatic tendencies yet they may not have an inhaler with them. Chest infections are common too. Noisy breathing (grunting or wheezing) is a sign of illness, and the breathing rate will give some indication of the severity. Flaring of the nostrils on inspiration suggests that the child is struggling to get enough air into the lungs. Whistling or high-pitched musical noises, mostly on breathing out, suggest asthma, while deeper sounds, mostly on breathing in, are most likely to be due to croup or obstruction above the level of the lungs. Remember that asthma and croup can kill so, if in doubt, or if the child is small, evacuate to a hospital.

Normal breathing rates

Newborn baby	—30–40 breaths/min (>60 suggests difficulties)
Child >2 months	—less than 30/min (>40 suggests significant problem)
Big kids and adults	—<20 breaths/min

First aid supplies

Those new to family travel tend to take too much. Probably the most important item is a knowledge base or book. Colourful dressings seem to have remarkable analgesic properties and so does chocolate: these are important items to have immediately to hand. Wound infections begin readily in hot climates and so an appropriate means of cleaning and dressing wounds is essential. Savlon® Dry spray is convenient, as are antiseptic wipes. For long periods in remote regions, potassium permanganate crystals are light, cheap, and portable; they are often available at the destination (make up to a rosé wine-coloured solution in water and use this to bathe wounds). Do not use antiseptic creams since these promote infection. Other medication will depend upon the level of knowledge of the carers or medic.

Suggested medical kit

- Insect repellent (up to 30% DEET can be used, with care, on children).
- Sunscreen 15–30 SPF, broad-brimmed hat and sun-protective clothes.
- Paracetamol and/or ibuprofen syrup. (NB. If bought locally may not be so palatable.)
- Digital thermometer.
- Steri-Strips™.
- Colourful sticking plasters.
- 'Savlon® Dry iodine spray or other drying antiseptic.
- Hydrocortisone or Betnovate® ointment (for itchy bites and eczema).
- Amoxicillin syrup (if confident in use of antibiotics).
- Motion sickness preparation if child troubled by this (hyoscine is best for rapid onset one-dose situations or an antihistamine like cinnarizine if multi-dosing is likely).

Summary

Diagnosing illness in children, especially in the under-3s, is difficult—even for paediatricians—and so any adult travelling to remote places with small children must be well prepared, well read, and have a good back-out plan. The commonest causes of problems in travelling children are accidents, scrapes and bumps, swallowing things they shouldn't have, traveller's diarrhoea, skin sepsis, and common infections as at home: tonsillitis, ear, and chest infections. The responsible adult should either be carrying the wherewithal to treat these problems or should know someone who can.

Further reading

Baby Check is at http://www.nicutools.orcon.net.nz/MediCalcs/BabyCheck.html

Morley CJ et al. (1991). Field trials of the Baby Check score card. *Archives of Disease in Childhood* **66**: 100–20.

Wilson-Howarth J, Ellis M (2005). *Your Child Abroad: a travel health guide*. Bradt/Globe Pequot. Chalfont St. Peter, UK.

Risk management

The concept of managing risk is to identify potential hazards and use control measures to reduce significant risks. This process is only effective if all members of the expedition understand the necessity for these control measures to be in place and are willing to behave accordingly.

Risk can never be completely eliminated, and different people have different thresholds of 'acceptable risk'. Therefore, it is essential to include all expedition members in risk management planning. This ensures that members are fully aware of the risks the expedition is likely to encounter and are able to make an informed decision as to whether to take part in the expedition.

Risk assessments

At the heart of planning a safe and responsible expedition is the process of compiling the risk assessment. (See http://www.rgs.org/medicalcell for a generic Expedition Risk Assessment form.) The concept is simple; hazards need to be identified and assessed for the severity of risk they represent to the people associated with the expedition (Tables 2.6–2.8).

Risks that are identified are ranked on the basis of the relationship between severity of impact and likelihood of occurrence; the significant risks are then accepted or reduced using appropriate precautions (control measures) such as those identified in Table 2.9.

Definitions (source UK Health and Safety Executive (2006))

Five steps to risk assessment. Health and Safety Executive publication ref: INDG 163 (rev 2) 06/06.

- A *hazard* is anything that may cause harm, such as chemicals, electricity, working from ladders, an open drawer, etc.
- The *risk* is the chance, high or low, that somebody could be harmed by these and other hazards, together with an indication of how serious the harm could be

---

Areas to cover in a risk assessment

- The group
- The environment
- The activity, e.g. glacier survey
- Travel and camp life
- Local people
- Health

The UK Health and Safety Executive refers to the process as '*5 steps to risk assessment*' (2006). These are as follows:

1. Identify the hazards and associated risks
2. Identify who is potentially at risk and how
3. Identify the precautions or control measures to minimize the risk, including any further action required to reduce the risk to an acceptable level
4. Record findings
5. Review the risk assessment periodically.

Table 2.6 Relationship between likelihood and severity of risk

LIKELIHOOD / PROBABILITY *	SEVERITY / CONSEQUENCE / HEALTH EFFECT **				
	NEGLIGIBLE	LOW	MODERATE	HIGH	CRITICAL
IMPROBABLE					
REMOTE					
OCCASIONAL					
PROBABLE	LOW	MODERATE	HIGH	HIGH	CRITICAL
FREQUENT					

LOW MODERATE HIGH CRITICAL

* Definition see table 2.7
** Definition see table 2.8

Table 2.7 Likelihood/probability of impact of health exposure

Descriptor	Description of probability or health exposure
Frequent	Possibility of repeated incidents
	Approximately once or more per week
	Health exposure: frequent contact with the potential hazard at very high concentrations
Probable	Possibility of isolated incidents
	Approximately once per month
	Health exposure: frequent contact with the potential hazard at high concentrations
Occasional	Possibility of occurring some time
	Approximately once per year
	Health exposure: frequent contact with the potential hazard at moderate concentrations
Remote	Not likely to occur
	Approximately once in 10 years or less
	Health exposure: frequent contact with the potential hazard at low concentrations
Improbable	Practically impossible
	Approximately once in 100 years or more
	Health exposure: infrequent contact with the potential hazard at low concentrations

Table 2.8 Severity/consequence of the impact or health effect

Descriptor	Description of severity/consequence or health effect
Critical	*Health:* life-threatening or disabling illness
	Examples: HIV/AIDS, hepatitis B
	Safety: any fatality or potential for multiple fatalities. Permanent disability
High	*Health:* irreversible health effects of concern
	Examples: noise-induced hearing loss
	Safety: serious injuries with potential for a fatality
Moderate	*Health:* severe, reversible health effects of concern
	Examples: back/muscle strain, repetitive strain injury, heat stroke
	Safety: extensive injuries, hospitalization
Low	*Health:* reversible health effects
	Examples: sunburn, heat exhaustion
	Safety: injury requiring medical treatment
Negligible	*Health:* reversible effects of low concern
	Examples: minor muscular discomfort, skin rash
	Safety: minor injury requiring first aid treatment

Focus on the serious risks

To ensure risk assessments are effective, it is important to focus on hazards that present a serious risk to the group. Many models exist but simply by considering the severity of probable illness or injuries, it is then possible to judge the likelihood of a risk occurring (see Table 2.6)

> *The five locations where injuries are most likely to occur are:*
> - Roads
> - Beach
> - Hotels
> - Remote locations
> - Ski slopes
>
> (Source: FCO, 2005)

Research

The best tool for compiling risk assessments is experience of similar expeditions to the same destination involving similar activities. Reports from past expeditions and networking with individuals who have relevant experience will be useful.

Sources of expedition reports include:

Royal Geographical Society with IBG	http://www.rgs.org/expeditionreports
British Mountaineering Council	http://www.thebmc.co.uk
BP Conservation Award	http://conservation.bp.com/projects/default.asp
Royal Scottish Geographical Society	http://www.geo.ed.ac.uk/rsgs/expedits/reports/

A record of incidents and accidents on expeditions, and near misses has been compiled by the Royal Geographical Society's Medical Cell http://www.rgs.org/medicalcell and is summarized in Chapter 1 (📖 p. 6).

Expedition participants

Participants themselves create risk, for example through pre-existing medical conditions and inappropriate behaviour. People travel to remote places for various reasons, often involved with the wish to escape the confines and constraints of life at home and to take more risks. The data on increased levels of unprotected sexual contact by individuals on overseas visits reinforces this; however, extra risk-taking extends to all activities whilst on an expedition. It is the experience of many large expedition organizations that accidents tend to occur more often on days when expeditioners are relaxing (R-and-R 'off-duty' days), after hard work, and after drinking alcohol.

Assess the threats

Assessment of threat (including insurrection, political turmoil, anarchy, and lawlessness) can be completed via consultation with specialists or those who know the destination well. There are a number of risk consultancies that can be used, such as Control Risks Group, Kroll Security International, and Salamanca Risk.

Travel-related risks can also be researched using information sources provided by government representatives:

UK—Foreign and Commonwealth Office	http://www.fco.gov.uk
Australia—Department of Foreign Affairs and Trade	http://www.dfat.gov.au
US—State Department	http://www.travel.state.gov
Canada—Department of Foreign Affairs and Trade	http://www.voyage.gc.ca
World Health Organization	http://www.who.int
Centre for Disease Control	http://www.cdc.gov/travel
MASTA—Medical advice site	http://www.masta.org
BBC website	http://www.bbc.co.uk
In-country contacts and agent	
Special interest clubs	
Local Tourist Board website	
Guidebooks	

Control measures

Once the serious risks have been identified, each one must be reduced to an acceptable level using a control measure (Table 2.9).

As the table outlines, personal protective equipment (PPE, e.g. helmets) is one of the least effective methods of preventing risk and should not be used in isolation. A behavioural solution, such as avoiding areas of loose rock, should be used in combination with PPE.

Many control measures can be put in place by an expedition. For example:
- Providing first aid training for all members
- Getting immunized before exposure to disease
- Preventing bites by disease-transmitting insects.

During the expedition more control measures may need to be implemented that were not identified in the planning process. Reactive plans should aim to reduce the consequence of the incident via effective incident management and good crisis management. (See www.rgs.org/medicalcell for a generic Expedition Risk Assessment form that includes risk management strategies.)

Table 2.9 Proactive and reactive risk-reduction measures

	Method	Description
Most effective	Elimination	Do not do the activity
	Substitution	Do it in a different way; consider a 'Plan B'
↓	Engineering	Implement mechanical solution to reduce risk
	Behaviour	Behaviour to minimize risk
	PPE	Reduce the severity and likelihood of injury using PPE (personal protective equipment)
Least effective	Reactive Plans	First aid and emergency response plans to reduce severity of incident

Educate the group

It is important to share the outcomes of the risk assessment with the participants. This also provides the background for participants to understand why control measures are in place.

Therefore, the pre-visit information should include the risk assessment or, as a minimum, the key risks and control measures in place to reduce them. Continual enforcement of control measures and frequent briefing of risks is considered good practice.

Employ sensible flexible control measures

The key to effective control measures is to be flexible. Unnecessary overuse of control measures will produce a negative response from expedition members.

The level of controls used must reflect the seriousness of the risk. For example, drowning is more serious than new boots causing blisters. However, both these hazards can be highlighted in different ways. For example, a note about new boots in the pre-trip information coupled with group observation would be an effective way of reducing the likelihood of blisters.

The severity of drowning would require a different approach. This would include gathering data on whether participants can swim, providing appropriate life jackets, ensuring competent supervision and, finally, having an emergency response plan in case of capsize.

See also Emergency Response Planning 📖 p. 132 and Crisis Management 📖 p. 130 for further information.

Medical insurance

Making sure that there is adequate and appropriate insurance cover in place for all participants is an essential part of pre-expedition planning and integral to the Emergency Response Plan (📖 p. 132).

Eligible travellers from the UK are entitled to receive free or reduced-cost medical care in many European countries on production of a completed EHIC form (available from local Post Offices or Department of Health website). The EHIC is valid in all European Community countries plus Iceland, Liechtenstein, and Norway. However, few EU countries pay the full cost of medical treatment, and travellers visiting Europe even for a few days should take out insurance.

Most overseas visits will require insurance for the following elements:
• Medical treatment and additional expenses
• Repatriation
• Personal accident
• Search and rescue
• Replacement/rearrangement
• Public/personal liability.

You might also want to consider insurance for:
• Cancellation and curtailment
• Loss of baggage and equipment.

When buying insurance
• Do not under-insure; the costs of in-country medical expenses and repatriation can be high.
• Disclose all activities and risks to the insurer—including pre-existing medical conditions. Failure to do so will invalidate your policy.
• Check the small print and make sure cover is in place for all aspects of the visit and what exclusions apply.
• Ensure that specific risks are mentioned which concern your trip; for example, death from exposure.
• If local staff are hired, make enquires as to your responsibilities to them. Many countries have requirements for workers' compensation in the event of an accident or injury.
• Ensure that your policy will not expire if your expedition over-runs.
• For a group policy, be certain that the insurer has not limited the number of individuals covered in a single incident.
• The insurer should provide a 24-h phone number which can be called when an incident occurs.
• Report all claims as soon as possible; late claim notices may be affected by a time bar on the policy.

Types of insurance
Medical and additional expenses
Medical insurance should pay for treatment and travel expenses incurred for individuals following accidental injury or illness. The insurance should have a 24-h contact number available for the insurer to guarantee payment to treatment centers or emergency services should their help be required. The level of medical cover for each member should be at

least £1million for Europe and £2million for the rest of the world (source: FCO). Any pre-existing medical conditions must be disclosed to the insurer.

Personal accident

This covers death and disablement due to an accident whilst on an expedition. An amount is paid to the injured party in the event of loss of use of limbs, eyes, disablement, or death.

Search and rescue considerations

Insurance may be found to cover a search and rescue situation. However, this is an expensive activity and the price of insurance will reflect this. Pre-training and good communication will reduce the chance of individuals becoming detached from the group. The majority of search and rescues around the world are carried out via a mixture of police, army, and volunteers. The Emergency Response Plan should have links to these organizations. Emergency funds may be required to initiate this process.

Replacement and rearrangement

Insurance is available to cover the cost of replacing a key team member in the event of an expedition member being disabled or killed. It should also be possible to cover the costs of returning the injured person to the expedition when they have recovered.

Public/personal liability

Insurance against any legal liability incurred on the group or an individual or to a group or individual in the event of an incident is advisable. Leaders and medical professionals and expedition organizers have greater responsibilities than other members of the expedition.

Professional indemnity insurance

Doctors and other medical professionals should confirm that their professional indemnity insurance company will cover them to work with members of the expedition and/or host country nationals (see Legal Liabilities 📖 p. 87).

Legal liabilities and professional insurance

Introduction

This section is based on UK law; please be aware that the laws of the country in which the expedition takes place may apply. When reading this section please take away the legal principles but seek further specialist advice.

To date, there have been no reported cases where an expedition doctor has been successfully sued in a UK court. In this increasingly litigious climate, however, no practitioner can afford to be complacent.

In 1997 a UK court held that a mountain guide's breach of duty of care resulted in the death of a client, and awarded damages to the client's infant son. More recently, in December 2005, *The Times* reported that a private prosecution for unlawful killing had been launched by the father of the youngest Briton to reach the summit of Mount Everest—the judge ruled that there was no negligence and stated in his ruling that high altitude mountaineering is a hazardous sport where the risks are well recognized.

Relevant medical law is more likely to be found in case law (where judgments provide precedents) than in statute (enacted through Parliament).

Negligence

Negligence for clinical practitioners under UK law requires a claimant to demonstrate the following (known as the 'Bolam test'):
- The plaintiff owed a duty of care
- There was an accepted standard of care
- The duty of care was breached
- The claimant suffered harm
- Causation (that is, that the breach of the duty of care led to, or materially contributed to, the harm that the claimant suffered).

This has subsequently been slightly modified by the Bolitho ruling in which the Judge ruled that any standard of care would have to withstand logical analysis in a courtroom and that, exceptionally, a court may decide that expert medical opinion was flawed.

Courts have also extended these tests for negligence by a doctor to other cases where a defendant owes a duty of care to a claimant: for example, in the case of the mountain guide discussed above and in the case of the standard of care expected from a volunteer first-aider.

Duty of care

In the UK, an individual has no legal duty to assist members of the public when acting privately. The situation may differ in other countries. In France, for example, there is a legal obligation on every person to give emergency assistance at the scene of an accident, and failure to do so has resulted in prosecutions, most notably in the case of the paparazzi who abandoned the scene of the car crash involving Diana, Princess of Wales.

There may, however, be a professional obligation to render medical assistance. Even when off-duty, the General Medical Council expects doctors to provide emergency assistance.

> *'In an emergency, wherever it arises, you must offer assistance, taking account of your own safety, your competence, and the availability of other options for care.'*
>
> Section 11, Good Medical Practice, November 2006

The Nursing and Midwifery Council has indicated in its professional Code of Conduct that it requires similar actions of its registrants.

These professional obligations do not carry the full force of law, but penalties for failing to comply may be serious (recently, for example, the GMC issued a formal reprimand to a doctor who failed to render assistance to an injured person at the scene of a road accident) and, in the absence of legal precedent, this may be taken as instructive by courts.

Any person treating a patient, advising a patient, or advising an expedition company has, in law, a clear duty of care.

Standard of care

Where a duty of care is owed, the obligation is to exercise reasonable care and skill in the circumstances. The case of Bolam v Friern Hospital Management Committee (1957) produced the following definition of what is reasonable:

> *'The test is the standard of the ordinary skilled man exercising and professing to have that special skill. A man need not possess the highest expert skill at the risk of being found negligent ... it is sufficient if he exercises the skill of an ordinary man exercising that particular art.'*

This definition is supported and clarified by the case of Bolitho v City and Hackney Health Authority (1993).

Courts have indicated that they will not allow inexperience as a defence in actions of professional negligence: if a doctor is unable to exercise reasonable care in carrying out a particular task then he should not undertake this. Should a practitioner hold himself out to be an expedition doctor (and as such having a 'specialist' skill), therefore, his actions would be judged against what might reasonably be expected of a competent expedition doctor even if this were the first time the individual had ever taken on such a role.

At present, there are no established standards of care for expeditions, but a court may accept the expert advice of other practitioners who provide similar services to members of expeditions in defining what would currently be considered 'reasonable'. In the future, qualifications such as the recently established Diploma in Mountain Medicine http://www.medex.org.uk/dimm_(mountain_medicine_diploma).htm may be cited as evidence of a standard to be expected of a doctor accompanying a mountaineering expedition (see First aid and medical training for expeditions 📖 p. 54).

Causation

A claimant must prove that the breach of duty caused the harm suffered. What has to be proved is illustrated by the case of Barnett v Chelsea and Kensington Hospital Management Committee (1969). A man was sent home from a hospital accident and emergency department after complaining of acute stomach pains and sickness. He died later that same day of what proved to be arsenic poisoning. The hospital admitted a breach of duty but the widow failed to recover damages because the patient would have died whatever the doctor had done, i.e. causation could not be demonstrated.

In the context of an expedition, the requirement to demonstrate causation may prove to be the main obstacle to a claimant trying to sue a doctor for negligence. For example, in the case of a patient who suffered an intracranial bleed secondary to a head injury, it would be a challenge to show that it was a doctor's failure to site burr holes that led to long-term disability rather than the injury caused by a falling rock.

Emergency situations

In an emergency, courts take into account the specific circumstances, such as the need to act with speed in a hazardous situation, and determine whether a practitioner had acted with reasonable care. A court will recognize the fact that medicine was being practised in a remote area and that medical resources would be limited. As one judge ruled:

> '... I accept that full allowance must be made for the fact that certain aspects of treatment may have to be carried out in what one witness [...] called 'battle conditions'. An emergency may overburden the available resources, and, if an individual is forced by circumstances to do too many things at once, the fact that he does one of them incorrectly should not lightly be taken as negligence.'

> Wilsher v Essex Area Health Authority

However, expedition members, as potential patients, must be informed of the skills and limitations of the expedition medic (such as equipment carried, distance to definitive care, evacuation times, etc.). Similarly, the risks that expedition members will be taking need to be clearly spelt out—the popular *laissez faire* attitude of years gone by is unacceptable.

Liability on commercial expeditions

Most of the medical indemnity organizations will provide 'Good Samaritan' cover for doctors acting in any part of the world. However, this would apply only where a team member just happens to be a doctor. It would certainly not cover a doctor receiving any form of inducement (for example, a 10% discount on the trip fee) that may imply the doctor has an official medical role on the expedition.

Particular caution is required where citizens of the USA or Canada are participating in the expedition. Indeed, it may be impossible for a UK-registered doctor to obtain professional indemnity insurance other than on a 'Good Samaritan' basis for treating or advising people who are ordinarily residents of North America. English courts have jurisdiction over the deaths of Britons wherever they occur and there is no formal time limit for criminal prosecutions for unlawful killing. There is little doubt that an American court would claim an analogous jurisdiction over the death of an American citizen.

Expedition companies have a responsibility in Common Law to ensure that any medic that they choose to employ is suitably experienced. In the event of a claim for negligence, any claim would normally be made against the expedition company but this would not cover the professional negligence of a doctor.

Expeditions departing without a doctor

Many smaller expeditions may not have the resources to be able to take a doctor into the field. However, the team will still require medical advice and the supply of a suitable medical kit. In these cases, doctors may be approached to perform various services:

- Provide advice on vaccinations or antimalarial chemoprophylaxis
- Advise on contents of a suitable medical kit
- Supply private prescriptions for an expedition (NB. Drugs may be used for the treatment of trip members previously unknown to the doctor)
- Medical advice by phone to expedition medics
- Delegate the responsibility for initiating treatment to a trip leader.

In these situations, the administration of medication should be via a written protocol or verbal consultation with a doctor (e.g. by telephone, satellite phone or email). All prescription medication should be accompanied by a letter from the prescribing doctor. It would also be prudent for the doctor to seek a written understanding from the person to whom prescriptions are supplied that the medication prescribed will only be used for the immediate treatment of expedition members while some distance from a hospital or clinic and not as a substitute for seeking professional medical advice where this is readily available.

Professional indemnity insurance

Most of the principal medical insurance bodies in the UK will extend the scope of their cover to include the practice of expedition medicine. However, this needs to be specifically requested (even if, depending on the grade and specialty of the practitioner, it were then provided at no extra cost) and, as mentioned earlier, may not extend to the care of North Americans.

Other factors to discuss with insurers would include:

- The scope of the treatment you propose to provide (especially if this were to fall well outside your normal full-time specialty)
- Whether you intend to extend this beyond your expedition members (such as to local workers employed by your team, other members of the local population, and perhaps other travellers not involved with your own trip).

Be aware of the differing organizational structures of the principal medical insurance bodies: the scope of their services may differ (one, for example, agreed to indemnify this author—free of charge—for providing a service that another would not offer indemnity against for a fee).

Summary

- Expedition medicine is an interesting and challenging vocation which needs to be practised with care.
- A clear written understanding of one's responsibilities as an MO is very important, but particularly so where charity or commercial expeditions are concerned.
- Drugs supplied to an expedition for administration or dispensing by non-medical personnel need to be prescribed via a written protocol or via a tele-medicine consultation.
- Finally, good specialist insurance cover needs to be actively sought, including professional indemnity insurance.

Food, water, and hygiene

Section editor
Shane Winser

Contributors
Jim Bond, Larry Goodyer, Paul Goodyer,
Christina Lalani, Akbar Lalani, Nick Lewis,
and James Moore

Accommodation

Clean water, good food, and a comfortable place to sleep are essential for a happy and healthy expedition. Tired and hungry people are significantly more prone to accidents and illness. Expeditions can base themselves anywhere from luxury hotels to bivouacs under the stars. Whichever type of accommodation is used it should offer:
- Refuge from the elements
- Security from personal attack or theft
- Protection from the local flora/fauna
- An acceptable level of comfort
- Privacy.

Camp location

When choosing the site for an expedition camp, consider:
- Weather
- Providing shelter from stormy weather
- Avoiding areas prone to snow accumulation
- Use of available shade and breeze in hot climates
- Avoiding areas at risk of lightning strike
- Floods
- Avoiding tidal regions and flood plains
- Dry river beds that may be liable to flash flooding
- Narrow valleys in areas of high rainfall
- Dangers from falling rocks and mud slides, avalanche (snow/ice), dead trees and branches, or animal attacks
- Not placing camp between animals and their watering holes
- Avoiding large animal mating and breeding areas
- Avoiding areas of insect infestation
- Avoiding routes of migration/travel.

Animal attacks are more likely during camp construction or new occupation, as humans initially invade the animals' environment. As the local fauna gets used to human presence, they may move closer to the camp to take advantage of food scraps, etc. During camp deconstruction the animals may again be disturbed, making a hostile response more likely.

Local permissions and environmental impact

Permissions may need to be obtained from the landowner.

Avoid placing a campsite in an area that has religious or spiritual significance for the local people.

Many cultures will readily offer supplies and hospitality even when this leaves them with shortages. Ensure that your presence does not deplete scarce local resources such as water, firewood, food, or fuel when these are in short supply.

Ensure that your campsites create no long-term ecological damage.

Storage

Supplies should be protected from:
- Animal invasion (e.g. bears, rats, weevils)
- Environmental and climatic damage
- Theft—many expeditions are supplied with food, equipment, and clothing costing more than the local village's annual income. Overt displays of wealth should be avoided.

Re-supply and casualty evacuation

Investigate the logistics of:
- Evacuating an injured casualty (📖 p. 136)
- Access to re-supplies of food, water, and fuel
- Reliable communications with local agencies and emergency services, or others upon whom you may rely for services.

Campsite identification

In unfamiliar surroundings or poor weather conditions, it is easy to become disorientated, even within the vicinity of base camp. To reduce the risk of members getting lost, clearly identify key areas such as:
- Camp entrances, exits, and boundaries
- Latrines
- Washing areas
- Refuse areas
- Communication facilities
- Medical and first aid facilities
- Fire extinguishing equipment and fire exits.

Once marked, ask the following question: 'Could I find who or what I need, in an emergency, in the dark or in poor visibility?'

Extreme environments

Those who intend to live in extreme environments may choose to construct their own temporary accommodation.

Tropical forest accommodation (see Chapter 23)

'A' frame sleeping platforms or 'Bashas' are popular in tropical forests. They elevate the individual above the forest floor, minimizing interference from insects and animals. Ensure:
- There is no deadfall above the selected site
- The ground is clear underneath the sleeping platform
- Equipment and bags are stored closed and off the floor
- Boots are up-turned and placed on sticks.

Desert and savannah accommodation (see Chapter 23)
A sleeping shelter is often not required in the desert environment—a simple roll-mat will suffice. Consider using a mosquito net to protect against crawling as well as airborne insects. Tents provide more robust protection against larger animals and the prying eyes of humans. Ensure:
• The ground is cleared of thorns and other sharp objects
• There are no spider/scorpion holes present
• Be prepared for surprisingly cold night temperatures in the desert.

Polar and mountain accommodation (see Chapters 19 and 20)
Expeditions to polar and mountain regions generally rely on good quality tents for shelter. These should be robust and able to withstand violent winds and heavy snowfall. Currently 'geodesic' designs offer the best combination of strength and lightness. Ensure:
• Maximum use of available shelter, if any
• Proper marking of tents and guy ropes, latrines, supplies, and hazards such as crevasses, icefalls, etc.
• A blizzard will cover supplies and make micronavigation almost impossible. Mark supplies using avalanche probes, skis or other posts.

Emergency shelters
Before embarking on an expedition, consider a contingency plan regarding accommodation. Ask yourself 'What if our shelter is lost or destroyed?' In many environments it is possible to construct a shelter from materials in the local environment. Examples might include:
• Snow holes
• Igloos
• Tropical shelters or 'lean-tos'.

Construction of these shelters should be learnt and practised prior to going into the field, so that the first attempts are not made amid the stress of an emergency.

Campfires

Sitting around a campfire is one of the most enjoyable aspects of being in the wilderness. Campfires provide:
- Warmth
- A place to cook
- A means to purify water and sterilize instruments
- A way to dispose of rubbish
- Security against animals
- A great camp atmosphere.

However, they can cause:
- Burn injuries through carelessness or horseplay (📖 p. 260)
- Damage to the camp
- Damage to the wider environment.

Positioning a campfire
- Designate a specific area for the fire at least 3 m from scrub, grass, or other potential combustibles.
- Beware of overhanging foliage. Animals living in a forest canopy, for instance, will soon descend when gassed by noxious fumes from a campfire.
- If possible, create a fire surround with non-porous rocks. Porous rocks can explode when heated.
- Make sure there is a sensible distance between the fire and any tents or supplies.
- Consider the wind direction and speed. If sparks are likely to fly, reconsider the appropriateness of an open fire.
- Keep the fuel stores well away from the fire and prevailing winds.
- Have a supply of water ready to extinguish the fire if required.

Fires that have been left to burn out or extinguished with sand have been shown to hold temperatures of 100°C 8 h later. In contrast, a fire extinguished with water has a temperature of 50°C only 10 min later.

Campfires can consume significant amounts of fuel in relatively short periods of time. Be careful not to exhaust wood supplies needed by local communities.

Finally... .

... never leave a fire unattended.

Animal and insect invasion

As soon as a camp is established, the local fauna will exhibit interest in it, and those within. Often there is a chain reaction leading to the appearance of animals of increasing size. For instance, crumbs of food attract insects, which attract mice, rats, and other small mammals. These in turn attract snakes. All constitute health hazards, from gastrointestinal upsets to unhygienic mouse droppings, through to potentially fatal snake bites.

Generally speaking, most animals tend to shy away from humans as our noisy behaviour appears threatening, but when attracted into a camp, it is usually for one of the following reasons.

Food
- Probably the biggest causative factor of animal invasion
- Food scraps and food wrappers should be disposed of properly
- Food should be stored in animal-proof containers distant from sleeping accommodation
- For more information on food hygiene, see 📖 p. 98.

Shelter
- Piles of firewood are an ideal habitat for snakes
- Boxes and containers provide potential rodent or snake accommodation
- Open rucksacks or sleeping bags are potential homes for insects, snakes, or other small creatures
- Boots can house scorpions, snakes, and spiders.

Territory
- Consider the animals likely to be present whilst setting up camp. How will their habitat be affected?
- Minimize interference with animal's natural food supplies
- Interfering with an animal's habitat might provoke a potentially fatal response for either yourself or the animal, e.g. disturbing a hornets' nest.

Curiosity
- Larger animals might find belongings to be perfect construction material for their home
- Equipment, shiny or dull, will be interesting to some animals and birds. If it is not packed away, it might be taken away.

Repellants

Widespread use of chemical repellents has environmental and ethical implications. However, the subtle use of personal repellents such as diethyl-toluamide (DEET) can help in the prevention of mass insect invasion. A few squirts on the strings of a hammock, or on the guy ropes of a tent will divert insects elsewhere. Note: DEET in high concentrations will dissolve manmade fibres.

Useful repellents
- Smoke from a campfire
- Insecticides such as permethrin
- Insect repellent coils
- Reducing the amount of artificial light used after sunset.

Causes of insect attraction
- Perfumed/strongly scented deodorant/antiperspirant
- Odorous feet/boots
- Poor personal hygiene.

See also Prevention of malaria, p. 474.

Kitchens and food preparation

One of the greatest contributing factors to the success or failure of an expedition is the standard of the food. Success depends not only on the provision of a nourishing and varied diet, but also on the prevention of diet-related illness and disease, probably the biggest cause of diarrhoea in travellers abroad.

The kitchen

The position and construction of a kitchen will vary according to the type, size, budget, and location of the expedition. The gold standard for a big base camp, one could argue, should be to reproduce a commercial kitchen, with all the regulations required to pass a health and hygiene examination. Ideally the kitchen should be located at least 30 m away from areas of possible contamination such as latrines, wash areas, and equipment stores. The kitchen should have the following:

- A clearly defined place in camp
- Facilities for handwashing: a can with holes in the bottom and a jug can be used to create running water
- Separate areas for:
  - Storage
  - Food preparation
  - Cooking
- A system for disposing of food and other waste
- A system of cleaning cooking and eating utensils.

Catering personnel

Some teams will employ local people for this role, whilst others will use expedition members and may opt for a rota system of cooking, cleaning, and washing up. It is important that everybody on the team is clear about their roles and responsibilities.

Beware of illnesses in all members of the expedition team. This might include chronic illnesses carried by locally hired staff such as:

- Diarrhoea or other gastrointestinal upsets
- Helminth infections
- Tuberculosis.

Ensure that both catering and expedition teams clearly understand what is required regarding:

- Standards of hygiene and cleanliness within the kitchen
- Regular handwashing with soap
- Use of equipment
- Disposal of refuse.

Basic kitchen rules

- If you are ill, do not go in the kitchen. Do not prepare food until at least 48 h have passed since last vomit or loose stool
- Wash hands regularly
- All cooking utensils should be washed, dried, and stored appropriately.

The kitchen should be kept scrupulously clean at all times:
- Clean work surfaces after use
- Clean storage areas daily and when required
- Clean and dry equipment immediately after use (including the cleaning equipment itself)
- Restrict the kitchen area to those involved in food preparation
- Look after the chef, and the chef will look after you.

Food storage

Proper storage of food is of paramount importance, as:
- It prevents gastrointestinal illness through contamination
- It provides protection against foraging animals
- Properly stored food lasts longer
- It is easier to track supply requirements.

Food needs to be accurately labelled and accounted for, preferably managed by a designated quartermaster. Remember to separate cooked foods from raw. If using a fridge, store cooked food above raw.

Cooking in tents

- Avoid cooking in tents or other small enclosed areas if at all possible
- Use great care when handling stoves in enclosed spaces—burns and scalds are common
- Ensure adequate ventilation
- Consider risk of carbon monoxide build up
- Plan escape route from tent if fire develops
- Hygiene
  - Handwashing is still vital
  - Consider alcohol-based hand rubs
- Keep food/cooking at opposite ends of the tent to boots/equipment
- Clean up after eating
- Consider refuse disposal—carry in/carry out.

Food preparation

Gastrointestinal upsets are the commonest illnesses to affect travellers. Problems can be minimized by ensuring that water is clean (📖 p. 106), and that food preparation is as hygienic as possible.

The saying 'if you can't wash it, peel it or boil it—forget it' holds true. Common sense dictates that it is not always possible to control the preparation of food whilst on expedition, but the further one strays from this advice, the greater the chance of succumbing to diet-related illness.

Safe food preparation lies in cleanliness:
- Surfaces should be cleaned prior to and after any food preparation

- Scrupulous handwashing should be maintained, including the scrubbing of nails
- Consider the use of alcohol-based hand rub
- Raw foods should not be prepared on the same surface as cooked foods
- Meat, poultry, and fish should be well cooked
- Vegetables should be boiled
- Cooked food should be eaten immediately
- Food should not be re-heated
- Food waste should be cleaned away immediately.

During meal times, refrain from sharing cutlery, bowls, and other eating or drinking utensils. Sharing is one of the fastest ways of spreading bugs and germs around camp. Note that many contagious diseases have an asymptomatic incubation period.

After eating:

- All cooking and eating utensils should be washed, dried, and stored cleanly and away from possible interference by insects and animals
- Try to use a two-bowl system for washing up, one for washing, the other to rinse
- Surfaces should be wiped clean, if possible with a disinfectant, as it will reduce the chances of bacteria/viral contamination or build-up.
- Floors should be cleaned of even the smallest crumbs of food
- Hands should be washed, again.

Dietary requirements

Most expeditions involve considerable physical exercise. A balanced and varied expedition diet is essential to enable expedition members to maintain health, fitness, and morale. The choice of foodstuffs will depend upon the:
- Duration of the expedition
- Environment: energy requirements are greatly increased in cold climates, while travel in hot climates will require increased fluids and electrolytes
- Availability of local foodstuffs
- Energy expenditure of the participants
- Levels of fitness: untrained individuals will take longer to complete a journey and hence have greater total energy expenditure
- Budget of the expedition
- Ability to transport food: backpack, porters, pack animals, vehicles or by air
- Availability of fuel and water.

Calorific requirements

The basic daily calorific requirement for a 75-kg person doing little physical work is 1500–1700 kcal; additional energy requirements are dependent upon the work undertaken. Fast walking burns 600–700 kcal/h, running around 850 kcal/h. The duration of a task must be considered; working at low intensity for several hours requires more energy than short bursts of high-intensity exercise. Remember the more food carried, the more energy is burnt in carrying food. Climbing carrying loads and man-hauling sledges are amongst the most energetic activities known, with around 10 000 kcal/day expended. On short expeditions, deficits in energy balance can be tolerated healthily; this is not the case on longer expeditions. Highly trained individuals can endure persistent energy deficits but at a cost of up to one-third of their lean body weight, and gradual decline in physical capabilities.

Dietary components

Dietary balance

Individuals tolerate novel food to different degrees, but providing the same menu each day will also discourage healthy eating. Simple sauces or condiments can make basic food more interesting. Where hunting is legal, the game taken may be an acquired taste, and it is sensible to have some additional staple foods for those that cannot face the evening meal. Fresh fruit and vegetables are always welcome, but are difficult to preserve without refrigeration. Jams and conserves are rich in vitamins and are worth taking. Additional calorie intake is less important in the short term than the quality of nutrition and the distribution of nutrients.

Table 3.1 Food types: pros and cons

Food type	Advantages	Disadvantages
Prepared food, e.g. sandwiches	Pleasing to the palate	Requires prior preparation
		Not practical on longer expeditions. Short shelf life
Tinned produce	Very long shelf life	Bulky and heavy
	High liquid content	Non-biodegradable waste product
	Can be eaten cold	
Local produce	May be readily available	Risk of infections and gastroenteritis
	Part of cultural experience of travel	Longer preparation time
Dried produce e.g. pasta and sauce	Pleasing to the palate	Time-consuming
		Requires large amount of fuel to prepare
		Bulky compared to finished product
'Boil in the bag' or MRE (meal ready to eat)	Easy to prepare	Expensive: £3–4 per meal
	Can taste good	Limited choice of meals
	Long shelf life	Lower energy density than dried products
	Can be cooked in dirty water or even eaten cold	
	Requires no pan washing	
Dehydrated meals	Some can be made with hot water added to bag and not prepared on a stove	Others require cooking over stove for 6–8 min
	Energy-dense	Uses significant amounts of water
Powdered synthetic foods, e.g. sports drinks	Easy to prepare. No cooking utensils required	Taste
	Energy-dense (several thousand kcal can be carried in under 1 kg)	Unbalanced diet, lack of fibre

Protein

Proteins enable muscle strength and allow repair and regeneration. Animal protein sources are better balanced than lactovegetarian sources; vegetarians can sustain high daily activity but their diet is bulkier. Protein intake should be greatest during rest periods and evenings, as protein consumed during exercise is largely burned to provide energy. Studies have shown that low protein consumption leads to a decrease in exercise potential over time. The recommended daily intake to minimize losses in lean body mass should be 1.5–2.0 g/kg. Roughly 15% of total calorific intake should be protein.

Carbohydrate

Carbohydrates are the main energy substrate for exercise. Simple sugars (sweets and glucose drinks) are rapidly absorbed, requiring little or no digestion. They should be consumed during exercise to provide the body with a constant source of energy. Complex sugars (pasta, rice, bread) are digested slowly, and must be metabolized to simple sugars before they can act as an energy substrate. Consuming complex sugars during exercise will have the detrimental effect of diverting blood flow to the gut from exercising muscle. They should therefore be ingested before and after exercise to replenish glycogen stores. Body glycogen stores are exhausted after just 2 h of strenuous exercise. In the absence of further intake, the body will begin to break down muscle and fat stores.

Fat

Fatty acids cannot be metabolized sufficiently rapidly to be used as an energy substrate during high-intensity exercise, but fats provide a useful substrate during prolonged low-intensity exercise. Fat is three times more energy-dense than carbohydrate and on expeditions a high fat diet reduces the bulk and weight of food needed. Fat metabolism pathways must be enhanced prior to departure; this process can be achieved by 1 or 2 h of low intensity (and hence low lactate production) training early in the day before breakfast, when glycogen stores are already depressed. Caffeine increases fatty acid utilization during exercise. Eating a high fat meal immediately after exercise delays glycogen store replenishment and muscle regeneration, and hinders recovery for the next day. In hot climates and at altitude, high fat diets can be unpalatable, but hungry travellers will enjoy a high fat content, high calorie diet in cold climates.

Vitamins and minerals (micronutrients)

Trace dietary constituents include magnesium, zinc, calcium, selenium, chromium, vitamins C and E, beta-carotene, and omega and fatty acids. These substances are needed to produce key substances in metabolic pathways. Vigorous exercise generates free radicals that can damage protein structures. Certain vitamins and trace elements (e.g. vitamin C) act as scavengers to prevent such damage. On prolonged journeys the correct balance of micronutrients becomes much more significant.

Water and electrolytes

While energy imbalances can be tolerated for days or weeks, water and electrolyte imbalances are poorly tolerated. Drinking large volumes of plain water for even a single day in a high humidity/high exercise situation can result in catastrophic hyponatraemia with muscle cramps, confusion, coma, and even death. In hot climates, additional electrolytes should be added to water to optimize rehydration (see Chapter 23). Thirst is a poor indicator of hydration; typically thirst indicates more than 2% loss of body fluids and this corresponds to a 10% loss of exercise performance. Raised resting heart rate, or a higher than normal heart rate for a given exercise load, can indicate dehydration. In cold dry climates dehydration can develop in the absence of obvious sweating or thirst, and manifests itself when returning to a warmed environment at the end of a day (see Chapter 19).

In hot humid climates exercise must be restricted until acclimatization has developed (see Chapter 23).

Factors necessitating increased fluid intake:

- Environmental temperature—above 30°C sweat rates can reach up to 2.5 l/h.
- Increased exercise load leads to an increase in fluid lost through sweating and imperceptible losses through increased panting and loss of water vapour in breath.
- Clothing choice—wearing many layers, using poor quality waterproofs, or wearing high wicking layers can increase fluid losses through sweating.
- Excessive diuretic consumption, e.g. tea/coffee.
- Blood loss—hypovolaemia though loss of circulating volume. (NB. Further treatment may be needed in addition to increasing oral intake; see relevant chapters.)
- Age and sex—testosterone and aldosterone have effects on the size of sweat glands and hence sweating rates.
- Fluid should be consumed before exercise (approximately 0.5 l), during (from 20 min into load and at a rate of 500–750 ml/h) and after (until passing clear urine).
- Consumption of sports drinks containing electrolytes in isotonic concentrations and carbohydrates at 5–8% has benefits during competitive events, but beware of excessive consumption of fluids during endurance events which may lead to hyponatraemic collapse (📖 p. 693).

Water purification

A safe water supply is essential. Adults in temperate conditions need to drink about 3 litres a day, but intake can rise to as much as 15 litres per day in hot climates; a further 4 litres of clean water per person per day will be needed for cooking and washing up. Sufficient safe water must be provided both at base camp and for use by field parties. Often water from taps and wells, as well as that from rivers, lakes, and ponds, can be contaminated. Spring water, i.e. clear 'pristine water collected away from human habitation' may be safer, but it is still sensible to treat this water source.

Water must be treated:
- To remove silt
- To remove harmful organic matter and other pollutants
- To kill all forms of organism.

Sediment must be removed initially if sterilization procedures are to be effective. Removing silt can pose considerable problems if you are trying to obtain supplies for a large expedition, and sedimentation tanks may be required. If the expedition is close to mines or factories, chemical pollution must be foreseen and appropriate filtration methods used.

Some methods of water purification are more suitable for the base camp and others for field workers. Before deciding on the system to use it is important to consider the likely infective organisms and the risk posed by them to the expedition.

Transmission of disease by water

Organisms such as bacteria, viruses, protozoa and other parasites (including schistosomes, guinea worm larvae and leeches) can transmit infections.

Giardiasis

This is caused by the protozoan *Giardia lamblia*, part of whose life cycle involves faecal–oral transmission. The organism is consumed together with contaminated food or water and then cysts, which are viable for a long time, are deposited from faeces into water or food to infect another host. Humans and animals, both domestic and wild, can host the infection and contaminate water; it only takes a few cysts to lead to a harmful infection.

The symptoms of giardiasis may be debilitating and develop 1–4 weeks after ingestion. Symptoms largely result from malabsorption of foodstuffs, and produce a frothy foul-smelling diarrhoea, in addition to nausea, abdominal discomfort, flatulence and bloating. Symptoms usually last for 1 to 2 weeks, but sometimes a persistent chronic disease develops.

Metronidazole or tinidiazole are effective treatments; in resistant cases albendazole has proven effective.

The cysts are relatively large and are quite easily removed by filter systems but are resistant to all but the highest doses of halogens and then still require prolonged contact times (📖 p. 108).

Cryptosporidium

Cryptosporidium spp. cause a very severe diarrhoea and, like *Giardia*, this organism is spread by the faecal–oral route, although ingestion of low numbers of cysts may not always result in infection. The organism is chiefly spread by humans and domestic livestock, either directly or through contaminated water. The spore of the organism can remain dormant in the soil for many years. The main danger for expeditions is when surface waters are used either close to human habitation that do not have effective sanitation systems or where water is washed from grazing fields. Cases have been reported after swimming in infected waters, as well as consumption of contaminated food and water. *Cryptosporidium* outbreaks occur from time to time in developed countries when sanitation systems break down.

Symptoms occur 2–14 days after contact and consist of a very profuse watery diarrhoea, abdominal pain, low grade fever, and cramps, which last around 7 days. Sometimes the disease relapses after about 14 days. The biggest danger is to those with impaired immune systems, e.g. those with HIV/AIDS or those taking immunosuppressive drugs, where complications can be fatal. The very young and the elderly may also be at greater risk. There is no specific treatment other than aggressive rehydration.

A complication for expeditions is that the cysts are resistant to the halogens so filtration remains the most viable option if this disease is perceived as a potential problem.

Removal of sediment and organic matter

If water is cloudy or contains suspended matter it must be cleared before further treatment.

Settling tanks

Cloudy water can be left to stand for some hours for solids to settle, either in a jerry can or in sedimentation tanks depending on the volume to be treated. Very fine particles, such as 'rock flour' in glacial outflow and mica flakes, are gastrointestinal irritants and must be removed by a ceramic filter. Simply clearing water does not sterilize it and further treatment will be needed before it may be drunk.

Millbank bag

A Millbank bag is a sock-shaped bag woven so that solids are retained but water flows by gravity through the weave. The bag can be left hanging over a receptacle with occasional top-ups to provide continuous production of filtered water ready for sterilization. The bag is robust and easy to clean. Millbank bags are available in two sizes: 2 l for personal use and 9 l for large quantities of water.

Coagulation–flocculation

Small amounts of certain chemicals can be added to cause an aggregation of particles which will sink to the bottom of the container. The flocculate is then strained off through a tight woven cloth or Millbank bag. A potential advantage is that larger organisms such as *Giardia* or *Cryptosporidium* are removed by this technique, although it is not as reliable as an appropriate mechanical filter. The most easily obtained chemical is alum, of which about an eighth of a teaspoonful is added to 4 l of water, more if it remains cloudy. The water is then stirred for 5 min and allowed to settle for 30 min.

Methods of water purification

Boiling

This is undoubtedly the best method, but is often inconvenient and wasteful of fuel supplies or natural resources. Water should be kept boiling continuously for 5 min, which is sufficient at any altitude, although some experts state that 1 min is adequate. The water must be covered when cooling to prevent recontamination.

Halogens

Chlorine

Chlorine is effective against a wide range of organisms, although it is less effective for amoebic cysts and *Giardia*, and is ineffective against *Cryptosporidium*. The effectiveness of chlorine is reduced by several factors that may not be easy to control, such as alkaline water, very cold water or the presence of organic matter—hence the need for prior filtering.

AquatabÔ tablets are the most widely available method of chlorination, and one tablet of the maxi size will treat 25 l. For very large tanks some expeditions prefer to use a substance called chloramine T, where 5 mg is added to each litre of water. Treated water should be left for at least half an hour before drinking and longer if it is very cold.

Sodium thiosulphate will improve the taste but will inactivate the chlorine, so it should be added by individuals only at the time the water is drunk. It should never be added to a storage receptacle such as a canteen or jerry can.

Iodine

Iodine is an effective chemical method most suited to individual treatment rather than groups. Its main disadvantage is that it is unsuitable for some people: those with a thyroid condition or iodine allergy, pregnant women and young children. There are also concerns about the long-term use of iodine-treated water. A further drawback is that the cheapest method involves the use of iodine tincture, which must be carried in glass containers that are messy and hazardous if they break. Iodine can only be stored in plastic bottles if the bottle has been fluorinated to stop the iodine reacting with the plastic.

Iodine is similar in activity to chlorine, but is sometimes claimed to be more effective against *Giardia* and amoebic cysts. Its chief advantage is that it is more tolerant to the presence of organic matter than is chlorine, although its activity will still be reduced if the water is not clear. Unlike chlorine, it is not effective at inhibiting the growth of algae which may grow in the storage tanks.

There is controversy about the exact amount of iodine to use. Commonly used doses are: five drops of 2% iodine tincture per litre of water, increasing to 12 drops if *Giardia* is suspected. It is always best to assume that *Giardia* is present and add 12 drops per litre when treating small amounts of water, or measure out 0.3–0.4 ml/l when treating large tanks. The longer the treated water is left to stand—the contact time—the better, 30 min being the minimum.

An alternative to iodine tincture is to use water sterilizing iodine tablets, but these are expensive and lose their potency after the bottle has been opened. Iodine tablets should always be crushed into the water; they can take time to break down if left whole, which can seriously affect the contact time.

Another method is to use iodine crystals (the Kahnn–Visscher method), but the method is rather fiddly and not suitable for preparing large amounts of water. It is, however, very economical. Between 6 and 8 g of iodine crystals should be placed in a 30-ml container and the bottle filled with water. After a short time (30–60 min depending on the water temperature) the relatively insoluble iodine forms a saturated solution. Fifteen millilitres of the supernatant should be placed in 1 litre of water to be purified and the water left for around 30 min before drinking. The iodine bottle can be refilled with water and used again after a further 30–60 min.

Ascorbic acid (vitamin C) can be added in small amounts to neutralize the taste of iodine-treated water. This should be done only at the time of use.

Silver compounds

Micropure™ tablets contain a compound called Katadyne silver that is ineffective against *Amoeba*, *Giardia*, or viruses. It does not impart a bad taste and it is claimed to be able to prevent recontamination by bacteria of water for many weeks. Micropure™ tablets should not be added to water previously treated with chlorine or iodine.

Filters and pumps

There are many mechanical devices available for purifying water (Table 3.2). Some devices employ a simple filtration method (microfiltration), in which water is pumped through tiny holes that organisms are unable to pass through. To remove organisms effectively the pore size must be less than 1 μm. Other devices employ both a filter and chemical treatment with an iodine resin which strains and sterilizes in one go. Choosing the right device is important, so here are some tips:

- Manufacturers often say how many litres of pure water a device will produce. However, this can be drastically reduced if the water is silty.
- If heavy use is expected, make sure that the purifier can be taken apart, cleaned, and reassembled in the field to prevent blockages.
- Check the pump rate as some can take a lot of effort to produce a small amount of water.
- Many manufacturers of pumps go to great lengths to state what they will remove, while keeping quiet about what is not removed. For example, pumps will not remove chemical effluent, such as mercury in the tributaries of the Amazon, without the addition of a carbon filter. For those visiting areas where there is mining or factories up-river this may be important.
- Water storage time is also important; ideally after sterilization the water should be used within 24 h.
- Although a filter plus iodine resin may appear the ideal solution for treating water in all circumstances, this system has been known to fail and, in the US, some have been withdrawn from the market.

Other potential methods of water purification
Coagulation–flocculation with disinfection
There has been recent interest in a new system developed by Proctor and Gamble, consisting of sachets containing chemical disinfectant and substances that cause flocculation of particles. This has been very effective in field trials and may also be useful against *Cryptosporidium*. The product goes under the name of 'PUR' but is not yet commercially available.

Chlorine dioxide
This is now widely used in water purification plants and is effective against *Cryptosporidium*. A formulation has been marketed which is suitable for personal use and is available in the US. All products have to be registered in the US with the Environmental Protection Agency (EPA) to prove their safety and efficacy. EPA approval has yet to be granted at the time of writing. If planning to use this product in an expedition it would be advisable to contact an expert source for the latest information.

UV radiation
There are a number of devices available that have claimed efficacy, including against *Cryptosporidium*. Water must be clear before treatment and power requirements may limit their viability.

Reverse osmosis filters
These are highly effective membrane filters that will remove all microorganisms and have the additional advantage of being able to desalinate seawater. The small hand pump versions are expensive but a useful survival aid at sea.

Drinking bottle filters
These are bottles with filters attached to the top. The most well known is the Aqua Pure Traveller™. The bottle is filled with the water to be treated and then squeezed into a drinking cup for purification. Drinking bottle filters are slightly misleading as they make it look as though you should be able to drink safe water straight from the bottle. By the addition of an iodine sleeve to the carbon microfilter, the Aqua Pure can be turned into a purifier so long as the water is left to stand for 15 min once it has passed through the system.

Choice of water purification system
The choice of technique will depend on the size and circumstances of the expedition.

If practicable a large pot should be put on to boil at the end of an evening meal to allow preparation of water for the following morning. In addition, all members should have some method of sterilizing their own drinking water. Boiling large volumes of water consumes considerable fuel.

If not relying on boiling, consider the sources of water likely to be used. Either mechanical filtration or halogenation can be used to purify clear pristine surface waters. However, near human habitation or agricultural areas a combination of methods may be required to give maximal protection. Filters are not as effective as the halogens at removing viruses, but on the other hand the halogens are not effective against *Cryptosporidium*. So, with potentially contaminated water one should either use a one-step device that incorporates both iodine resin and a filter, or use a two-step process involving both halogenation and filtration.

Possible methods include:

- For large groups: chlorination provided that the condition of the treatment tanks can be carefully monitored.
- For smaller groups: iodine, provided that everyone in the group can tolerate it.
- For smaller groups, particularly if on the move: strain water through a Millbank bag and provide members with their own small bottle of iodine or chlorination tablets to treat water after drawing it off into their own water bottles. The strained water could be used for boiling water, e.g. for beverages.
- Using one of the new generation of water bottles with a filtration/purification method attached (e.g. Aqua Pure™). Their ease of use helps the user to keep up a constant intake of water. However, there is a question of the contact time and it is suggested that the water be squeezed through and left to stand.
- Providing all field parties with small Millbank bags together with some method of chemical sterilization, or alternatively a portable filtration system.

Table 3.2 Personal water filters and purifiers available in the UK

Filter/purifier	Litres	Filtration time/litre (min)	Purification time (min)	Chemical/filter employed
Pocket travelwell	25	5	4	Filter/iodine
Millbank bag	Unlimited	5	n/a	Cloth filtration
Aqua Pure bottle	350	2	15	Filter/iodine
Trekker travelwell	100	2.5	4	Filter/iodine
Ranger travelwell	1000	5	4	
Katadyne mini filter	7000	2	Instant	Ceramic filter/silver
Katadyne pocket filter	10 000	1.5	Instant	Ceramic filter/silver
Katadyne Hiker	750	1	n/a	Microfiltration
MSRwater works	10 000	1	Instant	Ceramic

Note: purifying water using a pump filter can be fast, but organic matter may cause frequent blockages, making the process labour-intensive.

Camp water purification arrangements

Providing enough treated water from a natural source for a camp of 20 people is time-consuming, but exceedingly important. The best approach is to incorporate a strict regime from the start by appointing one person as 'water chief' to supervise the sterilization, safe storage, and use of the water. The appointed person should also make sure that every member of the expedition is capable of sterilizing his or her own drinking water.

Rigid plastic containers with a tap and handle are the best for water. These come in 10- or 25-litre sizes, but the larger size container is heavy when full of water so keep in mind distances to water source and terrain. If you do not have a method of removing the taste of chemicals, water will taste better when cold. Storing water in special canvas bags will keep it cool through evaporation from the small pores of the canvas. If they can be obtained, army surplus bags are excellent and come in sizes suitable for storage of large volumes in camp or for tying to the back of a vehicle.

If a daily average of 6 l per person is required for drinking and 4 l for cooking/washing up, containers holding 10 l per person per day will be required. Water treatment could be split into sessions if it is necessary to reduce the number of containers in use. To avoid confusion, have a good system of marking containers for the three different types of water treatment:

• Untreated for storage, sedimentation, or settling process
• Strained ready for treatment
• Fit for drinking.

Field parties

Each field party member should carry personal equipment for sterilizing water; metal cups are preferable to plastic as the latter often break. If using a filter system, a small Travelwell™ filter would be a good choice.

If travelling by vehicle, do not use one large container for storing water; a single puncture may have disastrous consequences. Jerry cans or the canvas bags previously described are the best option, but try to adopt the same system of markings as employed in base camp.

Sanitation and latrines

The health and hygiene surrounding the waste that we generate is as important to the prevention of illness as are the standards of cleanliness we apply to the preparation and consumption of food.

The management of waste on an expedition is a balancing act between factors such as location, available facilities, and personal adherence to standards or procedures, with an overall aim to minimize ecological and environmental impact.

A successful expedition is not only one which achieves its objectives, but when all is done and the members return home, the expedition location appears as it did before they arrived. The way in which sanitation and waste management are accomplished on expedition can have considerable impact on the environment for many years to come.

Latrines

The disposal of human waste on expedition can be separated into its two forms, with the provision of a place to urinate and a place to defecate.

Urine disposal

Unless infection is present, urine is sterile and therefore provides less of a problem in its disposal. However, large quantities of urine can smell offensive in a short space of time, and affect fragile ecosystems.

When siting a urinal:
- Choose an area 50–100 m from the camp
- Make sure it is downstream of any water collection point
- Avoid caves or other areas where urine will remain stagnant
- Avoid rocks or gravel, where urine lingers
- Clearly mark the path to the urinal and the urinal itself
- Re-site the urinal on a regular basis to avoid large collections of urine.

Latrine placement

The latrines have to be far enough from camp to pose no infection or contamination risk, yet close enough to be used with convenience. Thus:
- Place it 100 m from the camp
- Place it 100 m from any lakes, rivers, or streams
  - Look for high water marks
  - Consider local water tables
- Consider water run-off channels in the event of:
  - Heavy rain
  - Flash floods
- Mark a path to and from the latrine
- Include a system of notifying people when it is in use
- Identify latrine boundaries clearly
- Ensure that everyone is familiar with latrine etiquette.

Other options

Some national parks are now advocating urinating into fast flowing rivers or the saturated river banks. This avoids build-ups of unpleasant odours and damage to sensitive ecosystems.

The safe disposal of faeces and the levels of hygiene surrounding toilet etiquette constitute one of the most important barriers to stop the faecal–oral transmission of diarrhoeal disease. This transmission occurs through:

- Direct faecal contact
- Contact with faecal-infected hands
- Contact with faecal-infected water
- Contact with animals/insects that have been in contact with faeces.

Dealing with faecal waste in a safe clean way is influenced by factors including:

- Bacteriological activity within soil
- Soil type
- Climate
- Exposure to sunlight
- Permeability
- Hydrodynamics.

As human waste is made safe by two main mechanisms, bacterial decomposition or sterilization, there are three main options open to those in a wilderness environment:

- Bury it
- Treat it
- Carry it out.

Burying

This is only an option in environments where there is enough bacterial activity within the soil. Bacterial activity normally occurs only within the first 10 inches of topsoil, therefore only a shallow scrape is required.

When re-filling the scrape, use a stick to 'stir' in faeces, ensuring greater contact with soil enzymes, and then cover over with topsoil.

Group latrines should consist of a long trench, approximately 6 inches (15 cm) wide and 8 inches (20 cm) deep.

When the first trench is filled in, site another one.

If the environment is such that burying faeces is not an option, consider the alternative options.

Treating/sterilizing

Chemically treating faecal waste on expedition is a complicated process. It can be a potentially costly addition to the expedition budget, and requires equipment and proper faecal storage facilities.

In strictly limited circumstances where expeditions find themselves in remote locations away from human or animal populations, it is possible to use the sun's ultraviolet rays to break down faecal matter with a method known as 'frosting a rock' or 'icing a cake'.

The most favourable locations consist of hard-rock terrain or desert subject to intense sunlight and with an obvious dry season.

To use this method:

- Pick a rock which receives direct, day-long sunlight
- Deposit faeces
- Using a rock or stick, spread the faeces as thinly as possible over the rock.

This method is effective if used properly and with consideration for others but is not a suitable method for large groups of people on lengthy expeditions.

Carrying out

The last method requires a suitable container which should be:

• Either disposable or re-usable (and therefore cleanable)
• Durable
• Portable
• Appropriate size for expedition length
• Appropriate size for expedition population.

There should be a definitive plan regarding final disposal of effluent. 'Carrying out' is an appropriate option for those at forward camps in ecologically sensitive environments. On return to a base camp in a more hospitable environment, the waste can be disposed of appropriately.

Toilet paper

If storing toilet paper at the latrine, make sure it is kept in a container suitable for the conditions present, preferably animal-proof.

Toilet paper should be burnt. This can be on an individual basis, or stored and collected as part of the latrine rota, then burnt at the end of the day with other rubbish.

Sanitary towels/tampons

These should never be buried as they do not biodegrade effectively in the wild. Either store them separately from used toilet paper, then burn at the end of the day or carry out to dispose of after the expedition. For alternatives to sanitary towels/tampons see p. 403.

Hand hygiene

This is without doubt the most important part of personal hygiene.

At the latrine entrance there should be facilities for handwashing, which include:

• Water container/bucket with lid
• Water (clean but not sterile)
• Scoop or ladle
• Soap/disinfectant
• If possible, a nail brush.

Water should be scooped out with a ladle to prevent dirty hands contaminating the container. Hands should be washed and rinsed away from the container. In addition to soap and water, consider the use of an alcohol-based hand rub.

Latrine rota

Where possible, a latrine rota should be established. Tasks include:

• Digging new trenches
• Re-siting urinals
• The marking of new/old latrines
• Ensuring an adequate supply of toilet paper is available
• Replacing the handwashing water when required and on a daily basis
• Ensuring there is soap/detergent by the water
• Collecting and burning toilet paper.

Waste management

All teams should attempt to leave the expedition campsite(s) in the same or in a better condition than when they arrived. Any waste that remains once the expedition has departed needs to be both highly biodegradable in that environment and such that it does not pose any threat to local people or the surrounding ecosystem; alternatively, it should be burnable, with the residue ash disposed of in a safe manner

Waste that does not fall into these two categories should be carried out and disposed of appropriately.

Camp routines

An area in camp should be set aside for refuse. This can be separated into two parts consisting of:

- A burns pit
  - Approximately 50 m from the camp
  - Clearly marked
  - Dug and cleared of ignitable vegetation
  - Sufficient water to extinguish standing by
  - Lit at the end of the day
  - Never left unattended when lit
  - Covered at night
  - Burnable waste includes toilet paper and sanitary items and, unless going for recycling, food packaging. Tins should be opened at both ends, burnt, flattened then carried out.
- A slops pit
  - Approximately 100 m from camp
  - Clearly marked
  - Dug no deeper than the layer of fertile topsoil
  - Covered when not in use, especially at night
  - Slops waste includes food scraps, water used for cooking, e.g. pasta/rice water, water from tinned foods.

Animal considerations

Animals will be attracted to waste, digging up any buried foodstuffs.

Caution should be used when removing covers to both burns and slops pits. Snakes and other potentially harmful animals might be present.

Larger animals such as bears or big cats pose an obvious risk to humans. In this situation, placing waste further away from camp is advised. In addition, it would be advisable to visit the refuse pits in pairs and, where possible, only in daylight hours.

Personal hygiene

The routine surrounding personal hygiene can add an element of structure to the day and provide an opportunity for individuals to check themselves and each other for specific problems such as: frostbite in arctic conditions, ticks in temperate forests, foot rot, or leech bites in tropical conditions. Efforts to maintain good levels of personal hygiene will not only prevent disease and reduce the risk of transmitted infection but will also, by minimizing other factors such as unpleasant body odours and dirty clothing, improve the morale of the whole team, especially while living in close proximity to one another.

Washing area

A designated washing area should be identified and marked.

The wash area should be away from any water source to avoid soap contamination. If washing by a river, use an area far enough away to allow natural filtration by soil.

Privacy

If possible, consider separate areas for males and females. If this is not possible, rota male and female wash times.

Consider local people and customs/laws regarding modesty—especially, but not exclusively, amongst female members of the team.

If necessary construct screens/curtains.

Washing

- Use 'biodegradable' soap and detergent. This will break down after use.
- Limit use of soap—large amounts of biodegradable soap will also affect the environment.
- Use a bucket and scoop method to minimize:
  - Water use
  - Cross-contamination.
- Before swimming, consider washing off DEET to prevent chemical contamination of water sources.

Water supply

If using a water supply for both consumption and washing—do not waste water.

Do not balance washing/wash kits, etc. on the edge of a water supply. One bar of soap dropped into a well could have disastrous consequences.

Washing clothes

- Where possible, use a designated clothes washing area
- Use as little soap as possible
- Hang clothes on a line to dry them. This prevents:
  - Insect infestation
  - Clothes being swept away in flood-risk areas
- Consider how secure your clothes are from:
  - The environment
  - Animals
  - Theft.

After washing, consider carefully what deodorants/antiperspirants to use. Sweet-smelling or strong perfumed scents can attract insects such as bees, wasps, flies, and mosquitoes. You might smell nice but you will increase your chances of being stung or bitten.

Finally, clear away any washing utensils, soaps, or flannels as they are potentially harmful to flora and fauna.

Indigenous people

Understanding and learning from the life of the local inhabitants can be a very rewarding part of an expedition, and some researchers (e.g. ethno-botanists) rely almost exclusively for their data on what they learn from working with local people.

General approach

The wisdom of being open, honest, warm-hearted and respectful in your dealings with local people cannot be overstressed. All people hate it if they think you are trying to deceive them.

Local customs and hierarchy should be observed, e.g. not arriving at a village at daybreak, waiting to be properly introduced and accepted by the headman/elders, and seeking permission before taking any photos.

Put yourselves in their position:

- How would you wish to be treated by a group of wealthy foreign visitors who decide to come and spend some time in your community? Would you wish to be ignored, kept at a polite distance, or invited into their camp?
- How would you respond to their curiosity about your way of life?
- Would you prefer them to have at least mastered a few basic civilities in your language, such as greetings, 'thank you', 'delicious' etc.?
- How would you feel if they were overpaying staff and upsetting the economy of the village?
- Hospitality is very important to most societies and is never to be abused.

To treat or not to treat?

This is always a difficult question, so it is worth thinking about in advance. There are no hard and fast rules. In some communities, it appears to be the norm to walk up to anybody with a 'western' appearance and ask for medicines. The danger of reinforcing a culture of dependency by comply-ing with such a request is real. However, in a remote community, without easy access to medical care, it can equally seem churlish or even unethical for a doctor not to treat people who, strictly speaking, fall outside the scope of the expedition.

> **Three examples from remote expeditions in Madagascar**:
> - A villager with cerebral malaria.
> - An infant of a nomadic, forest people, with a severe chest infection.
> - A fisherman, stung by a stonefish, who had a necrotic dorsum of foot, requiring surgical debridement and antibiotics, to help it heal.

The examples in the box come under the 'Good Samaritan' category of care, i.e. emergency treatment to save life (or, in the third case, limb). When setting off to work in very remote communities, it may well be worth budgeting a little extra for such scenarios when preparing the medical kit.

Far more likely, however, is to be asked for treatment for 'headache', 'fever' (often just 'in case'), general malaise, abdominal symptoms, skin infections, infestations, etc. It is generally worthwhile seeing and examining each person who presents, if only to show willing and to reassure yourself and others whether it is a genuine emergency .

However, you should resist the temptation to reach into the medical kit to start treating minor or incurable ailments among the local population. The expedition medical kit is a finite resource, which has to serve the people for whom it was intended.

You also have an ethical duty to empower people, i.e. to manage their own illness, wherever possible, and to strengthen, rather than undermine, existing healthcare systems, including traditional healers (see below).

What if things go wrong?

As medical practitioners, we should be used to taking appropriate risks for our patients, with their full and informed consent. Good communication is thus paramount, particularly when warning of possible adverse effects. Know and admit your limitations—don't attempt heroic procedures when you're out of your depth. A useful maxim is 'always treat each patient as you would if they were a member of your own family'.

Public health

Occasionally, it may be clear that the whole population of a village or surrounding area could potentially benefit from an intervention to address a common threat to health, e.g. dirty water, malaria, trachoma.

Public health interventions, working with a local population, can appear seductively simple, but should not be undertaken lightly. They require a good deal of sensitive groundwork to work well. An ongoing project in the same area has many advantages over a 'one-off' expedition, by being able to build up trust and demonstrating commitment. It may be more empowering and effective in the long term to sow the seed of an idea, rather than to raise false expectations.

Working with local healers

Indigenous healers provide roughly 80% of the medical services used worldwide. Beyond their wealth of local knowledge, they usually have a strong sense of clinical duty toward their constituency, and a great deal of influence. This is an often overlooked potential resource, particularly in public health (see case study below).

As an expedition doctor, working in the territory of a local healer, one might anticipate that you could be viewed as competition, or worse, a threat. This should not put you off going the extra mile to seek out and pay one's respects to a fellow healthcare professional. You might be surprised at the reception and level of cooperation you subsequently receive for showing this simple courtesy.

Other expeditions

The same basic rules about ethical conduct apply when interacting with other expeditions; for instance, avoid negative criticism of another expedition's methods or style, etc.

In the field, your expedition will inevitably be scrutinized and compared with others by local people. Overt displays of friendliness towards another group, e.g. of the same mother tongue/nationality as your own, that is, different from your interactions with local people, will not go unnoticed.

Expeditions are not competitions. If you hear, in advance, that another expedition is planning something similar, or might coincide with yours, the 'right' thing to do is to take the initiative and start talking things over with them. You might find that the ground you are each planning to cover is actually somewhat different, or even complementary, from a research perspective. Aside from the possibility of sharing data, there may be the opportunity to pool certain resources, such as medical expertise or use of a satellite phone for CASEVAC. For obvious reasons, this kind of arrangement is preferably discussed in advance.

If another expedition has already set up camp at the site you had intended to use, normal etiquette would be for your, second group, to find another suitable location at a comfortable distance, if possible. Establishing good relations should be a priority, once local formalities have been completed.

Your interaction with other expeditions visiting the area may continue long after the expedition is over. Keep in contact, learn from each other's successes and mistakes, never misrepresenting others' efforts, and share your expedition findings.

Case study: Project Renala

Community-led TB treatment in SW Madagascar

On an ethnobotanical research project, working with the Mikea, an elusive, forest people, the expedition doctor/botanist was approached by local healers to advise on how to deal with an outbreak of tuberculosis, which was affecting their (apparently TB-naïve) population. Because of cultural differences, a nearby mission's TB programme was finding it hard to reach the Mikea people effectively in their forest home.

Over the next few years, the project helped to bridge the gap between the two health care systems, by providing backup and training. A special, fully ambulatory TB treatment regime/arrangement for the Mikea was worked out with traditional healers and other *notables* taking full responsibility for initial case detection, and treatment supervision in the forest, and the mission's health care workers confirming diagnoses and managing any complications.

In this way, a responsible DOTS-TB treatment programme was extended to include the Mikea on their terms, but without compromising their semi-nomadic, hunter-gatherer lifestyle, and without undermining the authority or undervaluing the clinical acumen of either set of healers.

Environmental impact

Environmental management on expeditions is simply a case of understanding, and then mitigating where necessary, the consequences of your actions. The size of an expedition is the major factor controlling the level of impact it will have. Reducing the number of members will minimize:

- The transportation requirements
- The amount of supplies that the expedition needs
- The number of local staff needed
- The amount of waste and sewage produced
- The cost of the expedition.

Environmental manager

Each group should appoint an environmental manager, whose responsibilities should include:

- Researching the environmental requirements of the host country
- Ensuring that these are taken into account during permit and grant applications
- Looking into the specific environmental issues of the expedition, including areas such as path erosion, sensitive areas, problems from existing waste accumulation, etc.

The environmental manager should work closely with the other members of the expedition to consider:

- Transport options to and from the destination—can public transport be used?
- Accommodation options—do the hotels or guesthouses subscribe to an industry environmental initiative?
- Local employment cooperatives—will the expedition's employees get the best deal?
- Expedition support agencies (guides, trekking companies, boat charters)—what is their environmental policy?
- Waste management procedures during the expedition, including the packaging on food and equipment, the type of waste handling structures available in the expedition area, and any documentation required for waste disposal in the country.

Everything should be considered from the point of view of reducing the amount of resources that the expedition will use. At the end of the expedition, it is the environmental manager's job to record the environmental section of the expedition report.

Assessing an expedition's environmental impact

When all the information is gathered, the environmental manager should be able to identify the following:

- The main environmental sensitivities and constraints of the expedition area, e.g. protected areas or species
- Those environmental aspects of the project which may result in potential impacts, e.g. overland transport, anchoring of vessels
- The potential environmental impacts of the expedition, assessed in basic terms.

An expedition may have several types of impact:

- Physical: the creation and erosion of paths and tracks, disturbance or destruction of various habitats and their dependent ecosystems, deforestation.
- Use of natural resources: water, local energy supplies, firewood, food.
- Pollution: engine emissions will impact air quality; soil and groundwater may be contaminated from poor waste and/or sewage disposal.
- Economic, social, and cultural: you will bring money and a different set of values into the area. These can negatively impact vulnerable local communities who may not possess the skills to deal with the changes they bring.

Making an environmental mitigation plan

An environmental plan needs to be drawn up to explain how the impacts already highlighted will be mitigated. The environmental plan should include the following:

- The expedition's environmental statement. Say what it is you are trying to achieve from an environmental point of view
- A summary of the environmental problems that may already be present in the area
- The impacts that will be generated by you
- How you will mitigate them, listing the different responsibilities
- The waste management options available to you
- What environmental permits or applications are required to visit your area
- Your arrangements for local employment: you need to educate any local expedition employees (e.g. cooks and porters) sympathetically and diplomatically about the importance of avoiding environmental damage. For example, use wood fires as little as possible, as deforestation is a serious problem in many expedition areas. Supply stoves and encourage their use
- Any reporting requirements upon completion of the expedition.

The plan should be short, succinct and easy-to-understand—try getting it onto one side of paper.

Crisis management

Section editors
Shane Winser, Chris Johnson

Contributors
Tina Birch, Iain Grant, Peter Harvey, Stephen Jones,
Charlie McGrath, and Marc Shaw

Medical crisis management

A medical crisis on an expedition can result from illness, injury, or accident to team members. The expedition planning team has a duty to foresee and try to prevent a crisis by developing a risk analysis and safety management system (RAMS). If an emergency develops, a comprehensive emergency response plan (ERP) will provide the team with the information and resources necessary to manage the situation effectively.

Medical aspects of the safety management system include:
- Organizing medical training for all participants (📖 p. 54)
- Providing appropriate medical kits (📖 p. 46)
- Organizing medical insurance with full emergency evacuation cover (📖 p. 82)
- Planning for evacuation and repatriation of a severely ill or injured person (📖 p. 136 and 146)
- Preparing a communication network in case of evacuation (📖 p. 133)
- Investigating medical facilities and support available both locally and remotely (e.g. using telemedicine, 📖 p. 148)
- Maintaining medical records and compiling accident reports.

During an emergency the team are likely to be involved in:
- Locating the ill or injured parties
- Preventing additional illness or injury
- Providing care to the ill or injured (📖 Emergencies—trauma p. 169)
- Expediting evacuations using effective logistics and communications
- Managing and supporting the rescue team
- Communicating accurately and effectively with key individuals
- Considering how to minimize long-term psychological effects on casualties and other team members (📖 p. 153).

Emergency response plan

Associated with each phase of the expedition should be an ERP, a reference document that includes information to enable any member of the team to respond appropriately to an emergency. Elements of an ERP are summarized in Figure 4.1.

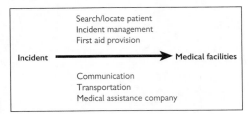

Fig. 4.1 Elements of an emergency response plan.

All these elements are important in expediting an evacuation. A rapid and timely response to a crisis may save a life; prior research, training, and resourcing are vital. Global communication is now relatively easy and satellite phones enable medical consultations from the field, so long as the medic has ready access to a medical specialist.

The most reliable source of help in an emergency is your expedition team. As far as possible be self-contained. Reliance on third parties in home countries is not robust and the best solutions are often local and simple. Therefore, do your research and know the transport, medical, search and rescue options for the region in which you are working. Once collated, everyone involved in the expedition should know the plan:
- All participants
- On-call contacts in the home country and host nation
- Support organizations (e.g. medical assistance company)
- Insurance company.

Components of an emergency response plan

An ERP should include as a minimum:

Section 1: roles and responsibilities in an emergency situation
This should clarify roles and responsibilities, focusing on the initial priorities as outlined below. Simplicity is critical. Consider who is trained and competent for each nominated role.

Table 4.1 Roles and responsibilities in an emergency situation

Role	Tasks
Leader	Overall coordination
Incident manager	Scene safety
Logistics	Evacuation/transportation
Communication	Radio/telephone links and information transfer
First aid	Provision of temporary immediate care

Section 2: initial response steps
Ensure that the initial response of the team is quick and effective. The generic steps outlined below can be applied to diverse situations:
- S.T.O.P.—Stop, Think, Observe, and Plan
- Manage the scene
- Remain calm
- Assess hazards
- Preserve life and prevent further injury
- Minimize damage to property/environment
- Delegate roles
- Inform expedition leader
- Ask expedition members not to call home
- Contact appropriate medical assistance company
- Contact on-call team with details, location, and contact number.

An example of an initial response plan is given in Figure 4.2.

Section 3: emergency services—contact numbers
This should contain important telephone, email contacts, and addresses, and include:
- All the expedition mobile/satellite phone numbers
- 24-h on-call contact details
- In-country contact details
- Emergency medical support company details
- Insurance companies
- Response organizations you may need to call on, such as air charter companies, the host country air force, police, air ambulance, local mountain rescue teams, coastguard, etc. The more information that is available, the better.

Section 4: medical facility information
This section should list in-country medical facilities to enable effective evacuation of ill or injured participants. Each facility should be listed with its name, address, directions (including maps), telephone numbers, capabilities, and hours of operation. Hospitals and clinics vary around the world and it is important to assess what capabilities exist in the area of your expedition. People are not always safer in a local clinic or hospital.

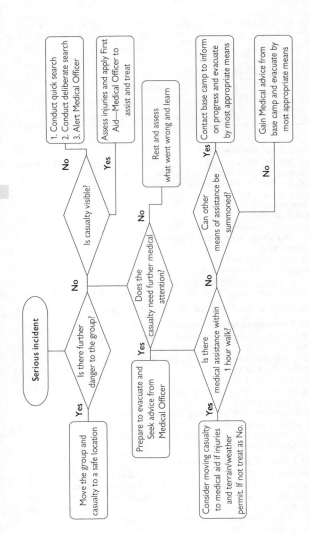

Fig. 4.2 Initial response plan.

Screened blood

In countries where adequate supplies of blood are not available or the standards of quality are unreliable, arrangements can be made to provide blood cover in an emergency. The Blood Care Foundation states that it is able to provide screened blood, in an emergency, to its members in any part of the world. Further information can be found at http://www.bloodcare.org.uk.

Section 5: trip itinerary and evacuation options

This section enables the on-call contact to locate the group if there is an emergency at home or a breakdown in communications. The itinerary should include enough detail and contact numbers to enable the on-call contact to locate the group. As a minimum this must include a list of dates of where the group will be staying, including addresses and phone numbers.

In addition, this section should briefly outline the emergency evacuation route for an injured participant from each phase of the expedition.

Section 6: participant emergency contact list

In emergency situations it may be necessary to contact a participant's next of kin. To enable this, each participant will need to supply a minimum of two contact names and numbers to be stored in the ERP.

Section 7: plans to deal with death or critical injury

These are discussed in later sections: the Initial response to an incident (📖 p. 170) and Death on an expedition (📖 p. 152).

Section 8: media plan

The media plan needs to establish the procedures and resources needed to respond to the press in the event of a serious incident and/or death. It might include a draft Press Release outlining the intentions and purpose of the expedition, the framework for reporting the incident and who to contact for further information.

Evacuation

Casualty evacuation (CASEVAC) is defined as the movement of a sick or injured expedition member to appropriate local medical facilities. Transfer may be by land, water, or air. Repatriation is the return of a casualty home following initial treatment. About 10% of expeditions will have to evacuate someone who requires medical assistance, while 3% will need to repatriate a team member.

Advance planning reduces the stress of a difficult situation and should allow an evacuation to proceed as smoothly and safely as possible, with minimum risk to casualty and rescuers. The aim is to get the casualty to the right care at an appropriate speed. Too much haste may increase hazard without benefit to the victim.

Many expeditions visit areas with sophisticated search and rescue facilities. If visiting such areas, determine the capabilities of the local rescue services and their requirements and costs.

Considerations in planning a specific evacuation

- Is the patient's condition time-critical?
- Can the patient receive further treatment in their current location?
- Can care be provided in a local clinic or hospital, or should they be transferred to a major hospital?
- Might they be able to rejoin the expedition after treatment?
- What is the capacity, availability, and suitability of procurable local transport?
- Could the patient survive a road/water journey or is air transport a better option?
- Is the patient safe to travel by air at the altitudes involved?
- Is medical supervision available for the journey?

The answers to these questions vary depending on the location of the incident, the nature of the casualty's injuries and the treatment required. A serious head injury, for example, will require a different response from a fractured finger.

Moving a casualty

Incidents often occur at locations remote from good transport links; initially the casualty must be transferred to a location from which evacuation is possible. Casualties in danger should be moved at once by whatever means possible. Patients not in immediate danger should first be stabilized and positioned to prevent aggravating their injuries during transport. Once a safe location is reached, fully assess the patient's condition to determine the urgency of evacuation.

Urgent movement

If an injured person must be moved immediately from a life-threatening situation (damaged building, fire, avalanche or rock fall), the greatest danger is the possibility of aggravating a spinal injury or compromising the airway. Try to pull the patient in the direction of the long axis of the body to provide as much protection to the spine as possible.

If on the ground, pull the patient's clothing in the neck or shoulder area. If available, log-roll the patient onto a sleeping bag, blanket, or air mattress (Fig. 4.3) and drag the material head first with the patient's head and shoulders off the ground to prevent further injury. If nothing is available to support the patient, place your hands under the armpits (from the back) and grasp the forearms to drag the patient (Fig. 4.4).

If not on the ground, move the patient by any means possible, but do not pull a patient's head away from the neck or the rest of the body.

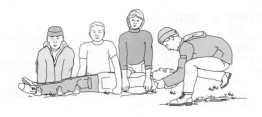

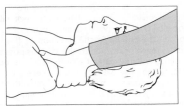

Always support the neck (never release)

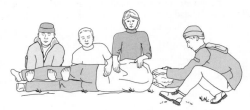

Everyone works together, with the person
at the head directing movement

Fig. 4.3 The log-roll method of turning a casualty with a suspected spinal injury.

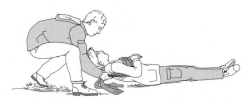

Fig. 4.4 Reverse drag.

Non-urgent movement

A variety of techniques can be used to transfer the patient to the nearest piece of appropriate equipment. Carrying a heavy human is exhausting, especially over rough ground, and the more people who are involved the safer it will be for everyone.

Single rescuer

A single rescuer is always at risk of injuring themselves, but there may nevertheless be circumstances where a lone rescuer seeks to move a casualty. Traditionally the way to carry an unconscious casualty is the fireman's carry, but there is a high risk of back injury to the rescuer and it should be avoided if the casualty has injuries involving the arms, legs, ribs, neck, or back. If the patient is able to assist a sling carry may be attempted (Fig. 4.5). Walking poles may assist with balance.

The tied hands crawl (Fig. 4.6) may be used to drag an unconscious casualty a short distance. This is especially good for crawling under low structures. The casualty's head is not supported.

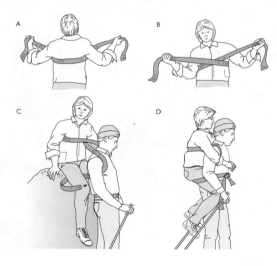

Fig. 4.5 Single person sling carry.

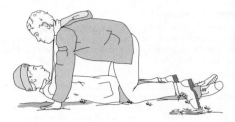

Fig. 4.6 Tied hands crawl.

The chair carry is good for going up or down stairs or down narrow passages. This should not be attempted in a patient with neck, back, or pelvic problems. Variations of this lift can be used without a chair with two rescuers.

Rope sling (Fig. 4.7) using two rescuers relieves some strain over longer distances, but increases the risk of falling in rough ground.

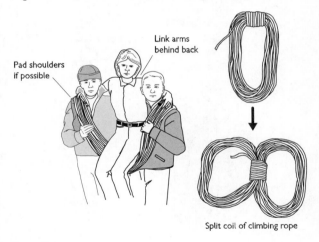

Link arms behind back

Pad shoulders if possible

Split coil of climbing rope

Fig. 4.7 Two-person sling carry.

Stretchers

Standard stretchers should be used if possible to transport a casualty. If none are available, improvisation may be necessary. Always ensure there are sufficient people to carry the stretcher so that you do not drop the casualty.

- Whenever possible, take the stretcher to the casualty instead of the casualty to the stretcher.
- Fasten the casualty to the stretcher so they do not slip, slide, or fall off.
- Use blankets, clothing, or other materials to pad the stretcher and protect the casualty from exposure.
- Try to splint broken limbs before movement and provide appropriate pain relief to minimize distress and reduce shock.
- Lay the casualty on their back for transport unless this may cause further injury.
- Ensure that the airway will remain open and unblocked.
- Move the casualty feet first so that the rear bearer may watch the patient for signs of difficulty or distress.
- Always brief the personnel carrying the casualty and the casualty themselves, if applicable, about the procedure to be employed.
Ensure one person is designated as team leader.

Improvising a stretcher

If a custom-made stretcher is not available, a stretcher may be improvised by using available materials such as boards. Always attempt to secure the casualty to the makeshift stretcher to prevent the risk of further injury. Other methods for manufacturing a stretcher include:

Blanket stretcher: the casualty is placed on their back in the middle of a blanket, tent or similar fabric material. Four people roll the side edges towards the casualty and lift.

Blanket and poles stretcher: a blanket may be wrapped around two poles (approximately seven feet in length) to make a stretcher that two persons can carry.

Jackets and poles stretcher: button or zip two or three jackets together and turn them inside out with the sleeves on the inside. Pass the poles through the sleeves after making holes in the shoulder areas to allow the poles to pass through (Fig. 4.8).

Most improvised stretchers give inadequate support to permit the evacuation of a casualty with fractures or extensive wounds.

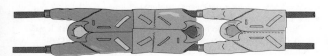

Fig. 4.8 Improvised jacket and poles stretcher.

Priority for evacuation of a casualty

A system commonly used to communicate the priority required for evacuation of the patient is outlined below (Table 4.2).

Table 4.2 Priority classification

Priority 1A	Immediate evacuation of the casualty required, if possible from the accident site
Priority 1B	Immediate evacuation required but the casualty can be moved from the accident site
Priority 2	Evacuation required within 12 h
Priority 3	Evacuation required within 12–24 h
Priority 4	Evacuation required but is not time-sensitive

Evacuation transport and considerations

Evacuation may be by:
• Air—fixed wing or helicopter
• Land—usually motor vehicle, but mules or porters can be better over rough ground
• Water—boat or raft.

Evacuation of a casualty by air

Advantages
• Casualty can be transported relatively long distances quickly
• Sophisticated medical care can be accessed quickly
• Air transport allows difficult terrain to be traversed safely
• Rotary wing aircraft can reach areas inaccessible to ground or water transport, especially if they have winch facilities.

Disadvantages
• Aircraft are very expensive to run
• They cannot fly in adverse weather conditions
• Fixed wing aircraft require a landing strip, while helicopters usually require a suitable landing zone (LZ), unless they are equipped with winching facilities
• Noise and vibration may make monitoring of and communication with the casualty impossible. Ear defenders for the patient and any person accompanying them are preferable. Diagnosis is difficult
• Air sickness can be a significant problem
• Helicopters work inefficiently at high altitude and trade payload for altitude. Do not rely on helicopter rescue from high altitudes; it will only be possible in ideal weather using the best available aircraft
• Altitude: As altitude increases and pressure decreases, air will expand. If air is trapped in a confined space, severe problems may result. At 18 000 ft the atmospheric pressure is half that of sea level, but the drop is not linear, with the decrease in pressure greater closer to sea level.

Creating a temporary helicopter landing zone (LZ)

- A LZ may have to be improvised if casualty evacuation by rotary wing (helicopter) aircraft is planned.
- Try to keep the LZ at least 150 m downwind of base areas or the casualty to prevent blowing dust and debris affecting the patient or operations. The LZ should be level and free of obstacles such as cables, wires, rocks, or ruts. Obstacles that cannot be moved should be clearly marked with items that cannot be affected by prop wash or gusting winds. Mark the wind direction to assist the pilot in landing into wind.
- Light signals should be planned. For example, the head lights of two downwind vehicles converging on the LZ, or four people with flashlights marking each corner of the LZ. The lights must be bright enough to be visible during the day, but not so bright they blind the pilot.
- A designated person should guide the aircraft in with land-to-air communication and direct the pilot by standing with their back to the wind and arms outstretched to indicate the LZ.
- Never approach a helicopter unless signalled to do so by the crewman. If a crewman is not on board, only approach in the pilot's field of frontal vision so they may indicate when and how to approach the aircraft.

Potential problems include:
- Development of tension pneumothorax
- Distension of gas in stomach or bowel
- Intracranial air expansion if pneumoencephaly
- Over-pressure of air in endotracheal tube cuffs
- Ambient temperature falls by about 2°C per 1000 ft increase in altitude
- Hypobaric hypoxia: the reduction in partial pressure of oxygen in inspired air produced by ascent to altitude is a serious potential risk during flight at high altitude, particularly if the patient's oxygenation is critical. (See 📖 p. 616 in Humans at altitude.)

Evacuation of the casualty by land
Advantages
Vehicles, either propelled mechanically or by animals, are usually more available than aircraft, and in locations with road access permit immediate evacuation to medical facilities. Vehicles can travel in conditions that impede boats and aircraft.

Disadvantages
Speed and range may be limited. Rough terrain and winding roads may prevent immediate access to the casualty and make evacuation a slow, painful or nauseating journey for the casualty.

Evacuation of the casualty by water
Advantages
In tropical forests and marine archipelagos, water is the main communication route. Evacuation by boat or seaplane becomes possible. Boat transport can be quite quick and smooth, with good access to the patient during transfer. Care must be taken to ensure that a restless or confused patient does not upset the boat or plunge overboard.

Disadvantages
Boats must be big enough and stable enough to be capable of transporting a patient. Weather, geographical, and biological hazards must be considered before the evacuation begins.

Helicopter evacuation from offshore craft
See 📖 p. 656 in Yachting section.

Documentation

It is desirable that a companion travels with a casualty to ensure that they are properly supervised and so that their condition can be communicated back to the expedition and to relatives at home. However, there are circumstances such as helicopter transfers where this will not be possible and it is essential that appropriate paperwork travels with the casualty. This should include:

- Passport and travel documents
- Insurance documents
- Next of kin details
- Copy of any medical documents (e.g. pre-expedition medical questionnaire, and any assessment notes). (See 📖 Chapter 5, Emergencies—diagnosis)
- Note any allergies or current medication
- Incident report
- Written instructions to personnel accompanying the casualty (if relevant).

Other considerations

- Ensure you know the whole evacuation plan, from the patient leaving your location to arriving at a facility that can offer adequate care. Make sure any escort is aware of the planned destination. If possible, try to confirm the arrival of the casualty at a medical facility
- If accompanying the patient, try not to do so alone. It can be a long and very tiring process. Try not to leave the casualty alone if medical facilities are basic
- Carry enough money or credit cards with you. You can always be reimbursed later
- Carry communications with you in the form of a radio or mobile phone if possible
- Take a translator with you if available and required
- Take a medical kit
- Take a snatch bag with food, water, spare clothes, and wash kit. This may make the journey more comfortable.

Repatriation

Repatriation, if required, may use a dedicated air ambulance or a commercial airliner. The patient will usually need to be escorted by an experienced aeromedical doctor or nurse. Such transfers are very expensive and it is essential that insurance covers this possibility.

Medical assistance companies

Because they will not start an evacuation or repatriation without guarantee of payment, most expeditions will initially contact a medical assistance company through their insurers. Most of the work of medevac organizations involves tourists and businessmen in destinations with good travel links rather than expeditions in remote regions, so their databases may not contain information on the capabilities of remote clinics/hospitals, or on the logistical solutions to remote evacuations. They should be relied upon as a third level of support after seeking help from the group's own medical expertise and the host country resources.

Expeditions should do their own research on local medical facilities and the logistics necessary to ensure a patient can get to an internationally recognized airstrip capable of receiving a medical team via Lear Jet.

These companies include:

- International SOS—http://www.internationalsos.com
- Medical Air Rescue Service—http://www.mars.co.zw
- Royal Flying Doctor Service of Australia—http://www.flyingdoctors.org
- AMREF—http://www.amref.org
- CEGA—http://www.cega-aviation.co.uk
- First Assist—http://www.firstassist.co.uk

Establishing a direct relationship with a medical assistance company is recommended, although this can be difficult as one normally is forced to negotiate through the insurance company. Once in direct contact, it is important to confirm the organization's capabilities and limitations. Check all contact numbers before departing on the trip and consider running a test to ensure the system works.

Telemedicine and communications

The literal definition of telemedicine is 'distance medicine'. Writing a letter about a patient and getting a reply is telemedicine, but the term is now usually taken to mean any medical consultation conducted where the patient and doctor, or two practitioners, are distant from each other and technology is used to facilitate communication or transmit data.

Telemedicine must be:
• Safe for the patient with minimal loss of accuracy
• As effective as it is practicable to be
• Acceptable to patient and practitioner
• Cost-effective.

Telemedicine is not necessarily:
• Technologically complex
• Very costly
• The solution to all problems.

Uses of telemedicine in expedition medicine

Probably the biggest single use is as back-up and reassurance for a relatively inexperienced expedition doctor or medical officer. Just knowing that there is someone else to call in an emergency can be very helpful. On larger expeditions, spending prolonged periods in the field, facilities for treatment may be relatively sophisticated. Remote telemetry, backed up by specialist advice, may avoid the need for an evacuation. Given the costs of evacuation, and the potential disruption caused by loss of key personnel, this can in some circumstances justify the high set-up costs. Where several remote parties will be working away from the expedition doctor, telemedicine can provide consultations and advice without the need for difficult travel.

Before departure

Direct medical advice from experienced doctors can be established using a medical assistance company or a personal contact.

Whoever is providing support should have the necessary experience and understanding of the circumstances you are likely to encounter and the facilities you have available.

Consider whether an agreement with a centre that does a lot of telemedical support would be sensible. Many centres will not charge for the privilege if the work rate is predicted to be very light. In general, costs are not that high, especially on a call-for-service basis rather than a retainer where you pay whether or not you use the service.

There are several telemedicine companies offering this service: e.g. World Clinic: http://www.worldclinic.com, Talk to a Doctor http://www.talktoadoctor.co.uk.

Check the communication equipment you are taking and ensure you can use it. Training has been identified in several studies as the key to successful telemedicine.

Check that the communication equipment is robust enough to cope with your demands on it. Check battery life and recharge facilities.

Train at least one other team member in using the facilities you have set up. It may be the doctor who is the patient.

Support at the centre must be available 24-h a day and the staff aware of the issues associated with wilderness travel.

Permits and licenses may be needed both to import and to use communications equipment.

If non-medics are going to be using the system, consider developing or using a field medical questionnaire to assist their questioning and examination of the patient (📖 see example on p. 158). Make sure they know the information you will need when they call you. There is enormous frustration in repeated waits while they respond to questions they have not prepared for in advance.

Maintaining clinical confidentiality is a significant issue. Security of transmitted data is improving all the time, and the risks from satellite communication are small; however, consider anonymizing any data you send, especially if it is of a sensitive nature. At the moment this limits the use of many internet-based communications systems as they are insecure. Clinical responsibility can also be an issue unless a formal contract is in place.

In the field

Test the system when you arrive in country and on a regular basis, to ensure you can contact the person you expect to contact, and that all the equipment is working. Keep good records of telemedicine consultations. Consider recording the call if you can do so. Note what advice was given and by whom. These are as important as any other clinical record.

It is good practice to pre-arrange the format of both routine and emergency reports back to a project base or home base so that communications can be efficient.

Arrange a time schedule for planned communications between groups or back to a project or home base.

Agree what action will be taken by your home base or in-country agent in the event that you miss a scheduled call in. Depending on the remoteness and level of risk associated with your activities, this could be a 24-h, 36-h, or 48-h response in the event of no contact.

Plan for a number of scenarios, including urgent and non-urgent medical evacuation, and itemize the information needed to create the format for the reports.

Agree 'prowords' to start pre-formatted reports so that the recipient knows what type of report is to follow.

Examples of prowords

- *Medevac*—Urgent assistance required for medical evacuation
- *Alpha*—Location including grid reference or latitude and longitude
- *Bravo*—Nature of injury
- *Charlie*—Name of injured person
- *Delta*—Treatment given
- *Echo*—Details and time of incident
- *Foxtrot*—Assistance required and when will they next communicate
- *Golf*—Date and time of report
- *Hotel*—Are the next of kin to be informed by project home base?

Technologies for telemedicine

Telephones—land line, mobile, and satellite (SATCOM). Telephones have the advantage of familiarity of use. Coverage is steadily improving.

Radio still has a place, though possibly less so with advances in telephony. It is very useful in short-range networks within a limited geographical area. It requires some training to be used effectively, and is not secure.

Digital cameras: unusual problems crop up quite commonly on expeditions, with tropical conditions, strange rashes, and bites from unknown creatures high on the list. Digital cameras are increasingly useful when there is a need to describe an injury, rash, or other sign.

X-rays: digital equipment and scanning are only available from relatively fixed locations, but even with low-cost methods of transmission using high compression, useful information can be obtained. Experience in the Antarctic has shown that simple digital photographs of plain X-rays can, with a minimum of training be successfully used to guide fracture management. The nuance of subtle changes on a chest X-ray may be lost in file compression.

Email and internet: may have a place from fixed base camps, or with improving satellite technology. Broadband technologies are enabling live video conversations and conference links.

Satellite phones

Satellite phones work in remote locations beyond the coverage of normal telephony and cellular networks. Satellite phones complement the use of international roaming on GSM cellular phones or the use of locally bought SIM cards to access in-country cellular networks.

Satellite phones work with one of three basic systems. A stationary phone can be aligned with a specific satellite (Inmarsat, R-BGAN); a mobile satellite phone can communicate with a specific satellite overhead (e.g. GlobalStar and Thuraya); or a mobile phone can transmit and receive to an array of orbiting satellites to give global coverage (e.g. Iridium).

Considerations before rental or purchase of satellite phones:

- Location: compare the coverage maps to see which system will work where you are going.
- Applications: decide what you need, from 2-way voice to email and video conferencing, and then see which are supported.
- Accounts structure: decide on pre-pay or on account options, and check how easy it is to top up a prepaid SIM card whilst you are away.
- Running cost: compare the airtime costs per minute.
- Power supply: plan a recharging system suitable for your planned area of usage, such as solar panels or lithium batteries in areas where mains electricity is not available.

Plan to protect your equipment from water, dust, and shock hazards with padded or waterproof cases. Pelican Products® cases and micro-cases are excellent.

If your project is dependent on satellite phone communications take more than one and spare ancillaries.

Improve the functionality of email over slow satellite phone connections by using a specialist Satellite Email Service such as UUPlus.

Emergency beacons

The joint American–Russian COSPAS-SARSAT 406 MHz System provides an international search and rescue network with global coverage for transmission-only emergency beacons. The technology has a different name depending on where it is used:

- Aircraft carry emergency locator transmitters (ELTs)
- Ships carry emergency position indicating radio beacons (EPIRBs)
- People on the ground carry personal locator beacons (PLBs).

When a beacon goes off its signal is transmitted to a network of Mission Control Centres and then on to a Rescue Control Centre near the beacon's location. In some cases no action will be taken so it is critical to ascertain what action will be taken and by whom in advance.

Along with location information, 406 MHz beacons transmit *information on* the type of beacon, the country code, and identification of the beacon. Using this information, search and rescue (SAR) bodies can access contact details and information on the aircraft/ship from a beacon database.

An earlier generation of 121.5 MHz beacons is being phased out of satellite reception. Most current beacons transmit on 406 MHz and model options include GPS.

406 MHz emergency beacons need to be registered before use. In the UK this is to the *EPIRB* Registry of the Maritime and Coastguard Agency. For countries that do not have a registration system, beacons can be registered at the International Beacon Registration Database (IBRD) at https://www.406registration.com.

PLBs should only be used for life-threatening emergencies, as no qualifying information can be added. They are a useful item of last resort as a back-up to satellite phones.

Death on an expedition

Although death during an expedition is rare, expeditions need to have a plan for this eventuality included in their ERP (📖 p. 132). If an expedition member should die, then it is important that the death is dealt with sensitively, expeditiously, and in accordance with the legislative requirements of both the deceased's home country and the country where the incident occurs. Local police and judiciary should be informed as quickly as possible—in some countries the location of an unexpected death will be considered to be a potential crime scene until the circumstances have been confirmed. Your local Embassy or Consulate may be able to offer support, advice, legal assistance, and communication links. The psychological sequelae following the death must be considered, with all the surviving team members involved in measures to prevent their long-term distress.

Following the death, a designated person within the group should coordinate the necessary actions:

- *Ensure there are no further injuries.* Make sure that the team are at no increased risk as a result of the death. If the death has occurred in a difficult physical location, then retrieval of the body may be necessary, but there should not be any undue risk to the rest of the team in attempting recovery of the body.
- *Find out what happened.* Record the details as they are given and then check with all available sources to establish any other details that are known or gradually learned, and compile these together into an accurate 'diary of events'.
- *Locate the body.* Take responsibility for locating the body and, if retrieval is possible, collect it and deliver it to the appropriate authorities to obtain a death certificate. This may involve packaging and transporting the body some considerable distance, a process that should be done quickly and with dignity. Other expedition members will be noting the response of the medical team to the event.
- *Prevent possible infection.* If the person died of an infectious (or potentially infectious) disease, or if the cause of death is unknown, handle the body in a manner that minimizes the risk of infection spreading to other members of the expedition.

Practical considerations following the death

Once death has been confirmed

A signal or message needs to be sent to the expedition's headquarters informing them of the tragedy. Importantly for the families of other surviving members of the expedition, the information needs to note that other team members are safe and well.

Other expedition members need to be informed of the death (see Breaking bad news 📖 p. 155).

The next of kin must be notified at the earliest opportunity. This should be done in person by two people representing the expedition; two people because the person advising of the death will need support and both together have a greater chance of giving support to the deceased's relatives. In many cases, police in their home country will inform the next of kin.

The family of the deceased should be offered immediate access to practical and social support; whether this be psychological to deal with the event, practical help with the funeral or, where possible, financial assistance.

Legal responsibilities

- Urgently inform the embassy or consulate representative of the deceased person of the circumstances surrounding the death.
- Inform the embassy or consulate representative of other expedition members' situation and safety.
- Inform the police, particularly if there are legal issues about the death.
- Obtain a police report, if necessary.
- Organize an autopsy, if required.
- Contact insurance companies.
- Issue an appropriate report on the tragedy, for insurance purposes. This will need to be done in conjunction with the expedition leader.
- Develop contacts between the insurance company and the local authorities who can organize repatriation.

Repatriation of the body

- Often the local embassy or consulate will assist with this process.
- It will include negotiations with local authorities, insurance, and transport companies.
- Keep an accurate diary of all events, the persons who were communicated with, and the times of these communications.
- Care for the expedition team members and their families.
- Consider the needs of the concerned outsider.
- Ensure regular opportunities for communication between team members and their families whilst on the expedition.
- After the expedition, ensure members are followed up to ensure that there are no adverse psychological responses.
- Screen for symptoms of depression, excessive arousal, avoidance behaviours, intrusive phenomena, and dissociation. The emphasis here is on recognizing 'at-risk' individuals.
- If involved in the care of the deceased, the medic may have particular feelings of responsibility, guilt, or failure that need to be recognized.

Dealing with the media

Prepare a statement or press release that can be used to respond to any media enquiries and prevent any incorrect reportage.

Psychological reaction by team members

When the tragedy becomes known to the expedition, team members may go through a variety of reactions: grief, guilt, acceptance and then resolution:

- 'This can't have happened.'
- 'I don't believe it.'
- 'This is ridiculous—he was only here in this camp an hour ago.'
- 'Tell me that again!'

Psychological debriefing is the generic term for immediate interventions following trauma (usually within 3 days) that seek to relieve stress with the intent of mitigating or preventing long-term pathology. In the first days after the death of a colleague, expeditioners are advised to:

- Talk about the dead colleague, talk about the death, talk about their positive and negative feelings for their colleague. Talk about the nightmares that may result, and what these nightmares are and how they were handled.
- In the first 8 weeks expeditioners should not try to push flashbacks, intrusive images, or nightmares away. These are all ways the psyche is trying to work through and make sense of an abnormal situation.
- Advice should be given *not* to drink 'more than normal', as alcohol impedes the brain's processing of the trauma.
- All within the group need to remind themselves that they are not going crazy (a common feeling) but that they are reacting normally to an abnormal situation.
- Avoidance of discussion of the incident is the single best predictor of post-traumatic stress disorder (PTSD). The whole group must slowly confront the situations that they are avoiding. In the early stages after the tragedy this involves talking about the event and about the dead colleague. Such discussion may include the need or desire either to continue with the mission or to return home, and may predispose into feelings of selfishness (that turn into guilt), selflessness, remorse, blame, and whether there is willpower to go on. Collectively the expedition should talk in terms of:
  - 'We were shocked.'
  - 'We thought we'd have to quit.'
  - 'We decided to continue to honour our fallen friend.'
  - 'This is what he/she would have wanted us to do.'
- Initial counselling should occur within the group. Symptoms of PTSD may develop several weeks after the event, and team members should then seek help through their GP or family doctor. The value of formal counselling in these circumstances is highly controversial; some experts feel it is essential, while others suggest it may make PTSD worse rather than better.

Breaking bad news

S—*Setting up* the interview:
• Prepare yourself
• Have as much information as possible
• Think about the questions the person will ask
• Ensure privacy, avoid interruptions
• Involve significant others
• Sit down
• Make eye contact

P—assess *Perception*:
• What do they already know?
• What do they think has happened?

I—obtain the person's *Invitation*:
• Gain permission to give more information, e.g. 'Can I tell you what happened this afternoon?' or 'I need to tell you what happened this afternoon.'

K—give *Knowledge* and information:
• Give a warning: 'I'm afraid I have some bad news for you.'
• Avoid blurting it all out—give information in small chunks
• Avoid excessive bluntness
• Check for understanding periodically
• Respect the level of knowledge the person wants, e.g. some will just want to know the person has died while some will want to know how and why

E—address *Emotions* with empathic responses:
• Observe for emotional responses
• Identify the emotion and the reason for it to yourself
• Empathize: e.g. 'I can see you are really upset.' 'This must be very difficult for you.' 'I'm so sorry this has happened.'
• Avoid 'I know how you feel': you don't
• Give time and respect silence
• Use touch if appropriate

S—*Strategy* and *Summary*
• Summarize what has been said
• Agree what should happen next for expedition members, e.g. does the person wish to stay on the expedition, or do they want to go home, or who would they like to 'buddy' them.

Adapted from a protocol for breaking bad news to patients with cancer. Baile WF, Buckman R *et al.* (2000). *Oncologist* **5**: 302–11.

Emergencies—diagnosis

Jon Dallimore, Charles Siderfin

This guide to the medical history-taking, examination, and measurement of vital signs is designed to assist someone without medical training to obtain the necessary information to communicate effectively with a doctor over the radio.

For information on the initial management of an injured person see Chapter 6.

For the initial management of serious medical conditions see Chapter 7.

History and examination— an introduction for non-clinicians

There are three important aspects to the assessment of the ill patient.
- History—an account of how the illness developed
- Examination—three modalities are used to examine:
  - Look
  - Feel
  - Listen
- Monitoring—a few 'vital signs' are used to assess an individual's progress.

History
- Patient details
- Clearly identify the patient and time of examination
- Main complaint
- Identify the central problems. Use the patient's own words. Avoid technical medical terms—there is a danger of them being used incorrectly
- Short history of the illness
- Chronological description of how the illness evolved. Start from when the patient was last completely well and relate each symptom to time. For instance:
  - Last completely well yesterday
  - Started to vomit 3 hours ago
  - Vomited 5 times—initially food
  - Last vomit 15 min ago—yellow fluid
  - Abdominal pain for 2 h
- Ask all the questions.

Apparently unrelated symptoms can be important in reaching a diagnosis. A list of useful questions can be found in the Illness assessment form below.

Examination
Answer these questions from your own observations, not by asking the patient. Prior to the expedition, obtain training in the techniques of examination. Practise examining normal individuals so you can recognize abnormality. Try not to feel shy or embarrassed—you will do a sick person no favours if you fail to spot an important sign or symptom. Examine the whole person carefully in the following order:
- General appearance
- Hands
- Face
- Neck
- Chest
- Abdomen
- Limbs
- Nervous system.

- Look
  - General wellbeing. A subjective assessment as to whether the patient is generally well or unwell. Expose the patient and observe. Compare the left and right side of the body for asymmetry.
- Feel
  - Examine with the hands flat. Warm your hands, be gentle but firm. Whilst feeling, watch the patient's face for signs of pain.
- Listen
  - Use a stethoscope or put your ear on the body to listen for breath and bowel sounds.
- Measure
  - You may be able to make simple measurements to indicate the patient's condition. These include measuring temperature and respiratory rate, taking the pulse and blood pressure, and observing capillary return time (see below).

General appearance
- Look
  - At patient's demeanour: in pain, anxious, frightened, confused
  - At body posture
  - Colour of skin
  - Whether they are sweating
  - Assess breathing effort
- Feel
  - Skin temperature and dampness

Hands
- Look
  - Sweating
  - Temperature
  - Tremor
- Measure
  - Radial (wrist) pulse for rate, rhythm, and character.

Face
- Look
  - For colour or swelling of face and lips
  - Inspect mouth and throat for ulcers, blisters, and redness
  - Look at condition of tongue.

Neck
- Look
  - At veins in neck for degree of distension
- Feel
  - For lymph nodes and swellings in neck, cheeks and back of head
  - For position of windpipe
- Listen
  - For abnormal sounds associated with breathing.

Chest
Examine front and back of the chest:
- Look
  - Breathing rate
  - Compare chest movement on both sides
  - Check for injuries to the chest wall
- Feel
  - Irregularities or crepitus (grating) of chest wall indicating injury
  - Chest wall tenderness
  - For lymph nodes in axilla (armpit)
- Listen
  - Place stethoscope under the collar bone and then outside each nipple. Compare each side
  - Sit the patient forward, with arms crossed to pull the shoulder blades apart. Place stethoscope just inside the shoulder blades and then lower down, comparing both sides

  Breath sounds:
  - Normal
  - Absent
  - Added sounds—wheeze or crackles?

Abdomen
Make sure that your hands are warm. Ensure the patient is relaxed, lying on his back, head on one or two pillows and the abdomen exposed:
- Look
  - Swelling, discoloration or bruising (especially over flank), scars
- Feel
  - Place hand flat on abdomen and gently apply pressure with all four fingers by bending at the knuckles, keeping the fingers flat and straight
  - Begin away from region of tenderness and move towards the area. Move methodically around the entire abdomen
  - Feel for tenderness whilst watching the patient's face. Facial expression will signal tenderness
  - Tensing of the abdominal muscles (guarding) occurs with tenderness
  - Ascertain if guarding is localized or generalized. In severe cases, the abdominal wall will be rigid, implying diffuse inflammation within the abdominal cavity (peritonitis) owing to bowel perforation
  - Test for rebound. Gently push fingers into the abdomen and then rapidly remove your hand, without warning. Pain with this procedure implies peritonitis
  - Be gentle but firm. If the patient is unable to relax his abdominal muscles, ensure your hands are warm and ask him to bend his knees up to relax these muscles
  - Feel in groin creases for enlarged lymph nodes

- Listen
  - Place the stethoscope 1 cm below the umbilicus (belly button) and listen for bowel sounds for 1 min
  - Normal—gentle gurgling a few times per minute
  - Increased—overactive bowel, e.g. diarrhoea or bowel obstruction
  - Absent—peritonitis.

Limbs
- Look
  - Areas of redness, swelling, or bruising
  - Deformity
  - Joint swelling
  - Pain on movement
- Feel
  - Tenderness
  - Creaking or grating sensations

Nervous system
- Look
  - Assess AVPU (awake, verbal, pain, unresponsive) and Glasgow coma scale (📖 p. 192)
  - Check both eyes can move in all directions
  - Assess pupils for size, asymmetry, and reaction to light
  - Test power and sensation in all limbs.

Clinical measurements

Taking the temperature (see also Chapter 23)
• Normal temperature 36.5–37.5°C
• Hypothermia <35°C.

Oral
Place a thermometer under the tongue for 3 min with the mouth closed. This is unreliable if the patient has recently eaten, drunk, is hypothermic, or breathing with an open mouth.

Armpit (axilla)
Place thermometer under the armpit for 3 min. This method is unreliable in patients with hypothermia. The temperature is 1°C lower than oral temperature.

Rectal
This is the most accurate site for measurement as it measures the core temperature. Lie patient on his side and insert a lubricated thermometer into the rectum. Hold in position for 3 min; *do not let go*. Clean thermometer with alcohol wipe—identify for rectal use only. A special low-reading thermometer is needed for hypothermic patients.

Taking the pulse

Press gently with the pulp of the middle and index fingers. Count beats for a timed minute or half a minute and multiply by two. Evaluate whether regular or irregular and comment on its strength.
• Normal adult pulse at rest 60–90 beats per min.

Radial (wrist) pulse
Feel on the thumb side of the wrist.

Carotid (neck) pulse
Locate the larynx (Adam's apple) with your finger tips. Move your fingers across the neck towards you until reaching the groove between the trachea (windpipe) and muscle edge. *Press gently*. Never feel the pulse on both sides of the neck at the same time as this will reduce the blood supply to the brain.

Femoral (groin) pulse
Press in the skin crease at the top of the leg halfway between the midline and the iliac crest (prominent bony lump on the edge of the abdomen at the top front of the pelvis in line with the navel).

Blood pressure

There is large variability in blood pressure between different situations and individuals. It is an important measurement for monitoring a patient's progress over time.

Use of the sphygmomanometer

Undo any restrictive clothing and wrap the sphygmomanometer cuff around the upper arm. Straighten the arm, palm up. Locate the brachial pulse on the inner aspect of the front of the elbow. Inflate cuff 20–30 mmHg above the point that the pulse disappears. Hold the stethoscope gently over the pulse. Listen for pulse and release cuff 3–5 mmHg per second.

- Systolic pressure = level when pulse first heard
- Diastolic pressure = level when pulse muffles and disappears.

Automated blood pressure measuring devices are reasonably inexpensive and widely available. Basic versions of such machines will struggle to measure the blood pressure if a patient has collapsed.

Estimating blood pressure using peripheral pulses

- Radial pulse palpable: systolic BP >80 mmHg
- Femoral pulse palpable: systolic BP >70 mmHg
- Carotid pulse palpable: systolic BP >60 mmHg.

Capillary refill time

Firmly press your thumb on a fingernail, toenail, or bony prominence for 5 s. When the thumb is removed, the area will appear white. If it takes more than 2 s for the colour to return, reduced circulation is implied. NB. This is not reliable when patient is cold (compare with your own finger).

Respiratory (breathing) rate

Count the breathing rate over 1 min. Pretend to take the pulse as the respiratory rate may alter if the patient is aware the respiratory rate is being measured.

- Normal adult respiratory rate at rest 12–18 per min.

Reduced level of consciousness

In the case of head injury the AVPU scale (📖 p. 192) is a rough initial assessment. To monitor a patient's progress chart the Glasgow Coma Scale (📖 p. 192). Minimum GCS score is 3, with maximum score of 15. Three areas of basic brain function are tested and scored: eye opening, speech, and movement:

- Use increasing level of stimulus to obtain response
- Speak
- Tap the shoulders gently
- Apply pain—press firmly over the inner aspect of the eyebrow along the eye socket
- For scoring see 📖 p. 192.

A fall in the GCS score indicates deterioration in the patient's condition. Causes include:

- Bleeding
- Swelling
- Infection.

Remember, if the patient deteriorates during your assessment *immediately* re-check the ABC and rectify any life-threatening problems.

Monitoring
- Keep timed, written notes of the patient's condition
- Chart vital signs hourly or more frequently. If very unwell monitor every 15 min
- Pulse
- Temperature
- Blood pressure
- Respiratory rate
- GCS—if previous head injury or concerns about level of consciousness
- A model chart is given in Chapter 7 (📖 p. 216).

Illness assessment form

- Date/time:
- Name:
- Date of birth:
- Main complaint:
- History of illness (in the patient's own words):
- Past medical history (serious accidents/illnesses, operations, high blood pressure, heart disease, diabetes, asthma, epilepsy):
- Drugs (including oral contraceptives, inhalers, antimalarials):
- Allergies:
- Family history (any significant illnesses in the family, causes of premature death, high blood pressure, heart disease, diabetes):
- Social history (tobacco, alcohol, recreational drugs, recent foreign travel and immunizations):

Direct questions
- Cardiovascular
  - Chest pain
  - Shortness of breath
  - Palpitations
  - Ankle swelling
- Respiratory
  - Cough
  - Wheeze
  - Sputum
- Gastrointestinal
  - Appetite
  - Weight
  - Nausea/vomiting
  - Indigestion
  - Abdominal pain
  - Bowels (blood, diarrhoea/constipation)
- Urogenital
  - Pain on passing urine
  - Need to pass urine frequently
  - Loin pain
  - Genital discharge
  - Date of last menstrual period.........................
- Nervous system
  - Headache
  - Eyes/ears
  - Weakness/numbness
  - Fits/faints

Examination
- General comments (unwell, abnormal skin colour, rashes, sweating, dehydration):
- Temperature...............................°C
- Pulse....................................../min
- Breathing rate............................/min
- Blood pressure................/........mmHg
- Chest
  - Laboured breathing
  - Symmetry of chest movements
  - Breath sounds (wheezes, crackles, normal, absent)
- Abdomen
  - Distended
  - Bowel sounds
  - Tenderness (indicate on diagram)
  - Guarding
  - Rebound tenderness
- Nervous system
  —Level of response
  - Alert
  - Verbal
  - Pain
  - Unresponsive
  —Pupils
  - Equal size
  - React to light
- Limbs
  —Movements
  - Right arm   Left arm
  - Right leg   Left leg
  —Sensation
  - Right arm   Left arm
  - Right leg   Left leg

Possible diagnosis
- 1.
- 2.
- 3.
- 4.

Management...
- Signed...Date....................

Emergencies—trauma

Section editors
Jon Dallimore and Chris Johnson

Contributors
Sundeep Dhillon, Stephen Hearns, David Lockey,
Charles Siderfin, and Julian Thompson

Initial response to an incident

The ABC approach to patient assessment ensures that the most important life-threatening conditions are dealt with in the correct order.
- Ensure safety of scene, self, and casualty
- Triage casualties if multiple victims
- Airway (and cervical spine control where appropriate)
- Breathing and ventilation
- Circulation
- Disability
- Environmental control and evacuation following proper preparation of patient for travel
- Rescuer safety.

Patients who have been injured are often in hazardous environments. The safety of the rescuers should have paramount importance. Stop and assess the risks of the situation. A minute spent on this task is vital for the safety and efficiency of the rescue operation, and the delay rarely leads to an adverse outcome for the patient.

In *steep ground* place a belay (anchor) above the incident to secure both patient and rescuers. Consider the potential for rock fall or avalanche.

At *road traffic collision* sites deploy two members of the team to stop the traffic in both directions. To protect rescuers from further collisions, park vehicles back from the site at an angled 'fend-off' position. Once the crash vehicle can be approached (danger of fire, explosion, rollover, etc.) the vehicle ignition should be turned off and the handbrake applied. Vehicle stabilization procedures should be improvised as soon as possible.

If there is a continuing significant risk to rescuers or patient it may be necessary to extricate the patient rapidly from the hazardous zone before a primary survey has been completed and, in some cases, before spinal immobilization has been optimized (📕 p. 190).

Scene management

Management of wilderness injuries may be complex and requires excellent leadership, teamwork, communication, and forward thinking. If sufficient resources allow, the expedition leader should stand back and coordinate the situation, including initiating and planning the different stages of evacuation while the patient is being initially assessed and managed. Only with this ability to think ahead to the next steps in the rescue will it be rapid and effective. The leader also has the role of dynamically assessing and managing hazards to those involved.

Equipment should be organized in a kit dump a few metres from the accident scene. This ensures the equipment is readily located when needed and does not present a trip hazard to those managing the patient.

The rest of the group will require care (particularly true with commercial and youth expeditions). Try to involve them as much as is safe and possible in the rescue. Ensure that they are in a safe position and kept informed of progress.

Triage

A major incident involving several casualties, for instance an avalanche or road traffic collision, stretches the resources of fully equipped emergency services. In the wilderness it is easy to feel overwhelmed and helpless. However, developing and practising an effective triage and treatment system will enable as many people as possible to be treated and give later reassurance that everything possible was done.

The triage process aims to prioritize patients according to their medical needs given the resources available. This approach ensures that those requiring immediate treatment receive appropriate care, but also that limited resources are not diverted to treating an irrecoverable condition at the expense of other casualties. Triage principles should be applied whenever the number of casualties exceeds the resources of skilled rescuers available. It is a dynamic process where the state of the patient may change and the environment will dictate the level of care available.

Priorities

Several systems are used internationally. The four priority groups are defined as follows:

- **P1. Immediate priority**—casualties who require immediate life-saving procedures.
- **P2. Urgent priority**—casualties who require surgical or medical intervention within 2–4 h.
- **P3. Delayed priority**—less serious cases whose condition can safely be delayed beyond 4 h.
- **P1 Hold. Expectant priority**—casualties whose condition is so severe that they cannot survive despite the best available care and whose treatment would divert medical resources from salvageable patients who may then be compromised.

Triage classifications

Priority	Description	Label colour
P1	Immediate	Red
P2	Urgent	Yellow
P3	Delayed	Green
P1 Hold	Expectant	Blue
Dead	Dead	White or Black

In some areas a 'T' (treatment) system is substituted for the 'P' (priority) system but the categories are exactly the same. Casualties should, if possible, be regularly re-triaged. Triage categories can change at any time and are not fixed.

Triage sieve

- This is a rapid, simple, safe, and reproducible method of prioritization based upon the Airway, Breathing, Circulation (ABC) approach of resuscitation.

Mobility
- Walking patients are initially categorized as **P3, delayed priority**
- If the patient is not walking then apply the **ABC** approach

Airway
- Patients who cannot breathe despite simple airway manoeuvres (e.g. chin lift/jaw thrust) are dead
- If breathing starts on opening the airway, the patient is **P1 Immediate**.

Breathing
- Check respiratory rate (RR). If RR >30 or <10 then patient is **P1, immediate**.

Circulation
- Check capillary refill time (CRT)
- If >2 s then patient is **P1, immediate**
- If CRT <2 s then patient is **P2, urgent**
- Cold conditions may prolong CRT and comparison with the rescuer's CRT will allow adjustment
- In extreme conditions or in the dark, CRT may be impossible to assess and a pulse rate of 120 beats per minute can be used as the circulatory sieve.

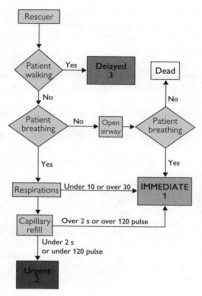

Fig. 6.1 Triage sieve.

Assessment of a casualty

Assessment of a casualty

Once the incident scene has been made safe, approach and evaluate the casualty. If you have the skills, follow Advanced Trauma Life Support (ATLS) guidelines. This text offers guidance to those without advanced resuscitation skills, and suggests courses of action appropriate to the wilderness setting.

Assessment of the trauma victim

The assessment and management of the seriously injured patient in remote wilderness environments is extremely challenging. Problems include:
- Lack of equipment
- Lack of skilled assistance
- Prolonged transfer times to definitive care.

It should be made clear to everyone in the expedition group that the clinical interventions possible in remote environments are extremely limited compared to those that one would expect in urban environments in a developed country.

The key to managing any pre-hospital trauma is to perform basic assessments and interventions well and then transport the casualty safely and rapidly to a centre capable of providing definitive surgical and critical care. A properly prepared evacuation plan will facilitate this process (📖 p. 136).

Airway

Assessment and management of the airway is the first priority in the management of an injured casualty, except in the rare situation of life-threatening haemorrhage from a limb, when bleeding should be controlled first (☐ p. 188).

The main causes of airway obstruction are:

• Loss of muscle tone owing to reduced conscious level, which can lead to the tongue falling back and blocking the throat.
• Blood and/or vomit in the airway.
• Anatomical distortion or swelling caused by direct facial trauma or burns.
• Trismus (tightly clenched jaw) during seizures.
• Initially ask the patient a question or get them to stick their tongue out. If they can speak or protrude their tongue then the airway is patent and protected; and usually no further intervention is required. If you think there is a problem with breathing:
  • Look
  • Listen
  • Examine.

Inspection of the chest and neck may reveal that the patient is working hard to move air through a partially obstructed airway. If the airway is seriously blocked, the casualty, particularly their lips, may appear blue from cyanosis.

When *listening* to the airway one may hear gurgling or stridor. If the airway is obstructed and the patient is unconscious the first thing to do is attempt to clear the obstruction with a jaw thrust. With both thumbs on the patient's cheek bones insert the index fingers of both hands behind the angle of the jaw. Firmly lifting the jaw upwards will move the tongue away from the back of the throat, opening the airway. Try to minimize neck movements during this manoeuvre.

Examine the airway. If there is fluid or vomit in the mouth or throat, this should be gently removed using a portable suction device. Alternatively, the patient should be log-rolled onto their side (see ☐ p. 138) whilst maintaining in-line cervical spine immobilization, to allow the fluid to drain with gravity. Inspect the mouth to see if there is foreign material in the throat.

Maintaining an open airway

Oropharyngeal airways (OPA)

Two types of basic airway adjuncts can be used to keep the airway open. The Guedel OPA is inserted into the mouth with the tip lying between the tongue and the back wall of the throat. An airway of this type is measured by placing it against the side of the patient's face before insertion. The length of the airway should be the same as the distance from the central incisor teeth (mouth in the midline at the front) to the corner of the jaw under the ear. Slide the curve of the airway over the tongue until the flange is against the lips. Do not trap flesh between teeth and airway. If the victim's mouth is dry it may be easier to insert the airway inverted, and then rotate gently as the tip reaches the back of the mouth. A size

2 (9 cm) is usually appropriate for adult females and a size 3 (10 cm) for males. A semi-conscious patient may not tolerate an OPA; do not persist in trying to insert the device as it may cause the patient to vomit. Consider removing the OPA and placing the patient in the recovery position, or use a nasopharyngeal airway instead.

Nasopharyngeal airways (NPA)

Such airways are ideal during seizures when the teeth are clenched, preventing the use of OPAs. A 6-mm internal diameter airway is appropriate for adults (use the diameter of the patient's little finger as a guide). The packet includes a safety pin which should be pushed through the NPA flange. Lubricate the tube well before insertion and apply gentle continuous pressure straight towards the back of the head, *not* upwards parallel to the ridge of the nose. Insertion can cause bleeding, but this will stop once the airway is in place. If one nostril seems very tight, try the other as nasal cavities are rarely symmetrical, or use a smaller size. Gentle rotation may help if the airway gets stuck at the back of the nose. Tape a safety pin to the skin to fix the NPA. Fears that the NPA will enter the cranial cavity via the cribriform plate are exaggerated and unfounded. The NPA is extremely useful in semi-conscious patients who will not tolerate an oral airway. Insertion of an OPA or NPA does not guarantee that the patient's airway will remain clear. Jaw thrust often has to be continued.

Endotracheal tubes and laryngeal mask airways

Airway manoeuvres and basic adjuncts help to maintain the airway in the majority of seriously injured patients, but do nothing to prevent aspiration of regurgitated stomach contents. *Definitive airway* maintenance and protection can only be achieved by the insertion of a cuffed endotracheal tube, or to a lesser extent by the insertion of a laryngeal mask airway. If an injured patient is so obtunded that an endotracheal tube or laryngeal mask airway can be inserted without the use of anaesthetic drugs, the patient's chance of survival is very low. Endotracheal tubes and laryngeal mask airway can be misplaced, lead to airway obstruction, spasm of the vocal cords, vomiting, bradycardia, and raised intracranial pressure.

Only personnel who both understand and can correct these problems should use these airway adjuncts.

Surgical airways

Surgical cricothyroidotomies, or tracheostomies, are indicated in patients whose upper airway obstruction cannot be relieved by other means, for instance victims of burns or serious facial injuries. Cricothyroidotomy should only be performed by appropriately trained personnel but its need can be anticipated in circumstances where the clinical situation typically deteriorates steadily, such as serious airway burns. An expedition medical kit is unlikely to include a cricothyrotomy kit; in dire circumstances the barrel of a ball-point pen or the sharp end of an intravenous fluid giving set could be used.

Platts-Mills, Timothy F, Lewin, Matthew R, Wells, Jesse Bickler, Philip. 2006: Improvised Cricothyrotomy Provides Reliable Airway Access in an Unembalmed Human Cadaver Model, Wilderness and Environmental Medicine Vol. 17, No.2, pp. 81–86.

Breathing

Chest injuries are common in serious trauma. Some are rapidly life-threatening but amenable to treatment if detected and acted upon in the early stages of resuscitation.

During assessment look for the following:

- Respiratory rate: one of the most important clinical indicators of significant chest injury. Count over 30 s and record regularly.
- General condition: severe respiratory distress suggests a tension pneumothorax. Look for cyanosis.
- Inspection: look for bruising, swelling, abrasions, wounds, flail segments. Examine the back as well as the front.
- Palpate the chest: in a noisy pre-hospital environment, palpation is often more practical than auscultation. Feel the back as well as the front for crepitus and tenderness over fractured ribs. Feel for surgical emphysema which could indicate pneumothorax.
- Tracheal position: deviation is difficult to feel and is a late sign in tension pneumothorax. The diagnosis is usually evident from other more reliable clinical features.
- Auscultation: listen in the axillae, not the front of the chest to compare air entry effectively. There is decreased air entry with pneumothorax and haemothorax.
- Percussion: dull with haemothorax. Hyper-resonant with tension pneumothorax.
- Saturation: if a pulse oximeter is available—should be above 98%, but decreases with increasing altitude.
- High flow oxygen (via a non-rebreather mask) should be administered to all patients with serious chest injuries if it is available. If a small supply of oxygen is available then lower inspired concentrations for a longer time are probably better than a short burst at high flow rates. Start with a high flow rate and then decrease until the reservoir bag is almost completely deflated at the end of inspiration.

Pneumothorax

This refers to air in the pleural space between chest wall and lung. Air leaks into the pleural cavity either from a damaged lung or through a hole in the chest wall. It is caused by blunt or penetrating chest injury, or barotrauma resulting from rapid ascent when diving (see Chapter 21). There is decreased air entry on the affected side. Chest drainage will be required if breathing is compromised and a chest drain must be inserted before aeromedical evacuation (📖 p. 146).

Tension pneumothorax

This is as above, but with ongoing increase in volume and pressure of trapped air. Pressure causes the opposite lung to be compressed and pushes the heart across the chest, compromising its venous inflow from the vena cava.

Clinical features:

- Severe distress—'air hunger'
- Increased heart rate

- Reduction in blood pressure, the pulse strength may vary with each breath
- Hyper-resonance on the affected side
- Cyanosis may develop when the condition is severe.

Tension pneumothorax requires urgent needle decompression followed by formal chest drainage.

Needle decompression of tension pneumothorax

Use a large bore cannula attached to a syringe partially filled with fluid. Insert the cannula at right angles to the skin, through the second inter-costal space in the midclavicular line, just above the third rib, so as to avoid the vessels and nerve that run immediately below the second rib.

Aspiration of air indicates that the cannula tip has entered the pneumothorax.

If no air is aspirated:
- Either the diagnosis was wrong
- Or the cannula has been occluded by a 'fat plug' (blow a few millilitres of air through the cannula).
- Or the chest wall is deeper than the needle is long. If the diagnosis is still suspected then try again in the fifth intercostal space in the anterior–axillary line.

After aspiration of air remove the syringe and tape the cannula in position. If available, insert a formal chest drain attached to an underwater seal or a Heimlich valve (Fig. 6.2).

A tension pneumothorax can often re-develop, especially when the patient is moved, and may require further decompression—leave the original cannula *in situ*.

Chest drain insertion (Fig. 6.3)

This procedure should only be undertaken by those with prior training and experience.
- Equipment required: local anaesthetic (lidocaine 1%), syringes, needles, scalpel, antiseptic solution, sterile gloves, artery forceps for blunt dissection, adhesive tape, chest drain (size 28–32), Heimlich valve or underwater seal set with water, suture material.
- Place the patient at 30–60° with patient's arm above head.
- Identify the site for incision—the fourth or fifth intercostal space in the anterior axillary line. Avoid breast tissue.
- Clean the skin and infiltrate local anaesthetic down to the pleura.
- Using the scalpel make a 3-cm incision directly above the rib.
- Bluntly dissect down to the pleura with artery forceps and insert a gloved finger through the pleura.
- While keeping the finger in the hole, slide the chest tube beside the finger (trocar removed). This is easier if the end of the chest tube is attached to one jaw of an artery forceps.

- Push the tube into the chest and direct the tip towards the apex of the lung. Ensure all the drain holes are in the pleural cavity.
- Attach the Heimlich valve or underwater seal. Look for condensation in the tube or swinging of water in the underwater seal apparatus.
- Fix the tube firmly to the skin using sutures. Avoid a purse suture which may cause unsightly scarring.
- Apply gauze swabs to the skin at the base of the tube and tape in position.

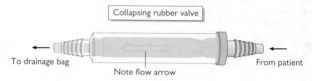

Collapsing rubber valve

To drainage bag

Note flow arrow

From patient

Fig. 6.2 Heimlich valve.

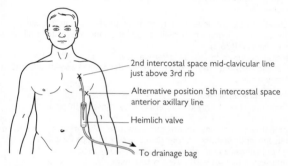

2nd intercostal space mid-clavicular line just above 3rd rib

Alternative position 5th intercostal space anterior axillary line

Heimlich valve

To drainage bag

Fig. 6.3 Chest drain with Heimlich valve.

Haemothorax

Following blunt or penetrating chest injury, blood leaks into the space between chest wall and lung, usually from damaged intercostal vessels. The bleeding often stops following formal chest drainage and re-inflation of the lung. The bleeding may be associated with a pneumothorax—the chest will be dull to percussion over the blood-filled area; bleeding can be massive and lead to hypotension.

Flail chest

If multiple adjacent ribs are fractured in two or more places there is a free-floating segment of chest wall that moves inwards with inspiration instead of outwards (paradoxical movement). This injury is typically caused by blunt chest trauma and is always associated with significant underlying pulmonary contusion.

Clinical features:
- Increased respiratory rate
- Visible flail segment (may not be obvious clinically)
- Palpable crepitus
- Painful breathing—use paracetamol and NSAIDs for background pain relief and titrate an opiate if available.

Splinting the flail segment with tape may improve both discomfort and breathing.

Urgent evacuation from the field will be required as bleeding and lung infection are common.

Sucking chest wound

This refers to an open wound through the chest wall as a result of penetrating chest injury. Air preferentially moves through the hole rather than the trachea with inspiration if the diameter of the hole is ≥2/3 of the diameter of the trachea (typically around 1 cm).

Clinical features:
- Sucking wound
- Decreased air entry on the affected side
- Severe respiratory distress.

Cover the wound with an occlusive dressing sealed on three sides to prevent tension pneumothorax developing.

Insert a chest drain then seal the wound completely.

All patients with suspected or actual chest injury will require evacuation. *All patients with a real risk of pneumothorax must have a chest drain inserted before air evacuation* (see above).

Circulation

Major haemorrhage in the seriously injured casualty can be from any of five places: 'blood on the floor and four more', i.e. external bleeding or bleeding into the chest, abdomen, pelvis, or thighs. Much can be done to arrest bleeding from wounds or closed long bone fractures but little can be done outside of the operating theatre to arrest haemorrhage in the other three sites. Rapid evacuation to a hospital with surgical facilities is therefore essential in these patient groups.

Assessment of circulatory status:

- Heart rate: may be raised with blood loss (≥120 bpm) but may be raised in the absence of blood loss due to pain or anxiety.
- Blood pressure: owing to compensatory mechanisms in young healthy adults, there may be significant blood loss before the blood pressure falls. Beware of a false sense of security with a normal blood pressure.
- Peripheral perfusion: very useful in a warm environment to indicate circulatory failure. Not as useful in cold environments as this may be a response to the environment rather than any blood loss.
- Peripheral pulses: absence of a palpable radial pulse indicates significant blood loss.
- Mental status: hypovolaemia leading to reduced cerebral perfusion leads to confusion and reduced conscious level.
- Bleeding source: look for wounds and haematomas. Examine chest, abdomen, and pelvis. Examine long bones, especially femurs. Don't forget the back and scalp.

All patients should receive oxygen if available. Minimize movement by planning the 'patient packaging' process in advance. Unnecessary movements may cause blood clots which have formed to dislodge, worsening haemorrhage. Most clotting factors are used in the formation of the initial clot. Give adequate pain relief and attempt to reassure the patient; this will reduce catecholamine release. Keep the patient warm. Hypothermia worsens clotting and increases haemorrhage.

Arrest external haemorrhage with direct pressure, dressings, and elevation (see box below). Wounds, especially scalp wounds, may require urgent suturing. In cases of life-threatening bleeding from limb injuries, initially apply very firm pressure over the wound but, if this fails to stem the flow, apply a proximal tourniquet such as the Combat Application Tourniquet (CAT®). A number of commercially available compounds are available which can be applied to wounds to promote clotting. They are currently in use with many military medical services and may be of use in certain remote expedition settings, e.g. QuickClot®.

Limb injuries should be splinted to promote clot formation and decrease pain. Femoral fractures can involve litres of blood loss. Traction splints act to reduce haemorrhage by reducing soft tissue damage and reducing the volume of the thigh compartment, hence increasing pressure and tamponading bleeding.

Open fractures should be reduced if possible. They should be covered with Inadine® dressings and broad spectrum antibiotics administered, e.g. co-amoxiclav or ceftriaxone.

Pelvic fractures can cause fatal haemorrhage. Examination and movement should be minimized to promote clot formation. A splint should be applied to stabilize the fracture. These can be commercially designed splints (e.g. SAM Sling®) or improvised with a sheet wrapped firmly around the pelvis. The aim is to return the pelvis to its normal anatomical position, not to tighten the splint as much as possible. The knees should be slightly flexed and tied together (with padding between). If a pelvic fracture is suspected it should be treated as such, splinted, and not re-examined until the patient reaches hospital.

Over the past decade there has been a shift away from routinely administering large amounts of intravenous fluids to injured patients. A normal physiological response to bleeding is for the blood pressure to fall, reducing flow through damaged vessels and tissues and so allowing clots to form. The remaining blood circulating has a high concentration of haemoglobin and may be sufficient in volume to allow perfusion of the vital organs if peripheral vasoconstriction has occurred. Administering intravenous fluids does not increase the oxygen-carrying capacity of the blood but does increase the blood pressure. This may dislodge clots which have formed, causing further loss of haemoglobin. Intravenous fluids, especially colloids, also adversely affect coagulation, again increasing bleeding.

UK accepted pre-hospital trauma management practice is not to administer fluids if the patient has a palpable radial pulse. If the radial pulse is not palpable, normal saline is titrated in 250 ml boluses until the radial pulse returns (NICE guidelines 2004). The evidence supporting this 'permissive hypotension' is mostly based in urban environments with short times from injury to definitive surgical care to arrest bleeding. Its use in remote environments is not proven but is likely to be appropriate when blood transfusion is not available and fluid supplies are limited.

Pre-hospital initiation of fluid replacement therapy in trauma. NICE Technology appraisal guidance 74. January 2004. http://www.nice.org.uk/TA074guidance

Control of haemorrhage

1. Direct pressure to the bleeding point

This should be tried first for all external bleeding and is effective in most cases. It may be ineffective if the bleeding vessel is not 'within reach' of pressure (e.g. deep in a wound). In this case, consider 'packing' the wound firmly from the base upwards using gauze/sterile bandage material.

2. Elevation of the affected limb/site of bleeding may also slow flow

Elevation helps less if bleeding is arterial rather than venous and is less effective when big vessels are damaged. Avoid raising legs if there are suspected pelvic, lumbar spine or leg fractures/injuries.

3. Pressure upon a direct arterial pressure point upstream of the site of bleeding

For bleeding from leg wounds, use the femoral pulse (middle of the groin); for arm wounds, grip the brachial artery firmly over the middle of the medial surface of the upper arm.

4. Using a tourniquet

A tourniquet is indicated when direct pressure to a bleeding point may be ineffective for any reason (above). It can be used to 'free hands' from having to apply such sustained direct pressure. It is generally used when major arteries have been severed and have retracted beyond reach or where the area of tissue disruption in a limb is extensive (e.g. avulsions or ballistic injury).

Always apply above the knee (for lower limb injuries).

You can increase efficacy by helping apply directed pressure (i.e. a packed pad over the artery).

Always pad a little beneath the tourniquet to prevent skin damage.

Use a commercial tourniquet or improvise:

- A strip of cloth 5–10 cm wide
- Tie around limb loosely, and tie a half-knot
- Slip to 5–10 cm above the wound (and above the joint if the injury is distal)
- Put a stick over the half-knot, and complete the tie
- Rotate the stick as a 'windlass' until the bleeding stops
- Leave on for at least 30 min. Use this time to try to identify the bleeding point and directly pack/compress. Do not 'dig and dab'; clot must be left to stabilize.
- Slowly release the tourniquet and observe. If bleeding continues, reapply the tourniquet.

Cervical spine immobilization (see Chapter 9)

- In a patient, conscious or unconscious, who has experienced sudden deceleration or a blow to the head, there is a risk that the spine could be damaged and that movement could produce spinal cord injury and paralysis. In these circumstances the cervical spine needs to be immobilized, and care of the cervical spine should run in parallel to airway management, although it should not delay extrication from a life-threatening situation.
- One member of the expedition should have the job of holding the patient's head to immobilize the cervical spine—the medic should not undertake this role as it prevents him or her from doing anything else.
- Only once the primary survey is complete and the patient is ready to be prepared for transport should a cervical collar be applied. Complete spinal immobilization is possible only if a properly fitted cervical collar is used, together with sandbags on each side of the head, and tapes to fix position relative to the two sides of the stretcher.
- Cervical collars come in a variety of sizes. In the pre-hospital environment clothing can impair collar application. Clothing should ideally be cut or removed to facilitate optimal operation of the collar. In the expedition setting it is appropriate to carry one adult multi-size collar such as the Stifnek select™. This reduces weight and cost.
- If a vacuum mattress is being used it may be acceptable to dispense with a cervical collar as an appropriately fitted vacuum mattress with forehead tape can provide adequate immobilization. This also prevents the discomfort of wearing the collar and the potential for raised intracranial pressure owing to neck vein compression by the collar.

Disability

- Assess the casualty's level of consciousness (disability) using the AVPU scale
  - **A**wake and alert
  - **V**erbal—responds to voice ('Squeeze my hand')
  - **P**ain—responds to pain
  - **U**nresponsive—no response to painful stimulus.

To monitor a patient's progress chart the GCS (see box). Minimum GCS score = 3, with maximum score of 15. Three areas of basic brain function are tested and scored: eye opening, speech, and movement. Use an increasing level of stimulus to obtain a response:

- Speak
- Tap the shoulders gently
- Apply pain—press firmly over the inner aspect of the eyebrow along the eye socket (supraorbital nerve).

A fall in the GCS score indicates deterioration in the patient's condition. Causes include:

- Bleeding
- Swelling
- Infection.

Remember, if the patient deteriorates during your assessment *immediately* re-check the ABC and rectify any life-threatening problems.

Glasgow Coma Scale	
Eye opening	**Score**
Open spontaneously	4
Open to verbal command	3
Open to pain	2
No response	1
Verbal response	
Talking and orientated	5
Confused, not orientated	4
Inappropriate words	3
Incomprehensible sounds	2
No response	1
Motor response	
Obeys commands	6
Localizes pain	5
Flexion/withdrawal	4
Abnormal flexion	3
Extension	2
No response	1

Exposure and environmental control

It is important both to examine the patient thoroughly and protect them from exposure to the elements.

A seriously injured patient, especially one with a reduced conscious level, may have life-changing injuries which are not obvious during the initial stages of resuscitation. This is because pain from them may be masked by more serious injuries, or the clinician involved is concentrating on immediately life-threatening problems. Such injuries might include peripheral joint dislocations or eye injuries which may lead to lifelong disability if not detected and corrected in the early stages. A systematic head-to-toe examination is necessary to seek and identify these injuries.

At this stage it may be appropriate to insert a urinary catheter if the patient is to be transferred by stretcher. Remember to exclude possible injury to the urethra by seeking signs: scrotal bruising, blood from the tip of the penis, and a high riding prostate on rectal examination.

Following the head-to-toe examination or 'secondary survey' the patient should be adequately insulated and protected from the external environment.

Continuing care

Subsequent care will depend upon:
- Magnitude of the injuries
- Condition of the patient
- Urgency of evacuation
- Ease of evacuation.

Isolation or adverse weather conditions will mean that the expedition may have to care for a casualty for several days. During this time consider:
- Regular observations to give warning if patient's condition deteriorates and they develop shock (📖 p. 214)
- Pain relief
- Personal needs and hygiene
- Good nursing to avoid pressure areas
- Psychological support for the casualty (📖 p. 504).

Emergencies—serious illness and collapse

Section editors
Jon Dallimore and Chris Johnson

Contributors
Sundeep Dhillon, Mike Grocott, Stephen Hearns, Hugh Montgomery, Julian Thompson, and David Warrell

The collapsed patient

Management of injured patients follows a well established sequence (see Chapter 6). However, when an individual suddenly becomes unwell ('collapses'), their life must be supported, a diagnosis made, the appropriate treatment instituted, and the patient stabilized before evacuation can be considered.

Collapse in young adults is very rare, but is generally very serious; infectious disease or environmentally induced conditions are the most likely cause. In older travellers the likelihood of cardiovascular disease increases.

Medical emergencies

Before attempting to examine any seriously ill person look for life-threatening hazards so as to avoid further injury to the patient and any injury to the rescuers. If necessary, rapidly and carefully move the casualty to a place of safety.

Rapid primary assessment and resuscitation

This is the simultaneous assessment, identification, and management of immediate life-threatening problems. Rapid primary assessment should follow the ABC model.
• A Assessment whilst approaching the casualty
• A Airway (with neck control if there is a history of injury)
• B Breathing
• C Circulation (control bleeding and manage shock)
• D Disability of the nervous system
• E Exposure and environmental control.

Primary assessment should be repeated following any change in the patient's condition.

Assessment and approach

When it is safe to approach, check the casualty's level of responsiveness. Tap or gently shake the shoulders and say 'Are you OK?' If there is no response call for help and proceed to check the airway.

Airway

Assess without moving the neck if possible—particularly if the patient has fainted or fallen and might have injured the head or neck.
    Open the airway using chin lift or jaw thrust (📖 p. 180).
    Look for, and remove any obvious obstruction, consider the use of airway adjuncts such as nasopharyngeal or oropharyngeal airways (📖 p. 180). Remember that oropharyngeal airways can provoke vomiting.

Breathing

• Once the airway has been checked and opened, assess breathing
• Look, listen, and feel for breathing (10 s)
• Give oxygen if available, particularly to those who are shocked, bleeding, or who have breathing difficulties
• If respiration is absent, impaired or inadequate, commence CPR (📖 p. 202)
• Is the breathing rate normal?
• Can the patient count to ten in one breath?
• If you suspect a chest problem, examine the chest for chest movements and breath sounds; normal, crackles, wheeze, or absent?

Circulation care with haemorrhage control

The aim is to detect and treat shock. Look for and control any external bleeding (consider direct pressure ± elevation). Consider the possibility of internal bleeding.

- Look at the patient's skin colour and assess the skin temperature
- Measure pulse rate and assess pulse character (normal, thready or bounding)
- Estimate the blood pressure:
  - Carotid pulse (neck)   Systolic blood pressure >60 mmHg
  - Femoral pulse (groin)   Systolic blood pressure >70 mmHg
  - Radial pulse (wrist)   Systolic blood pressure >80 mmHg
- Capillary refill should be less than 2 s in a warm casualty (📖 p. 163)
- Treat shock. If low cardiac output shock:
  - Lie the patient flat, elevate legs on pillow or rucksack
  - Keep warm and reassure
  - Consider iv fluids.

For management of other causes of shock see 📖 p. 214.

Disability

- Briefly assess the patient's neurological status using the AVPU scale:
  - **A** Alert
  - **V** Responds to verbal command
  - **P** Responds to pain
  - **U** Unresponsive
- Pupils—assess size and reaction to light
- Look for neck stiffness
- Check for blood glucose if possible
- If the patient is fitting, place them in the recovery position.

Exposure and environmental control

Where possible, examine the patient in a warm, light environment such as a tent or group shelter. Be *gentle*; unnecessary roughness may aggravate the problem. Undress the patient but be aware of hypothermia which can worsen shock. Measure body temperature and look for a rash.

Rapid history

The patient or bystanders may be able to give brief details to aid diagnosis:
- Events leading up to the illness, any history of injury
- Past history, particularly known cardiac or respiratory illness, diabetes, epilepsy, alcohol/drug abuse, head injury
- Medication taken on a regular or occasional basis
- Allergies.

Secondary assessment

Secondary survey is a methodical search for all signs of disease which may be present. On an expedition this should be delayed until the casualty is in a warm, dry environment such as in a tent or building or under a group shelter, lying on a mattress, airbed or sleeping bag.

History-taking and examination are covered in Chapter 5.

Basic life support (CPR)

'For any seriously ill or collapsed patient it is important to assess for level of response rapidly and to start cardiopulmonary resuscitation (CPR) if breathing is abnormal or there is no palpable pulse.' (From the Resuscitation Guidelines December 2005).

Initial management of adult patients (Fig. 7.1)

- Check for a response:
  - Gently shake the shoulders. Ask loudly 'Are you alright?'
- If patient responds:
  - If the individual is able to speak the airway is open and maintained
  - Leave him in the position you find him, provided there is no further danger
  - Stabilize the head and neck if there is a possibility of injury (📖 p. 290)
  - Find out what is wrong and get help (ideally via radio, telephone or written message), if available
  - Reassess regularly

Adult basic life support

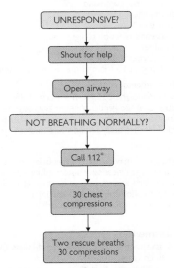

*Or national emergency number

Fig. 7.1 Basic life support algorithm.

http://www.resus.org.uk/guide.htm

- If patient is unresponsive:
  - Shout/call for help
  - Turn the casualty on his back, whilst maintaining neck control
  - Institute life support measures.

Assess, open, and manage the airway as described on 🕮 p. 180.
  If the casualty is not breathing normally start cardiopulmonary resuscitation (CPR; Fig. 7.2):
- Start with 30 chest compressions at a rate of 100/min (a little less than two compressions/second):
  - Kneel beside victim
  - Place heel of one hand in centre of victim's chest
  - Place heel of other hand on top of the first hand
  - Interlock fingers of your hands and ensure pressure is not applied over the victim's ribs, upper abdomen or bottom end of the bony sternum
  - Position yourself vertically above the victim's chest and, with straight arms, press down on sternum 4–5 cm
  - Release pressure without losing contact between your hands and the sternum. Compression and release should take equal time.
- After 30 compressions give two rescue breaths:
  - Open airway with chin lift and head tilt
  - Pinch soft part of the victim's nose closed with the index finger and thumb of your hand on his forehead
  - Allow his mouth to open whilst maintaining chin lift
  - Take a normal breath and place lips around his mouth. Ensure a good seal
  - Blow steadily into his mouth for about 1 second and watch the chest rise
  - Maintaining head tilt and chin lift take your mouth away and watch for the chest to fall as air comes out
  - Take another normal breath and blow into the victim's mouth to give two effective rescue breaths. Immediately return your hands to his sternum and give a further 30 compressions
- If rescue breaths do not make the chest rise and fall, before next attempt:
  - Check victim's mouth and remove any visible obstruction
  - Recheck there is adequate head tilt and chin lift
  - Do not attempt more than two rescue breaths before returning to 30 chest compressions
- Chest compressions: rescue breath ratio 30:2.

Continue CPR until:
- Normal breathing resumes
- You become exhausted
- A more experienced doctor tells you to stop.

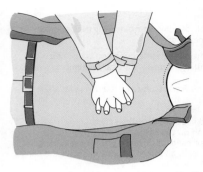

Fig. 7.2 Hand position for CPR.

Core rules of CPR

- Call for assistance
- Push hard (effective cardiac compressions)
- Push fast (maintain regular cardiac compressions)
- Breath slow (excessive ventilation unnecessary)
- Don't stop (gaps in compression reduce survival)
- Obey automated defibrillator (if available)

Resuscitation in the wilderness

Survival from cardiac arrest is most likely when the event is witnessed, when early cardiopulmonary resuscitation is started, and defibrillation and advanced life support are instituted at an early stage. In an expedition setting it is unlikely that advanced life support will be available. If attempts at resuscitation are not successful after 30 min the chances of success are very low.

The exception to this is when the victim is hypothermic; in this situation CPR should be continued until the victim is warm (📖 p. 597). For victims of avalanches, initiating CPR depends on whether the victim has been buried for more or less than 35 min.[1] There are other important exceptions: where a victim has been struck by lightning, or has been immersed in cold water, after certain snake bite envenomations, or in paralytic shellfish poisoning. In these cases successful resuscitation has occurred after several hours.

Remember the safety of other expedition members must remain the priority, and resuscitation efforts should be abandoned if their safety is jeopardized.

Do not initiate CPR
- If there is danger to the rescuers
- Obvious lethal injury, e.g. decapitation
- Rigor mortis.

Discontinue CPR
- If spontaneous pulse and breathing return
- Rescuers become exhausted
- Rescuers are placed in danger
- Patient does not respond to 30 min of resuscitative efforts *except* in cases of lightning strike, cold water immersion, paralytic shellfish poisoning, or snake envenomation

Dangers of resuscitation

There is understandable concern about the possibility of transmission of bloodborne diseases during resuscitation—particularly HIV and hepatitis. Although viruses can be isolated from the saliva of infected persons, transmission is rare and there are few cases of CPR-related infection in the literature. Three cases of HIV have been reported and were acquired during resuscitation of infected patients; on two occasions from a needle stick injury and in the third after heavy contamination of broken skin. To minimize the risk of acquiring infection, rescuers should wear gloves and use barriers whenever possible, and great care must be taken with sharps.

---

1 Brugger H, Durrer B (2002). On-site treatment of avalanche victims. ICAR-MEDCOM recommendations. *High Alt Med Biol* 3: 421–5.

Choking

Recognition

Foreign bodies may cause either mild or severe airway obstruction. The signs and symptoms enabling differentiation between mild and severe airway obstruction are summarized below. It is important to ask the conscious victim 'Are you choking?'

General signs of choking
- Attack occurs while eating
- Victim may clutch his neck

Signs of mild airway obstruction
Response to question 'Are you choking?'
- Victim is able to speak, cough, and breathe.

Signs of severe airway obstruction
Response to question 'Are you choking?'
- Victim unable to speak
- Victim unable to breathe
- Breathing sounds wheezy
- Attempts at coughing are silent
- Victim may become unconscious.

Management

Mild airway obstruction
Encourage him to continue coughing, but do nothing else.

Severe airway obstruction
- Give up to five back blows
- Stand to the side and slightly behind the victim
- Support the chest with one hand and lean the victim forwards
- Give up to five sharp blows between the shoulder blades with the heel of your other hand.

If five back blows fail to relieve the airway obstruction, give up to five abdominal thrusts:
- Stand behind the victim and put both arms round the upper part of his abdomen
- Lean the victim forwards and clench your fist and place it between the umbilicus (navel) and the bottom end of the breastbone
- Grasp hand with your other hand and pull sharply inwards and upwards. Repeat up to five times
- If the obstruction is still not relieved, continue alternating five back blows with five abdominal thrusts.

If the victim becomes unconscious:
- Support the victim carefully to the ground
- Begin CPR (see above).

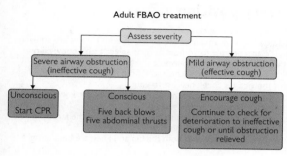

Fig. 7.3 Adult foreign body obstruction treatment algorithm.

Recovery position (Figs. 7.4 and 7.5)

- Remove the victim's spectacles, if worn
- Kneel beside the victim and make sure that both his legs are straight
- Place the arm nearest to you out at right angles to his body, elbow bent with the hand palm uppermost
- Bring the far arm across the chest, and hold the back of the hand against the victim's cheek nearest to you
- With your other hand, grasp the far leg just above the knee and pull it up, keeping the foot on the ground
- Keeping the hand pressed against the cheek, pull on the far leg to roll the victim towards you onto his side
- Adjust the upper leg so that both the hip and knee are bent at right angles
- Tilt the head back to make sure the airway remains open
- Adjust the hand under the cheek, if necessary, to keep the head tilted
- Check breathing regularly.

If the victim has to be kept in the recovery position for more than 30 min turn him to the opposite side to relieve the pressure on the lower arm.

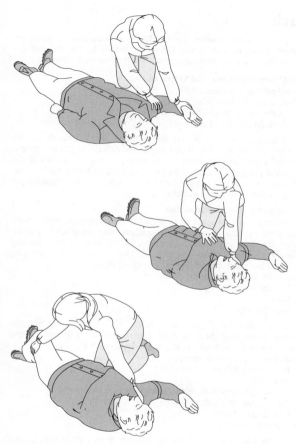

Fig. 7.4 Turning into the recovery position.

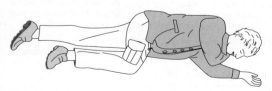

Fig. 7.5 The recovery position.

Shock

Shock is said to occur when the circulation is inadequate to meet the metabolic demands of the body. When key organs such as the kidneys, heart, and brain are relatively underperfused their function fails.

Clinical presentation and types of shock

All 'shocked' patients may exhibit:
- Cerebral effects—irritable, drowsy, yawning
- Gastrointestinal effects—nausea, vomiting
- Renal effects—reduced urine output, >0.5 ml/kg/h being 'normal'.

Other findings will depend on the type of shock. Shock is usually accompanied by hypotension (low blood pressure). Arterial blood pressure is governed by the combination of cardiac output driving the blood into the arteries and peripheral vascular resistance resisting its forward flow. Thus low blood pressure may result either from a reduction in cardiac output or from a fall in peripheral resistance.

Shock caused by low cardiac output

A fall in cardiac output leads to a reflex increase in sympathetic activity, and so to an increase in heart rate, respiratory rate, peripheral vasoconstriction, and sweating. Cold clammy skin, fast pulse, and rapid breathing will be common to all underlying causes. Underfilling of the main pumping chamber of the heart, the left ventricle, may result from:
- Loss of fluids from the body:
  - Diarrhoea
  - Vomiting
  - Haemorrhage

Skin turgor (elasticity of the tissues) is low, the mouth is dry, and the patient is thirsty. If whole body water is low, sweating is limited (i.e. the skin isn't 'clammy'). With blood loss alone, sweating is expected.
- Loss of fluids into tissue spaces:
  - Burns (including severe sunburn)
  - Anaphylaxis
  - Profound hypoproteinaemia (as may occur in dysentery)
  - Obstruction to cardiac filling
  - Pulmonary embolus
  - Cardiac tamponade.

When fluids have been lost from the body or moved into tissue spaces, neck veins will be empty: when there is obstruction to blood flow from pulmonary embolism or cardiac tamponade, the neck veins will be full and jugular venous pressure will rise with inspiration. Breathlessness may be most profound with pulmonary embolism (as hypoxia contributes).

Shock caused by low peripheral resistance

This occurs in anaphylaxis, or any major systemic inflammatory response, including:
- Severe infection (septic shock)
- Toxins (stings, venom) and/or anaphylaxis
- Severe sunburn.

Blood vessels vasodilate, peripheral resistance decreases, and therefore blood pressure falls. The inflammatory response directly affects the peripheral blood vessels and so the compensatory sympathetic response cannot cause the blood vessels to tighten up again; blood pressure remains low. The skin may be warm, hot, or 'patchy'. In sepsis, such 'patchiness' may alter with time (legs freezing one minute, and warm the next). Neck veins will be collapsed, and the skin may sweat due to fever but will not be 'cold and shut down' (i.e. clammy). Pulse rate and cardiac output will be high.

Catches in the wilderness

The young and fit can maintain blood pressure for a very long time through sympathetic activity. Indeed, blood pressure may not fall until around 50% of the circulating volume has been lost.

Underlying dehydration may be common.

Urine output may already be low.

Sweating responses may be reduced—sweating thresholds are altered by acclimatization to ambient temperature and to exercise loads (📖 p. 688).

In the heat, most people are vasodilated. In 'heat stroke' (📖 p. 684), severe inflammation coupled with volume loss may lead to a 'shivering clammy' patient, despite a very high central temperature.

In the cold, most are vasoconstricted.

Management of the shocked patient

- Identify the type of shock.
- As for all major emergencies—make sure that the environment is safe, summon help, and attend to Airway, Breathing and then Circulation (see Chapter 6).
- Control the source of any massive haemorrhage first. Apply direct pressure to the bleeding point and/or directed focal pressure to the arterial supply. Tie off or clamp large bleeders. Use a tourniquet where necessary (📖 p. 188). Pack deep large wounds and bind firmly.
- Treat anaphylaxis at once (📖 p. 220). Look/listen for signs of airway obstruction such as wheeze, stridor, facial and neck swelling, or/and urticarial (nettles-type) rash.
- If the patient is more than mildly unwell, establish venous access at once. You may find it a lot harder later!
- Stop the losses and treat the causes:
  - Stop all sources of loss (e.g. use antidiarrhoeals, antiemetics, cooling with sponging and fanning, keeping in the shade, light-reflective clothing if sun unavoidable).
  - If septic, seek the source (including the rare, but missed, retained tampon) and treat at once with broad spectrum antibiotics.
  - Give fluids. Most wilderness victims will be depleted of intravascular volume, as will most with shock of any cause (see above). Most will thus require intravenous fluids. The rate and route will be determined by a number of factors: if you have an uncontrolled source of blood loss, internal or external, give fluids cautiously until the source of bleeding is controlled. Raising pressure by rapid resuscitation will make bleeding worse. If fluid supplies are limited, use 'permissive hypotension' (maintain a just palpable radial pulse).
  - If the patient is conscious and able to swallow (without GI tract injury), let the patient drink as a means of conserving iv fluids.
  - No data, beyond anecdote, support the rectal administration of fluids in this context. However, this may be considered in the absence of other means of resuscitation.[2]
  - Consider intraosseous administration if oral or venous routes are unavailable, and you have the kit (and are trained to use it!).
  - During fluid resuscitation, give fluids by 'bolus' of 250 ml, and observe response, especially heart rate. For maintenance, calculate losses (blood loss, diarrhoea, vomiting, from skin in burns), including insensible losses (sweating and breathing, 10–20 ml/kg/day). Once resuscitated with boluses, spread this 'maintenance' over 24 h.
- Treatment endpoints:
  - Control of fluid losses.
  - 'Organ survival and function': urine output >0.5 ml/kg/h; patient is alert and orientated.
  - Improvements in observations—heart rate within normal range and respiratory rate falling, blood pressure rising.

2 Grocott MPW, McCorkell S, Cox ML (2005). Resuscitation from hemorrhagic shock using rectally administered fluids in a wilderness environment. *Wilderness and Environmental Medicine* **16**(4): 209–11.

Additional specific treatments depending upon the type of shock are described below.

Remember to put this treatment in the context of what is available to you. If you have only 2 l of iv fluids, then you must use them with care to resuscitate fast (e.g. if massive bleed now stopped) or gently (e.g. minor hypotension with continuing losses).

Remember, too, to call for help/evacuate fast. Prompt and sustained resuscitation is vital to survival.

Monitoring shock in the wilderness

Blood pressure may be well maintained at first. Look for trends over time and any postural drop (measured while lying then sitting or standing). If in doubt, use sitting blood pressure as standing can provoke loss of consciousness.

- Signs of compensation. Are heart rate and respiratory rate rising?
- Signs of low perfusion. What is happening to:
  - Skin perfusion (skin colour/temperature?)
  - Brain (alert/orientated?)
  - Gut (nausea/anorexia?)
  - Renal function (urine output?)
  - Breathlessness (reflecting sympathetic activity, and clearance of lactic acidosis through respiratory compensation)?
  - Consider a urinary catheter (if you have one) and measure hourly urine output
  - Record the above on a chart to give a visual display of changes (Fig. 7.6).

Prevention and preparation

- You cannot prevent a fellow traveller becoming seriously ill. However, you can take appropriate equipment
- Decide on the volume of fluids you will carry, depending on logistic constraints (weight, bulk), duration of trip, evacuation times
- Take antibiotics for infections and epinephrine, steroids, and antihistamines for anaphylaxis
- Find out how safe or dangerous local blood sources may be
- Avoid gastrointestinal tract infection if possible (📖 p. 380), and all the other recognized environmental causes
- Know the arterial pressure points
- Make sure your cannulation skills are not rusty

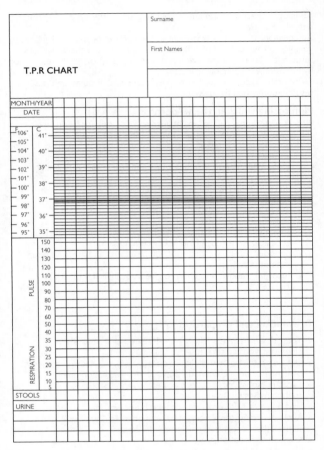

Fig. 7.6 Observations chart.

Types of shock

Hypovolaemic shock

Causes

- Blood loss:
  - External and visible (e.g. external wound)
  - Internal and invisible (e.g. into gut, into muscle around a fractured bone, into chest or abdominal cavity, into tissues behind abdominal contents)
  - Low fluid intake (usually when combined with high losses)
- Loss of fluid from the body:
  - Gut (diarrhoea, vomiting)
  - Skin (extensive grazes, burns)
  - Sweat (fever, environmental heat)
  - Breathing (dry air, high respiratory rates)
- Loss of fluid into tissues:
  - Anaphylaxis
  - Crush injury
  - Severe systemic inflammation and sepsis.

Signs

- Those of 'low cardiac output shock' (☐ p. 212).

Specific treatment

- Stop losses, fluid challenges of 250 ml iv, calculate daily maintenance and administer over 24 h.

NB. *Crush injury* leads to loss of volume into the tissues, and low output shock. Tissue damage may worsen the inflammatory state. Muscle damage worsens kidney function. Maintain a high urine output if possible. Do not use diuretics (as this will worsen volume depletion). Check for compartment syndrome (as this may be causing low perfusion every bit as much as a fall in systemic perfusion pressure). Fasciotomies may be needed but beware: fluid losses will be massive. Have you enough intravenous fluids to keep up?

Septic shock

Causes

- Infection in the bloodstream. Sometimes this may be from a wound that is hard to see. In women, ask about possible retained and infected tampons. Urine infection may be a source.

Signs

- Those of 'low peripheral resistance shock' (☐ p. 212): tachycardia, high volume pulse, warm skin (or patchy skin temperature distribution which changes), low blood pressure, ± sweating/sweats. Rigors (severe 'bone-shaking' shivers) may occur.

Specific treatment

- Intravenous fluid challenges of 250 ml iv to resuscitate; calculate daily maintenance and administer over 24 h
- Administer iv broad spectrum antibiotics (e.g. ceftriaxone 1–2 g iv twice daily)
- Evacuate as soon as possible.

Cardiogenic shock

Causes

- Acute impairment of heart contractile function. In expedition staff, most commonly an acute myocardial infarction.

Signs

- Generally preceded by history of classic cardiac pain (tight across chest, to shoulders, jaw, or down arm(s) (📖 p. 352)
- Signs are those of 'low cardiac output shock': tachycardia, low volume pulse, cold clammy skin, low blood pressure. Breathlessness. Inspiratory crackles at bases, spreading throughout lungs. (NB. At altitude consider high altitude pulmonary oedema, 📖 p. 622.) Neck veins may be elevated if right side of heart involved (NB. Consider pulmonary embolus; see below.)

Specific treatment

- This is life-threatening. Arrange evacuation at once. Give oxygen if available
- Sitting upright may help relieve breathlessness
- Fluids only if jugular venous pressure not elevated and chest clear (suggesting isolated right heart infarct). Unguided iv fluids may make matters worse
- If stabilizes over time, may need cautious fluids (100 ml challenges maximum)
- Powerful analgesics to relieve chest pain
- Aspirin 300 mg may reduce progression of infarct
- A diuretic drug, if available, may relieve breathlessness if the jugular venous pressure is raised.

Pulmonary embolus

Blood clot impacts in pulmonary arterial circulation. Most commonly originates in leg veins, often after prolonged flight/coach journey/immobility. The risk rises when blood viscosity is high (dehydration, altitude).

Signs

- Those of 'low cardiac output shock': tachycardia, low volume pulse, cold clammy skin, low blood pressure. Neck veins may be distended. Look for unilateral (occasionally bilateral) lower limb swelling—may be confined to calf.

Specific treatment
- Intravenous fluid challenges of 250 ml iv to resuscitate
- Unfractionated heparin at treatment dose (e.g. dalteparin subcutaneous once daily by weight):
  - <46 kg, 7500 units daily
  - 46–56 kg, 10 000 units daily
  - 57–68 kg, 12 500 units daily
  - 69–82 kg, 15 000 units daily
  - >82 kg, 18 000 units daily.

Neurogenic shock

Neurogenic shock is a very rare situation, in which severe damage to the spinal cord disrupts the transmission of 'tightening up' nerve impulses to the small arteries. The blood vessels therefore dilate, and 'low resistance shock' results.

Causes
- Spinal cord injury (usually trauma, although inflammatory/infective causes are possible).

Signs
- Those of 'low peripheral resistance shock': tachycardia, high volume pulse, warm skin, low blood pressure. Casualty may develop priapism—an involuntary erection of the penis in males. Other signs of spinal cord injury (sensory loss, weakness or paralysis).

Specific treatment
- Intravenous fluids (as the gut usually 'goes on strike' with high spinal cord injury) using 250 ml fluid challenges. Calculate daily maintenance and administer over 24 h. Evacuate as soon as possible. May need a nasogastric tube. Remember pressure area care and immobilization of the entire spine.

Anaphylaxis and anaphylactic shock

Anaphylaxis is a rapidly evolving and often dramatic clinical syndrome, usually precipitated by recent exposure to a substance (allergen) to which the patient is allergic, e.g.
- Drugs: any, especially penicillins
- Foods: any, especially nuts, fruits, sea food
- Environmental factors: animal venoms (e.g. wasp, hornet, bee, ant, or snake), plant substances (latex).

Examination

Anaphylaxis is characterized by one or more of the following features in any combination:
- Rash and/or mucous membrane involvement: urticaria ('hives', 'weals', 'welts'), flushing, itching, generalized erythema and swelling owing to massive extravasation of fluid ('Michelin man') and swelling of the lips, tongue, gums, and uvula

- Life-threatening circulatory collapse ('anaphylactic shock') caused by vasodilatation and/or hypovolaemia: premonitory symptoms include dizziness, loss of vision, tachycardia, falling blood pressure, and loss of consciousness
- Life-threatening airway obstruction: lower airways—bronchoconstriction/asthma or, less often, upper airway—angioedema of the larynx. The signs include wheeze, tachypnoea, stridor ('croup'), and cyanosis
- Gastrointestinal symptoms (vomiting, diarrhoea, retrosternal pain, abdominal colic).

Patients look and feel severely unwell, are usually anxious, and may have a feeling of impending doom. In extreme cases, they may collapse and lose consciousness within minutes of allergen exposure. Some present with shock and hypotension alone.

Worrying features
- Upper airway obstruction
- Wheeze
- Systolic BP <90 mmHg.

Differential diagnosis
- Asthma
- Heart attack or pulmonary embolism (chest pain, shock, respiratory distress)
- Faint, panic attack, breath-holding in children
- Vasovagal attack precipitated by injections, stings or sharp trauma (but this will be associated with bradycardia).

Prevention and risk management
- Those with known allergy should carry an epinephrine (adrenaline) auto-injector such as EpiPen® or Anapen®
- Companions should know the location of the EpiPen® and how to use it (Fig. 16.8, 📖 p. 537)
- Ensure cooks are aware of food allergies.

Further treatment (Fig. 7.7)
- Maintain blood pressure >90 mmHg systolic. Give iv fluids as required
- *If bronchospasm is severe/persistent* despite adrenaline, give bronchodilator by inhalation (salbutamol, ipratropium) or iv (aminophylline)
- *If cardiac arrest occurs:* follow guidelines for cardiopulmonary resuscitation. Early advanced life support essential. Intramuscular adrenaline is unlikely to be beneficial in this setting so try an iv route or intraoral/intra-airway
- *If the diagnosis is uncertain:* keep a sample of clotted blood for mast cell tryptase
- Monitor urine output
- Continue chlorphenamine 4 mg/8 h PO
- Consider a short course of steroids—prednisolone 40 mg/24 h for 5 days to prevent recurrent anaphylaxis.

The patient may require evacuation for further investigation.

Useful websites

Resuscitation Council UK—http://www.resus.org.uk
European Resuscitation Council—http://www.erc.edu
Association of Anaesthetists of Great Britain and Ireland—http://www.aagbi.org
European Academy of Allergology and Clinical Immunology—http://www.eaaci.net
British Society for Allergy and Clinical Immunology—http://www.basci.org

Heat injury

Remember, severe hyperthermia may present with a shivering 'shut-down' patient. They need active cooling and sometimes a lot of fluid (see Chapter 23).

Environmental fluid loss: dehydration is common in all wilderness environments, owing to the effects of the heat, exercise, and sweating, high breathing rates (particularly in cold, dry air). Fluid intake is further reduced if the water supply is not potable and has to be treated with chlorine or iodine, which reduces the palatability.

Summary

Unless appropriately treated, shock of any cause is a very dangerous condition indeed. Identification of the cause and rapid appropriate treatment are crucial. In every case, rapid evacuation is indicated. This should be considered even if anaphylaxis rapidly resolves: it is hard to know that the environmental challenge (whatever it was) won't occur again (even if a bee sting); avoidance is the best option.

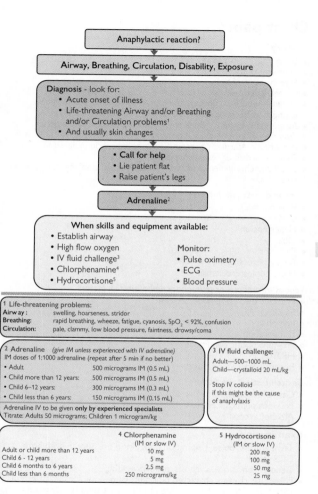

Anaphylactic reaction?

Airway, Breathing, Circulation, Disability, Exposure

Diagnosis - look for:
- Acute onset of illness
- Life-threatening Airway and/or Breathing and/or Circulation problems[1]
- And usually skin changes

- **Call for help**
- Lie patient flat
- Raise patient's legs

Adrenaline[2]

When skills and equipment available:
- Establish airway
- High flow oxygen
- IV fluid challenge[3]
- Chlorphenamine[4]
- Hydrocortisone[5]

Monitor:
- Pulse oximetry
- ECG
- Blood pressure

1 Life-threatening problems:
Airway: swelling, hoarseness, stridor
Breathing: rapid breathing, wheeze, fatigue, cyanosis, SpO_2 < 92%, confusion
Circulation: pale, clammy, low blood pressure, faintness, drowsy/coma

2 Adrenaline *(give IM unless experienced with IV adrenaline)*
IM doses of 1:1000 adrenaline (repeat after 5 min if no better)
- Adult   500 micrograms IM (0.5 mL)
- Child more than 12 years: 500 micrograms IM (0.5 mL)
- Child 6–12 years: 300 micrograms IM (0.3 mL)
- Child less than 6 years: 150 micrograms IM (0.15 mL)
Adrenaline IV to be given **only by experienced specialists**
Titrate: Adults 50 micrograms; Children 1 microgram/kg

3 IV fluid challenge:
Adult—500–1000 mL
Child—crystalloid 20 mL/kg

Stop IV colloid
if this might be the cause
of anaphylaxis

	4 Chlorphenamine (IM or slow IV)	5 Hydrocortisone (IM or slow IV)
Adult or child more than 12 years	10 mg	200 mg
Child 6 - 12 years	5 mg	100 mg
Child 6 months to 6 years	2.5 mg	50 mg
Child less than 6 months	250 micrograms/kg	25 mg

Fig. 7.7 Anaphylaxis algorithm.

Chest pain

History

- *Site* of main pain and any radiation to arms, neck, jaw, or back
- *Character* of pain—heavy, sharp, tight, pleuritic
- *Severity*—out of ten
- *Onset*—at rest or during exertion
- *Nature*—whether constant and aggravated by exertion, position, eating, breathing, or relieved by analgesics, antacids or GTN
- *Associated symptoms*—sweating, dyspnoea, nausea, palpitations
- *Trauma*—nature of injury if present
- *Past history*—cardiac or respiratory problems, acid indigestion
- *Drugs*—cardiac or respiratory drugs, antacids
- *Social and environmental factors*—alcohol/drugs, smoking status, recent stressors.

Cardiac disease risk factors

- Previous IHD
- Smoking
- Hypertension
- Obesity
- Diabetes
- Family history of IHD
- Hypercholesterolaemia.

Venous thrombosis or pulmonary embolism risk factors

- Previous thromboembolic disease
- Smoking
- Immobility
- Dehydration
- Pro-thrombotic conditions
- HRT/OCP
- Recent surgery/long travel.

Gastrointestinal risk factors

- Gastro-oesophageal reflux disease (GORD)
- Previous peptic ulceration
- Alcohol excess.

Examination

- Temperature, pulse, respiration rate, blood pressure in both arms, GCS score
- General condition—cyanosis, pallor, sweating
- Pulse rate, rhythm, character, blood pressure, look for elevation and dilatation of the neck veins, listen to the heart sounds (any murmurs?), look for signs of cardiac failure (basal crackles in the lungs and swelling of the ankles), look for calf swelling/redness/tenderness
- Feel for position of windpipe, and assess for chest wall tenderness
- Feel the abdomen for localized tenderness or a pulsatile mass (abdominal aortic aneurysm)
- Check blood glucose.

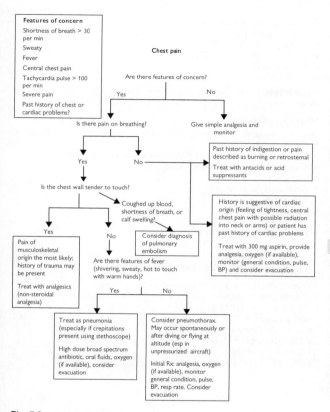

Fig. 7.8 Diagnosis of chest pain.

Differential diagnosis

Originating from the chest

- Myocardial infarction/angina (☐ p. 352)
- Tension pneumothorax (☐ p. 182)
- Pulmonary embolism
- Pneumonia (☐ p. 358)
- Pleurisy (☐ p. 358)
- High altitude pulmonary oedema (☐ p. 622)
- Chest wall pain
- Gastro-oesophageal reflux disease (☐ p. 370)
- Pericarditis
- Herpes zoster.

Originating from the abdomen
- Aortic aneurysm
- Cholecystitis (📖 p. 370)
- Peptic ulceration (📖 p. 370)
- Pancreatitis (📖 p. 371)
- Sickle cell crisis.

Make a 'best guess' diagnosis and treat accordingly. Observe the patient closely, record the details on a TPR chart, and monitor urine output.

Worrying features

Urgent evacuation for investigation and treatment is indicated if any of the following develop:
- Tachycardia—heart rate >100 persistently or irregular rhythm
- Bradycardia—heart rate persistently <50
- Hypotension
- Elevated respiration rate
- Reduced GCS
- Sweating
- Vomiting
- Pain radiating to jaw, arms, or back.

Urgent treatment (of chest pain)

Assess ABC. If the patient is unresponsive and there is no respiratory effort and/or no palpable pulse, commence CPR (📖 p. 202).

If the patient is conscious:
- Sit patient up
- Give high flow oxygen if available
- Consider aspirin, glyceryl trinitrate (GTN) and iv analgesia if cardiac cause seems likely (Fig. 7.8)
- Monitor pulse, blood pressure and respiratory rate (RR)

Shortness of breath

History

- *Dyspnoea*—speed of onset, cough, wheeze
- *Sputum* (colour, quantity, any blood)
- *Chest pain*—characterize any pain (see chest pain above, 📖 p. 224)
- *Associated symptoms*—sweating, nausea, palpitations
- *Trauma*—nature of injury if present
- *Past history*—cardiac or respiratory problems
- *Drugs*—inhalers, respiratory drugs, cardiac drugs
- Allergies
- *Social/environmental*—smoking status, travel history (📖 p. 242)
- *Risk factors for PE/DVT*—previous thromboembolic disease, smoking, obesity, immobility, dehydration, high altitude, pro-thrombotic conditions, HRT/OCP, recent surgery/long travel.

Examination

- Temperature, pulse, respiratory rate, blood pressure, GCS score
- General condition—confusion, cyanosis, pallor, cool peripheries, sweating, tremor, use of accessory muscles. Count to 10 in one breath?
- Pulse rate, rhythm, blood pressure, look for elevation and dilatation of the neck veins. Measure peak expiratory flow rate if possible, look for tracheal tug/deviation, percuss the chest, listen for air entry and breath sounds—normal, crackles, wheezes or nothing. Look for calf swelling/redness/tenderness or ankle swelling (DVT)
- Feel the abdomen for localized tenderness or a pulsatile mass (abdominal aortic aneurysm).

Differential diagnosis

Wheeze present:
- Asthma or chronic obstructive pulmonary disease (📖 p. 362)
- Anaphylaxis (📖 p. 220).

No clinical signs:
- Pulmonary embolism
- Hyperventilation (📖 p. 299)
- Diabetic ketoacidosis (📖 p. 239).

Crackles audible:
- High altitude pulmonary oedema (📖 p. 622)
- Pneumonia (📖 p. 358)
- Heart failure.

Stridor present:
- Foreign body (📖 p. 208).

Absent breath sounds:
- Pneumothorax (📖 p. 356).

Make a 'best guess' diagnosis and treat accordingly. Observe the patient closely; record the details on a TPR chart.

Worrying features

Urgent evacuation for investigation and treatment are indicated if any of the following develop:
- Respiratory rate >30 breaths/min
- Tachycardia or bradycardia
- Core temperature >39°C
- Hypotension
- Reduced GCS (📖 p. 192)
- Exhaustion.

Urgent treatment of shortness of breath

Assess ABC. If the patient is unresponsive and there is no respiratory effort and/or no palpable pulse, commence CPR (📖 p. 202).
If the patient is conscious:
- Sit patient up
- Give high flow oxygen if available
- Monitor pulse, blood pressure, and respiratory rate

Coma

Unrousable unresponsiveness.

History (from bystanders)

- How/where found
- Sudden or gradual onset
- Seizure
- Any trauma
- Recent illness—headache, chest pain, palpitations, fever, confusion, depression, sinusitis, seizures, vomiting
- Past history—cardiac, respiratory, diabetes, hypertension, psychiatric illness
- Drugs—overdose?
- Social/environmental—alcohol, illicit drugs, travel to malarial area.

Examination

- GCS score
- Check pupil responses frequently
- Smell the breath—alcohol, ketones
- Rashes, signs of dehydration, cyanosis, pallor, needle injection marks
- Signs of external head injury—bruising, haematoma, cerebrospinal fluid from ears/nose
- Neck stiffness
- Localizing signs such as increased tone in limbs, asymmetrical reflexes
- Heart/lung for murmurs, rubs, wheeze, crackles
- Abdomen for organomegaly, aortic aneurysm, bruising, melaena.

Differential diagnosis

- Hypoxia
- Hypotension
- Hypoglycaemia (📖 p. 238)
- Overdose
- Epilepsy (📖 p. 297)
- High altitude cerebral oedema (📖 p. 626)
- Hypothermia/hyperthermia (📖 p. 596/684)
- Sepsis
- Meningitis/encephalitis (📖 p. 468)
- Malaria (📖 p. 474)
- Carbon monoxide poisoning (📖 p. 586)
- Subdural, subarachnoid, stroke.

Treatment

Treat any identifiable cause. Monitor vital signs and urine output. If full recovery does not occur, evacuate for further investigation and treatment. Remember pressure area care, maintenance fluids, and temperature control during evacuation. Catheterize if possible.

Urgent treatment

- ABC
- Consider oropharyngeal or nasopharyngeal airway
- Give high flow oxygen, if available
- Stabilize the cervical spine if there is a history of trauma
- Measure blood glucose and body temperature
- Obtain venous access and consider iv fluids
- Control seizures, treat hypoglycaemia (BM<4)
- Treat life-threatening infection if suspected
- Check observations: pulse, blood pressure, respiration rate

Headache

History
- Headache—severity, location, character, speed of onset, nausea/vomiting, head injury?
- Direct questions—dizziness, blackouts/fits, visual changes
- Past history—previous headaches, migraine
- Drugs—recent change in medication
- Social/environmental—alcohol/drugs, recent stressors, post-diving or change in elevation.

Examination
- Temperature, pulse, blood pressure, blood sugar, GCS score
- Evidence of head injury? Neck stiffness, photophobia, Kernig's (fully flex hip and passively extend knee. Positive if painful in head or neck). Look for any focal neurology—weakness/paralysis or changes in sensation
- Check whole body for purpuric rash
- Look for signs of URTI, including ear infection or sinus tenderness.

Differential diagnosis
- Tension headache
- Migraine (📖 p. 302)
- Dehydration
- Acute mountain sickness (📖 p. 620)
- High altitude cerebral oedema (📖 p. 626)
- Carbon monoxide poisoning (📖 p. 586)
- Sinusitis
- Dengue fever
- Malaria and other febrile illnesses (📖 p. 474).

If signs of meningism:
- Meningitis/encephalitis (📖 p. 468)
- Subarachnoid haemorrhage

Decreased conscious level/localizing signs:
- Meningitis/encephalitis (📖 p. 468)
- Subarachnoid haemorrhage
- Stroke
- Malaria (📖 p. 470)
- High altitude cerebral oedema (📖 p. 626)
- Post-traumatic (extradural, subdural) (📖 p. 292).

Treatment
- If reduced GCS, see Management of coma (📖 p. 230)
- Focal neurology or possibility of meningitis/encephalitis: give oxygen, broad spectrum antibiotics such as ceftriaxone iv or ciprofloxacin PO, evacuate urgently
- Give fluids and regular analgesia. Advise rest. Observe closely.

Delirium/confusion

- Delirium: acute onset of confusion with hallucinations
- Confusion: acute deficit in orientation, thinking, and short-term memory with reduced awareness.

History (from bystanders)

- Sudden or gradual onset
- Any trauma
- Recent illness—headache, photophobia, chest pain, dysuria, cough, fever, seizures, vomiting, dizziness, incontinence
- Past history—diabetes, cardiac, respiratory, epilepsy, psychiatric illness
- Drugs—overdose, sedatives/hypnotics, mefloquine, steroids, psychiatric medication
- Social/environmental—alcohol, recreational drugs, usual state.

Examination

- GCS score
- Check pupil responses frequently
- Smell the breath—alcohol, ketones
- Rashes, signs of dehydration, cyanosis, pallor, needle injection marks
- Signs of external head injury—bruising, haematoma, CSF from ears/nose
- Neck stiffness
- Localizing signs such as increased tone in limbs, asymmetrical reflexes
- Abbreviated mental state score (see opposite)
- Check temperature
- Heart/lung for murmurs, rubs, wheeze, crackles, or injuries
- Abdomen for tenderness, signs of injury, melaena, organomegaly
- Test the urine and check blood glucose.

Confusion—differential diagnosis

- Hypoxia
- Hypoglycaemia (📖 p. 238)
- Head injury (📖 p. 292)
- Alcohol/illicit drugs (📖 p. 512)
- Sepsis
- Meningitis/encephalitis (📖 p. 468)
- Intracranial bleed
- CVA
- Drug toxicity
- Malaria (📖 p. 470)
- High altitude cerebral oedema (📖 p. 626)
- Post-ictal (📖 p. 297).

Treatment

Treat any identifiable cause. Do not leave patient alone. Sedate only with great caution: lorazepam 1–2 mg PO/im/iv. This may allow more detailed examination if the patient is very agitated/confused. Observe closely and evacuate for further investigation/treatment if complete recovery is delayed.

Abbreviated mental test score (AMTS)	
Age	1
Date of birth	1
Repeat 42 West Street	0
Year	1
Time (nearest hour)	1
Current location	1
Recognize two people	1
Year World War II ended	1
Name of the monarch	1
Count backward from 20 to 1	1
Recall 42 West Street	1
Total	10

Convulsions

Urgent treatment

- Airway: roll patient into the recovery position, protect from further harm but do not restrain. Consider oxygen and a nasopharyngeal airway
- Breathing: if no respiratory effort commence CPR
- Circulation and drugs: attempt venous access. Measure blood glucose; if <3.5 mmol/l give 100 ml glucose 10% by infusion. Recheck levels subsequently. Give lorazepam 4 mg iv over 2 min or diazepam 10 mg PR if no iv access
- If fits continue for >20 min, consider diazepam by infusion 100 mg in 500 ml of 5% dextrose; infuse 40 ml/h. Phenytoin is unlikely to be available
- If seizures continue, make arrangements for urgent evacuation

History

Get a detailed description of the seizure or fit:

- Onset—activity, position, warning, tonic, starting in one limb?
- During fit—sounds, cyanosis, breathing, eye, facial and limb movements, incontinence, duration
- Post-fit—tongue injury, post-ictal, limb weakness, muscle pain/injuries, headache
- Preceding illness—headache, chest pain, palpitations, dyspnoea
- Past history—previous seizures, diabetes, alcoholism, pregnancy, cardiac, respiratory or renal disease. Head injury
- Drugs—antiepileptics, oral hypoglycaemics, medication compliance
- Social/environmental—alcohol/drugs, recent feverish illness, post-diving, high altitude.

Examination

- Temperature, pulse, blood pressure, blood sugar, GCS score
- Evidence of head injury? Sweating, neck stiffness, photophobia. Look for any focal neurology—weakness/paralysis or changes in sensation
- Check whole body for injury—posterior dislocation of the shoulder is often missed (check for full, pain-free movements of both shoulders).

Convulsions—possible causes

- Epilepsy (📖 p. 297)
- Hypoglycaemia (📖 p. 238)
- Hypoxia
- Alcohol withdrawal
- Metabolic (low calcium, hyponatraemia/hypernatraemia)
- Head trauma (📖 p. 292)
- Meningitis/encephalitis (📖 p. 468)
- Malaria (📖 p. 470)
- Drug overdose
- Hypertension/eclampsia.

Treatment after convulsion
- If reduced GCS see Management of coma (see 📖 p. 230)
- Focal neurology or possibility of meningitis/encephalitis evacuate urgently
- Otherwise give fluids and regular analgesia. Advise rest. Observe closely. If a first fit, evacuate for hospital investigations.

Diabetic emergencies

Hypoglycaemia

- Coma or low GCS with BM <4mmol/l
- Can occur in non-diabetics—sepsis, alcohol excess, liver failure, malaria, quinine therapy.

History

- Sweating, hunger, anxiety, exercise, seizure, last meal, previous hypos, usual blood sugar levels
- Past history—diabetes, liver disease
- Drugs—insulin dose, oral hypoglycaemics
- Social/environmental—alcohol excess.

Examination

- Check observations: pulse, blood pressure, respiratory rate
- Glasgow Coma Scale score
- Pallor, sweating, tremor, slurred speech, acute confusion/aggression, focal neurology, convulsions
- Examine for cause of sepsis: see Fever 🕮 p. 242
- Consider card test for malaria such as Rapimal®.

Urgent treatment of hypoglycaemia

- Protect the airway
- Give high flow oxygen, if available
- Obtain venous access
- Give iv glucose (200 ml of 10%, 100 ml of 20%, 50 ml of 50%)
- Consider glucagon 1 mg sc/im/iv if access fails
- GCS should return to 15 in <10 min if hypoglycaemia is cause
- When GCS 15:
  - Encourage patient to eat or drink something sugary
  - Commence 1 l 10% glucose/4–6 h
  - Monitor BM

Treatment

Diabetes

Most likely cause is excess insulin, particularly if the patient has been undertaking unusually high levels of activity on the expedition. If hypos are recurrent consider reducing insulin doses. Monitor BMs regularly, preferably before each meal.

Alcohol

Hypoglycaemia may recur if further excess alcohol is taken. Monitor BMs until patient is sober and eating/drinking normally.

Other causes

Evacuate from the field for further investigations/treatment.

Diabetic ketoacidosis

High blood sugars in a diabetic patient with poor glycaemic control may be secondary to infection or steroids. The classical clinical description of diabetic ketoacidosis (DKA) is of a comatose or pre-comatose patient who is dehydrated and hyperventilating.

History

- Tiredness, thirst, polyuria, frequency, dysuria, weight loss, vomiting, breathlessness, cough, sputum, fever, chest/abdominal pain, skin infections, teeth problems
- Past history—diabetes, date of diagnosis, complications such as neuropathy, ulceration
- Drugs—insulin dose, oral hypoglycaemics, steroids
- Social/environmental—alcohol consumption, change in usual diet—often a problem on expeditions, particularly while travelling.

Examination

- Check BM glucose
- Check observations: pulse, blood pressure, respiratory rate, and temperature. Blood pressure may be low. GCS score. Record on chart
- Look for facial flushing, dry mouth, and rapid breathing (Kussmaul respirations), 'pear-drop' smell of ketones on breath
- Examine chest, abdomen, and skin for signs of infection (see Fever 📖 p. 242). Look for evidence of dental infection
- Test the urine for ketonuria or evidence for infection.

Ongoing treatment

Mild hyperglycaemia will not necessitate evacuation from the field, provided that the patient is eating and drinking and blood sugars normalize with increased doses of insulin and rehydration. If the patient does not respond rapidly to treatment, evacuate urgently; limited amounts of iv fluids will be available on most expeditions. Change to sc insulin when eating and ketonuria <1+. Continue to monitor BMs regularly, preferably before each meal.

Urgent treatment of diabetic ketoacidosis

- Protect the airway and give high flow oxygen, if available
- Obtain venous access
- Insulin: give 20 units soluble insulin im followed by 10 units im/h. When patient has improved and is eating change to insulin sc
- Fluids: give 500 ml 0.9% saline stat, then 500 ml/h for 4–6 h
- When BMs <15 mmol/l change to dextrose 5% 500 ml/2 h for 4–6 h (continue insulin 10 units im/h)
- Potassium chloride: give none for first hour, then 20 mmol/h for 3 h, then 10 mmol/h for 2 h
- Start a fluid balance chart and measure urine output
- Start antibiotics if any cause for infection identified
- If available give heparin 5000 units/8 h sc until mobilizing
- Monitor BMs hourly

Gastrointestinal bleeding

History
- *Vomit*—colour, quantity, blood mixed in, frequency, onset, pain on vomiting
- *Stools*—onset, quantity, colour (red, black, clots), pain on opening bowels, constipation, diarrhoea, change in bowel habit
- *Other*—appetite, dysphagia, weight loss, dyspnoea, palpitations, tiredness, dizziness, fainting, sweating, abdominal/chest pain
- *Past history*—previous bleeding, clotting problems, inflammatory bowel disease, liver disease (varices?), peptic ulceration, heartburn/indigestion
- *Drugs*—aspirin, NSAIDs, steroids, warfarin, iron
- *Social/environmental*—alcohol/drugs, smoking status, recent stressors.

Examination
- Temperature, pulse, blood pressure, blood sugar, GCS score
- Look for ongoing bleeding, evidence of shock, abdominal distension/tenderness/rebound/masses. Bowel sounds. PR examination for fresh blood/melaena/palpable mass/haemorrhoids.

Gastrointestinal bleeding—differential diagnosis
Upper GI
- Gastroduodenal ulceration (📖 p. 370)
- Mallory–Weiss tears (📖 p. 378)
- Oesophageal varices
- GI malignancy

Lower GI
- Haemorrhoids/anal fissure (📖 p. 379)
- Inflammatory bowel disease
- Diverticular disease.

Treatment
- Keep nil by mouth for 24 h. Maintain blood pressure >90 mmHg systolic by cautious use of fluids. Give analgesia as required (not NSAIDs or aspirin!). Monitor urine output. Consider PPI/antacids. Avoid spicy food. Observe regularly and evacuate for further investigation.

Urgent treatment
- Place the patient supine with legs elevated. If vomiting, place in the recovery position
- Give high flow oxygen
- Check observations: pulse, blood pressure, respiratory rate, and temperature
- Obtain venous access
- Consider intravenous saline depending on pulse and blood pressure

Fever

History
- *Fever type*—high swinging, low grade, periodic (i.e. every 2 or 3 days in malaria), association with rigors
- *Respiratory/ENT*—cough, wheeze, stridor or croup, sputum or nasal catarrh, haemoptysis, dyspnoea, chest pain, otalgia, sore throat, altered voice, facial pain, or tenderness (sinusitis), coryzal illness
- *Urinogenital*—frequency, dysuria, haematuria, loin pain, genital discharge/ulceration, suprapubic pain
- *Neurological*—headache, photophobia, neck stiffness, impaired consciousness
- *Skin/mucous membranes/joints*—rash, petechiae, skin infections such as bites/ulcers/sores, mucosal lesions, arthralgia, swollen joints
- *Gastrointestinal*—vomiting, haematemesis, abdominal pain, bloating, diarrhoea, blood in stools or melaena, foul/excessive flatus
- *Other*—changes in appetite, aching, night sweats, weight loss
- *Past history*—previous similar symptoms, immunocompromise, diabetes mellitus
- *Drugs*—steroids, antimalarials taken regularly, antipyretics, antibiotics, etc. as cause of fever
- *Social/environmental*—infectious disease contact, detailed travel history, adequacy of pre-travel vaccinations.

Travel history
- Which countries and which parts of the countries?
- When? Length of trip, date of arrival, and departure (estimate possible incubation period)
- Purpose of travel—business, pleasure, family visit, military, airline crew, expedition, emigration?
- Type of travel, hotels, safari, backpacking
- Special activities (climbing, diving, caving)?
- Insect bites/stings (tsetse, ticks, fleas)
- Animal contact
- Swimming in fresh water lakes
- Sexual or other infectious disease contact
- Antimalarials taken/immunizations received pre-travel
- Illness among other members of the family or party.

Examination
- Temperature (chart if possible), pulse/respiratory rate, blood pressure, GCS score, urine output
- Warm or cool peripheries, capillary refill time (📖 p. 163), sweating, rash, mucosal lesions, wounds, abscesses, insect bites, ulcers, eschar, buboes, cellulitis, or other focal skin infection (examine the entire body surface, including the scalp, axillae, and perineum). Look up the nose and at throat, tonsils, tongue, and buccal mucous membrane. Look in the ears with an auriscope. Examine chest for breath sounds and heart murmurs; abdominal tenderness, bowel sounds, lymphadenopathy; joint pain or swelling, external genitalia and rectal examination if relevant.

Investigations

- Usually impossible. The macroscopic appearance and odour of vomitus, stool, and urine may be helpful (e.g. obvious blood; cloudiness and foul fishy smell of urine suggests infection). Consider dip testing urine, microscopic examination of blood, sputum, urine, stool (experience required). Rapid antigen tests for malaria (see Malaria 📖 p. 474).

Possible diagnoses

- *Upper respiratory tract infection*—viral coryza, sinusitis, otitis media, tonsillitis, 'strep' throat
- *Chest*—bronchitis, pneumonia, tuberculosis
- *Gut*—gastroenteritis, dysentery
- *Urinary*—UTI, pyelonephritis
- *Neurological*—meningitis/encephalitis
- *Tropical infections*—malaria, typhoid, legionella, leptospirosis, hepatitis, rabies, typhus/other rickettsiae, viral haemorrhagic fevers.

Treatment

- If reduced GCS, see Management of coma (📖 p. 230)
- Focal neurology or possibility of life-threatening sepsis: give oxygen, broad spectrum antibiotics, evacuate urgently
- If malaria is a possibility treat urgently (📖 p. 474)
- Reduce fever with regular paracetamol and/or ibuprofen
- Encourage oral fluids and monitor urine output; start a fluid balance chart
- Advise rest in a cool place. Observe closely, evacuate if not improving
- Empirical antibiotic therapy
  - *Urinary tract infection*—trimethoprim 200 mg/12 h PO (or ciprofloxacin 250 mg/12 h PO)
  - *Cellulitis*—flucloxacillin 1 g/6 h iv + benzyl penicillin 1.2 g/6 h iv
  - *Wound infection*—flucloxacillin 500 mg/6 h PO
  - *Meningitis*—ceftriaxone 2 g/12 h iv
  - *Septic arthritis*—flucloxacillin 2 g/6 h iv
  - *Pneumonia*—amoxicillin 500 mg/8 h PO or erythromycin 500 mg/6 h PO
  - *Intra-abdominal sepsis*—cefuroxime 1.5 g/8 h iv + metronidazole 500 mg/8 h iv.

Skin

Jon Dallimore and David Warrell

Solar skin damage

Introduction

For many expeditioners one of the unstated aims of the expedition is to obtain a 'good' tan. However, excessive exposure to solar radiation is damaging and may cause skin cancers:

- Basal cell carcinoma
- Squamous cell carcinoma
- Malignant melanoma.

In the UK, incidence of all skin cancers has increased—doubling between 1980 and 1990, with a 5% annual increase in tumours. Chronic sun exposure is also associated with skin thickening, pigmentation, and increased wrinkles. A number of skin conditions are triggered by exposure to sunlight and some people are sensitive to the effects of sunlight.

Solar radiation

Sunlight is the commonest source of ultraviolet radiation (UVR). UVR is subdivided into UVA (320–400 nm), UVB (280–320 nm), and UVC (100–280 nm). UVC is potentially very damaging to human skin but is normally absorbed by ozone in the earth's atmosphere. UVB plays an important role in sunburn, carcinogenesis, skin ageing, and vitamin D synthesis. UVA is responsible for tanning, ageing changes, and may be involved in carcinogenesis. Between 10 and 20 times more UVA reaches the earth's surface than UVB.

Intensity of sunlight increases nearer the equator, at increasing altitudes, and in polar regions; this is especially true for UVR, where the protective atmospheric ozone layer may have thinned. It is also greatest when the sun is highest in the sky, between 10 am and 3 pm. UVR is reflected by water, white surfaces (such as snow and sand), and glass.

Sunburn

This follows acute, excessive exposure to UVR. It is an important risk factor for the development of malignant melanoma. Mild sunburn is characterized by skin redness, local heat, and pain. Severe sunburn may result in swelling, blistering, and generalized symptoms such as malaise, nausea, and rigors.

Treatment of sunburn

Sunburn is much easier to prevent than treat. Anti-inflammatories and paracetamol can be used for pain relief. 'Aftersun' creams containing aloe vera may help. Hydrocortisone 1% cream also helps to reduce inflammation but should not be applied to large areas or to broken skin. Blisters should not be drained unless very large.

Susceptibility to solar damage

People with different skin types are more or less likely to burn in the sun. A classification system has been developed (see box).

Susceptibility to solar damage

Skin type	Response to sunlight
1	Always burns, never tans
2	Usually burns, sometimes tans
3	Sometimes burns, usually tans
4	Very rarely burns
5	Mediterranean-type skin
6	Darkly pigmented skin

Generally, those with pale skin, red hair, blue or green eyes, and freckles are most susceptible to solar skin damage. Those with a personal or family history of skin cancer should be particularly careful to avoid excessive sun exposure.

Prevention of sunburn

- Avoid mid-day sun
- Use natural shade
- Cover up with hats and clothing (some have a sunlight protection factor rating)
- Use a sunscreen that protects against UVA and UVB, is water-resistant and has a sun protection factor greater than 15 (see below).

Sunscreens

There are two main types of sunscreen:

- Physical
- Chemical.

Physical sunscreens contain zinc oxide or titanium dioxide. They are highly visible on the skin and may be cosmetically unacceptable. However, they are very effective at blocking UVA and UVB.

Chemical sunscreens contain para-aminobenzoic acid or cinnamates, and protect against UVB. Some newer compounds also protect against UVA. Chemical sunscreens sometimes cause allergic or irritant reactions.

SPF (sun protection factor)

This is a guide to the strength of a sunscreen in protecting the skin from UVB. A star system, 1–4, where 4 is the strongest, indicates the capacity to block out UVA. In theory, the SPF increases the amount of time that can be spent in the sun by the factor quoted. However, variables such as the time of day, the amount of cloud cover, time of year, and the amount of reflection all affect the protective ability of the sunscreen.

Wounds

Minor wounds are common on expeditions but some wounds are life-threatening. An ABC approach should be used (see Chapter 6). All wounds need careful assessment, thorough cleaning, then closure and dressing. Wounds that involve tendon, nerve, or blood vessel injuries cannot be managed in the field. The patient will need to be evacuated.

Immediate assessment and treatment

See 🕮 p. 409 in limb section.

Take a focused history:

- How did the injury occur? (Mechanism is all important; was it an insect or mammal bite?)
- Where did it occur (clean or contaminated environment)?
- When did it occur? Old wounds >12 h should not be sutured and are more likely to be infected.
- Was the wound caused by broken glass? (Will need careful examination or preferably X-ray.)
- Was the limb trapped or crushed? (Swelling and compartment syndrome are possible; see also crush injuries 🕮 p. 257.)
- When was the last tetanus booster? (Particularly for deep, penetrating wounds.)
- Is the patient allergic to anything?
- Does the patient take any medication?

Examine the wound:

- Measure wounds and consider drawing or using a diagram (Fig. 8.1).
- Look for contamination and foreign bodies.
- Check for signs of infection (red, hot, swollen, painful, tender, crepitus, lymphangitis, enlarged regional lymph nodes, fever).
- Check for pulses and capillary refill time (🕮 p. 163).
- Re-examine carefully for signs of nerve damage—change in sensation, weakness, or paralysis.
- Look for evidence of damage to deep structures—examine the wound, preferably under local or regional anaesthetic.

General wound care

All wounds should be managed using the following principles:

- Stop bleeding.
- Clean carefully to reduce the risk of infection.
- Dress the injury to maintain cleanliness.
- Promote healing and restore function.

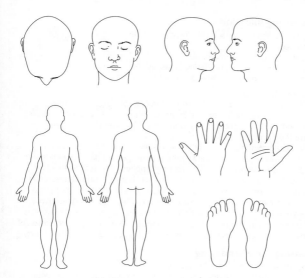

Fig. 8.1 Diagram of body for noting injury or skin feature.

Stopping bleeding
All wounds bleed to a greater or lesser extent. In some cases, bleeding may be life-threatening.
- Apply direct pressure over the wound with a clean dressing.
- Lay the casualty down.
- Raise the limb above the level of the heart.
- Apply a further dressing to control the bleeding on top of any original pad. If bleeding persists, remove the dressing, open the wound, and apply pressure deep in the wound (see below).
- Bandage firmly to hold dressing in place.

All wounds swell to some extent; watch for tourniquet effect.

When there are very deep wounds it may not be possible to control bleeding by applying pressure on the surface of the skin. The only way to stop severe, persistent bleeding from deep inside a wound may be to remove the dressings, open the wound, remove clots and debris, and to pack the wound open with sterile gauze. The use of artery forceps should be avoided as they may damage important structures such as tendons and nerves.

In torrential haemorrhage, for example following a landmine injury or traumatic amputation, it may be necessary to use other techniques such as a tourniquet (which should be released and reapplied every 30 min) or the use of pressure points.

Preventing infection

- Clean all wounds with purified water, sterile saline, or antiseptic solution.
- Remove any foreign material.
- Cover wound with a non-stick dressing.
- Bandage to hold the dressing in place.

Consider:
- If foreign bodies are deeply embedded and cannot be removed easily, they should be left and removed surgically. If an object remains embedded, the surrounding wound should still be cleaned carefully and then dressed.
- During an expedition it may be necessary to care for wounds for days or even weeks. Wounds should be inspected daily (maybe twice daily in the jungle) and clean dressings applied. Any pus or exudate should be gently removed but do not scrub the wound or use strong antiseptics which may damage healing tissues. If dressings stick, soaking in warm clean water will allow easier removal. Deep, contaminated, penetrating wounds are prone to tetanus infection. If the casualty has definitely been immunized against tetanus in the past, give a booster of toxoid. If no prior immunity, consider giving tetanus immunoglobulin.

Dressings and bandaging

Wounds should be dressed in layers:
- Use non-stick sterile dressing on the wound (such as non-adherent tulle dressings (e.g. Melolin or paraffin gauze).
- Sterile gauze swabs to absorb any pus or exudate from the wound.
- Next, apply a crepe bandage or other elasticated bandage to hold dressings in place.
- The bandage should hold the dressing in place without producing pressure or constriction.

Promoting healing and restoration of function

Wound healing is aided by a healthy diet and rest. Any significant wound will heal more quickly with an increase in oxygen at altitudes below 3000 m. Rest is needed initially, but prolonged splinting leads to stiffness and muscle wasting. Joints adjacent to a wound or burn should be kept mobile. See section on physiotherapy 📖 p. 447.

Notes on wound types and management

Lacerations

Are caused by a blunt injury and the skin is torn with irregular wound edges. There is often evidence of bruising in the surrounding tissues.

Cuts

Cuts or incised wounds are a result of sharp edges such as knives or glass. They have cleancut edges. Stab wounds are deep and slash wounds are long and shallow.

Closing cuts and lacerations

Gaping wounds will heal more quickly and result in a better scar if the skin edges are brought together.

Steri-Strips™

Steri-Strips™ are paper stitches that come in a variety of lengths and widths. They are placed across a laceration and, if left in place for a week or so, result in a clean, neat scar (Fig. 8.2). Steri-Strips™ do not stick near moving joints, on the palms of the hands and soles of the feet, or on the scalp. However, they are excellent for finger lacerations and facial wounds. In humid or wet environments, such as the jungle or at sea, consider applying tincture of benzoin (Friar's Balsam) to the skin—this helps the Steri-Strips™ to stick.

Suturing (Fig. 8.3)

Steri-Strips™ should be used where possible. If Steri-Strips™ will not close the wound, suturing should be considered. Only clean wounds that are less than 12 h old are suitable for suturing. Deep wounds should be closed in layers by an experienced surgeon in an operating theatre because of the risk of wound infection. If this is not possible, clean the wound, pack with sterile gauze soaked in saline, and re-dress daily until definitive care is reached. Sutures should never be used to close deep or dirty wounds, particularly animal or human bites. Suturing should only be attempted by those who are adequately trained.

Important points when suturing a wound

- Most inexperienced people use too many stitches, too tight, too close
- Lay the wound edges together to allow healing to occur—do not use tension
- Use toothed forceps to hold the skin edges and pass the needle close to the part of the skin which is being held with forceps
- Match up wound edges with strategically placed sutures along irregular wounds then close the gaps
- Do not be afraid to remove sutures and try again

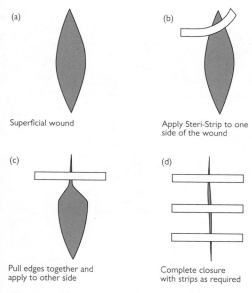

(a)

Superficial wound

(b)

Apply Steri-Strip to one
side of the wound

(c)

Pull edges together and
apply to other side

(d)

Complete closure
with strips as required

Fig. 8.2 Applying Steri-Strips™.

Choice of suture material: the skin should be closed with non-absorbable suture material such as Prolene or nylon on a curved cutting needle. Experienced operators may consider carrying absorbable suture material (such as Vicryl) to close deep tissue layers, and this will help to reduce the risk of haematoma formation. Vicryl can also be used to close wounds inside the mouth. Use 4/0 sutures for most parts of the body, 5/0 on fingers and the face.

Removal of sutures: sutures should be removed after 7–10 days except on the face where earlier removal results in better healing with less scarring when the foreign material is removed. Sutures can be replaced by Steri-Strips™ after 3–4 days.

Staples

These are easy to use with minimal training and may be used in particular to close scalp wounds rapidly. If carried, a staple remover must also be available.

Tissue glue

May be useful for superficial face and scalp wounds, particularly in children. When bleeding is controlled, clean and dry the wound edges and place glue on the skin edges, not in the wound. Hold the wound edges together for 1 min to let the glue set.

1

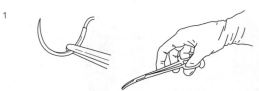

How to hold the needle and surgical instrument

2

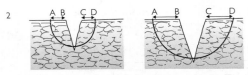

Distance from needle entry/exit points to would edge. The greater the distance from the would edge to the needle entry point, the deeper the bite of the needle. AB must equal CD, otherwise a step will occur

3

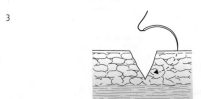

Depth of suture. Aim to close the wound fully by placing the suture to the deepest part of the wound

4

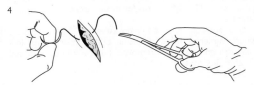

Istrument tie knot. Starting position, needle in left hand, needle-holder in right hand

Fig. 8.3 Skin suturing technique.

5

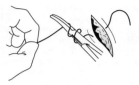

Wrapping the suture around the needle-holder.
Do this TWICE

6

The first throw: take the loose end of the suture in the
jaws of the needle-holder

7

To tighten the first throw, cross the hands, needle-holder
going to the left, and the left hand going to the right

8

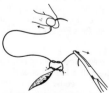

The second throw: the suture has been wrapped over the
needle-holder in the opposite direction and this time the
hand does not cross when tying the suture

Fig. 8.3 (Contd.)

Abrasions

These are grazing injuries where the top surface of the skin is removed. Abrasions should be cleaned carefully and a non-adherent dressing applied. Ingrained dirt, if not removed, will result in tattooing and makes wound infection more likely. Dressings may need to be changed once or twice daily in some environments such as the jungle. If dressings stick they can be soaked off with warm, clean water or saline.

Puncture wounds

Infection may occur at the base of deep, penetrating wounds. Tetanus is a significant risk in anaerobic conditions found deep in puncture wounds, and all expedition team members should be immunized before travel (see Chapter 2). Clean puncture wounds by encouraging bleeding and then irrigate the wound using a syringe. The skin surface should be prevented from sealing over by placing a small wick made from sterile gauze into the wound. This allows healing to occur from the bottom of a puncture wound upwards otherwise abscess formation may occur. Deep infection in a puncture wound will need evacuation for surgical exploration and cleaning.

Bites (animal and human)

Human bites carry a high risk of bacterial infections such as *Staphylococcus aureus* and *Eikenella corrodens*. Mammal bites should always raise the question of rabies (☐ p. 42 and 456) and there is a range of other special pathogens such as *Pasteurella multocida* (dog and cat bites), *Capnocytophaga canimorsus* (dogs), *Bartonella henselae* (cats), and *Streptobacillus monili-formis* and *Spirillum minus* (rodents). Bites should be cleaned as a matter of urgency with liberal amounts of soap and water followed by an antiseptic such as alcohol or iodine. Tetanus risk should also be considered. (See Animals capable of severe trauma ☐ p. 522.)

Bruises

Contusions or bruises are caused by a blunt force applied to the tissues. Bleeding under the skin gives the bruise its characteristic coloured appearance. Large muscle haematomas may cause hypovolaemic shock. Rest, ice, compression, and elevation (RICE) all help to reduce swelling and pain. Compression may be achieved by applying a crepe bandage firmly around the affected area. Anti-inflammatory drugs such as ibuprofen or aspirin may also help. After a day or two the affected part should be mobilized to reduce stiffness. (See Physiotherapy ☐ p. 447.)

Blisters

Blisters are best prevented. Ideally, stop walking and cover any 'hot spots' before they develop into blisters. If a blister does form, the fluid may be drained using a clean (sterile) fine needle and the area covered with an adhesive plaster. Moleskin®, Compeed®, and Spenco Second Skin® are dressings designed to relieve the discomfort. Blisters may become de-roofed; in this case treat with a non-adherent dressing. A thin application of Friar's Balsam at the edge of a blister or swathes of zinc oxide tape over the dressings may help to keep protective coverings in place. Healing is rapid if friction at the blister site can be eliminated. Where possible, leaving the blister uncovered will assist healing by allowing the area to dry out.

Crush injuries

Large amounts of tissue may be damaged in crushing injuries and the potential for infection is high. The crushed part should be carefully cleaned and then elevated. Swelling in the affected part may cut off the blood supply to the limb beyond the injury. If the injury is severe there may be a risk of losing the limb and renal failure. Evacuate the casualty for expert assessment; try to ensure casualty maintains a good urine output during the evacuation (📖 p. 136).

Amputation

A digit or limb may be replaced by microsurgery if the patient and the amputated part can be delivered to a surgeon in less than 6 h. The amputated part should be kept cool, preferably in a container with ice, but not in direct contact with the ice. In an expedition setting it is highly unlikely that such surgical facilities will be available; in this case, treat the bleeding with direct pressure and elevation. The stump should be cleaned gently and then covered with a non-adherent dressing such as paraffin gauze. People with these injuries need to be evacuated to allow surgical treatment to shorten any bone ends and cover the stump with a flap of skin so that healing can take place. Knife injuries that remove a chunk of palmar tissue such as the finger pulp are best treated by re-applying the excised tissue to the wound under a firm dressing or taking the tissue with the casualty as described above.

Splinters

Splinters can usually be removed using a fine pair of tweezers (the ones on Swiss Army knives are good) or a sterile needle. For more stubborn splinters, soaking may help. Spines from sea urchins are easier to remove after a couple of days when the wound becomes inflamed, or after softening the skin by soaking or applying salicylic acid ointment (see Chapter 16—Risks from animals).

Wound infections

Any wound can become infected; bites, dirty wounds, and deep wounds are more likely to become infected. Signs and symptoms of a wound infection are: pain, redness, heat, swelling, and loss of function. In the later stages, red lines may be seen running from a limb wound up towards the trunk (lymphangitis). Lymph nodes in the armpit, groin, or neck may become enlarged and fever may develop.

Abscesses

An abscess is a collection of pus or a 'boil', and is usually caused by a bacterial infection (see 📖 p. 274–80, Chapter 16, p. 542). As pus accumulates, the skin over the abscess thins ('pointing'). Once the pus discharges through the skin the throbbing pain rapidly resolves. If an abscess develops during an expedition, applying local heat and oral antibiotics (e.g. flucloxacillin) may help. However, once pus is present it is quicker and kinder to drain it. Exceptions include those affecting the face, genital and anal areas, and breast—these abscesses should be referred for specialist treatment. Local anaesthetic is less effective in the presence of infection because of localized high tissue acidity. Regional nerve blocks such as a digital nerve block may provide good analgesia (📖 p. 566). An elliptical cut over the abscess must be large enough to let the pus drain. A small piece of gauze soaked in saline inserted into the incision will act as a wick and stop the roof of the abscess healing over before all the pus has drained. In this way the abscess cavity will heal from the bottom upwards. The wick should be changed daily until the abscess has healed. If there is evidence of spreading infection, antibiotics should be considered.

Cellulitis

Cellulitis refers to a bacterial infection of the skin (usually staphylococcal or streptococcal). There may not be an obvious source of infection but the signs are the same as for a wound infection; that is, circumscribed redness, heat, pain, swelling, and fever with rigors which may precede the appearance of the skin lesion. Look for lymphangitis and lymphadenopathy. Treat with oral antibiotics initially (penicillin and flucloxacillin or co-amoxiclav). Consider intravenous antibiotics if the infection is spreading or there are other features of generalized infection such as fever and rigors.

Burns

Burns may be caused by dry heat, chemicals, electricity, friction, or hot liquids. On expeditions, open fires and fuel stoves commonly cause injuries, particularly when people refuel lighted stoves or burn rubbish with petrol.

Assessing the severely burned patient

Use an ABC approach:

- Ensure a safe approach for rescuers. Disconnect the electricity supply in electrical burns. Smother flames with a blanket or roll the victim on the ground. Remove any source of heat and remove any clothing that is not adherent to the skin.
- *Airway*—look for signs of potential problems—hoarse voice, burning or soot around mouth and nose, difficulty swallowing, singed nasal hair. A surgical airway may be necessary (p. 181) but the outlook on an expedition is likely to be very poor if evacuation times are long.
- *Cervical spine*—there may be other injuries, particularly if the patient jumped from a building to escape the fire. Immobilize the neck and spine if suspected.
- *Breathing*—severe circumferential burns on the chest may require rapid surgical treatment (escharotomy) and are likely to be fatal in a very remote area.
- *Circulation*—shock is a feature of severe burns and large quantities of fluids may be needed. For fluid resuscitation see below (see also Shock p. 214).

History

Establish:

- Did the fire occur in an enclosed space?
- What was the burning material, if known?
- Was the patient unconscious at any time?
- Was there an explosion?

Examination

Assessing burns

The severity and extent of burns is often underestimated, even by doctors and nurses, and extensive burns need specialist assessment and treatment. The 'rule of nines', which divides the surface area of the body into areas of approximately 9%, is one method used to calculate the proportion of the body which is burned and so helps determine treatment (see Fig. 8.4). It may be easier to remember that the patient's palm (excluding the fingers and thumb) represents approximately 1% of the body surface area.

Burns may be divided into superficial and full thickness burns.

- Superficial burns: characterized by redness, swelling, and pain (first degree). Deep partial thickness burns (second degree) are blistered and do not blanch on pressure.
- Full thickness (third degree) burns: characterized by pale, leathery, and sometimes charred skin with a loss of sensation. There are no blisters.

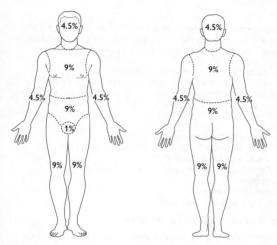

Fig. 8.4 Burns rule of nines.

Consider:

- On an expedition it is important to differentiate between deep partial thickness and full thickness burns, although this may be difficult initially. Full thickness burns need skin grafting, so evacuation to specialist medical help will be necessary.
- Fluid resuscitation for patients with >15% burns.
- Insert a cannula away from the burned areas and give 2–4 ml 0.9% saline/kg per % body surface area burned (excluding areas of erythema). This is the total volume to be given in the first 24 h; half of this volume should be given in the first 8 h.
  Example:
  - 70-kg man with 30% burns
  - $4 \times 70 \times 30 = 8400$ ml/24 h. Give 4200 ml in the first 8 h.
  - Cover burned areas with clingfilm.
  - Monitor pulse, blood pressure, respiratory rate, and body temperature.
  - Measure urine output.
  - Arrange urgent evacuation to hospital.

Treatment of severe burns and scalds

- Ensure scene safety to prevent other people becoming burn victims
- Remove the patient from the burning environment
- Halt the burning process and relieve pain by applying cold water and cover burned areas with cling film or clean sheets
- Irrigate chemical burns with copious tepid water
- Leave any adherent burnt clothing
- Give oxygen and iv analgesia if available.

Management of minor burns

As with severe burns, minor burns should be treated promptly to prevent the burning process, to cool the burn, control pain, and apply a suitable dressing.

- *Stopping the burning process*—the heat source should be removed. See Assessing the severely burned patient, above.
- *Cool the burn*—immerse in tepid water or irrigate. Cooling large areas of skin can cause hypothermia. Chemicals, particularly alkalis, need prolonged irrigation.
- *Control pain*—covering and cooling burns reduces pain. Strong painkillers such as tramadol or opiates may be required initially; later co-codamol or ibuprofen may be sufficient.
- *Suitable burn dressings*—clingfilm is ideal and has many other uses on an expedition. Clingfilm is essentially sterile if the first few centimetres are discarded. It is transparent, stretchy, and impermeable. Hand burns may be treated in a plastic bag. Cooling gels such as Burnshield® are useful to cool the burn and provide good pain relief.

Key facts for burns

- Burns to significant areas such as hands, feet, face, genitalia should be assessed by a specialist
- >10% body surface area burns need evacuation as many burns become infected
- Full thickness burns will almost certainly require skin grafting and should be evacuated early
- Blistered burns: do not de-roof; however, large blisters may be aspirated with a sterile needle and syringe
- In general, avoid prophylactic antibiotics
- Bactroban® or silver sulphadiazine (Flamazine®) creams help to prevent infection during evacuation and can be placed under clingfilm or inside a plastic bag in the case of hand burns. Paraffin gauze is very useful to dress burns as it is less likely to adhere to the burn
- Granuflex® (a hydrocolloid dressing) is adhesive and waterproof, and may be used for awkward areas which are difficult to dress. Change every 3–5 days
- Elevate limb burns to reduce swelling
- Early physiotherapy helps to maintain mobility (📖 p. 447).
- Regular ibuprofen is usually sufficient analgesia for a dressed burn
- On an expedition, burns should be re-dressed every 24–48 h. Look for signs of infection (📖 p. 258). Healed burns should be protected from the sun for 6–12 months

Insect bites

Bites by blood-feeding insects such as mosquitoes, midges, black flies, sand flies, tabanid flies (horse deer and stable flies), tsetse flies, and triatomine 'kissing' bugs pose a common irritation and nuisance during expeditions. These 'micro-predators' make brief blood-sucking attacks on humans and animals which can result in persisting medical problems. (See also Insect stings 📖 p. 536.)

Clinical features

Consequences of bites:
- Allergic reactions.
- Secondary infection of the bite site.
- Acquisition of systemic infections transmitted by the insect (see Chapter 14).
- Bites may be immediately painful and traumatic (horse flies) but the commonest problem is delayed local swelling and itching from hyper-sensitivity to insects' salivary allergens incurred by previous exposure. A small, intensely itchy, reddish lump with a central (haemorrhagic) punctum develops immediately or after a delay of 24–48 h. A papule, urticarial weal, blister, or bulla may develop (e.g. after 'Blandford fly' (*Simulium posticatum*) bites in Oxfordshire, UK), or bites may provoke a more generalized erythema multiforme or, especially in children, papular urticaria. Systemic anaphylaxis may be provoked (📖 p. 222). Scratching may lead to secondary infection, an inflamed, painful pustule or carbuncle (e.g. after Lord Carnarvon's fatal septicaemia from an infected mosquito bite on his cheek near the tomb of Tutankhamun), or a demarcated, hot, bright red, raised area of erysipelas or cellulitis. Causative bacteria include *Staph. aureus* and *Strep. pyogenes*. The risk of secondary infection seems to be higher under humid tropical conditions. Triatomine bug bites are usually multiple, often near the eye or angle of the mouth, and are painful, swollen, ooze blood, and may be surrounded by black staining from the bug's faeces (see Chagas' Disease 📖 p. 484).

Treatment

- Apply a cooling antiseptic solution, cream, or ointment (e.g. triclosan, hydrogen peroxide, Savlon®) to sooth irritation and prevent secondary infection.
- Reduce itch with counter irritants such as crotamiton (Eurax®) cream/lotion, with or without hydrocortisone.
- Topical corticosteroids (e.g. hydrocortisone 0.5% cream or ointment) can be tried but topical antihistamines are not recommended as they may be light-sensitizing.

- For severe pruritus use oral antihistamines. Try full dose, non-sedating anti-H₁ drugs such as cetirizine (adult dose up to 10 mg twice a day) during the day and chlorphenamine (Piriton®) 4 mg at night.
- Early systemic symptoms of anaphylaxis should be treated with adrenaline (epinephrine) 0.1% (1:1000) 0.5 ml by intramuscular injection (adult dose). This dose may be repeated after 5 min if there is no response (📖 p. 222).
- If inflamed pustules develop, apply a topical antibacterial such as mupirocin (Bactroban®). Multiple infected bites may warrant a course of oral antibiotic such as flucloxacillin or erythromycin.

Prevention

Be prepared for insect bites, not only in tropical rain forests and beaches but also in the arctic and in cool mountainous terrain such as the Californian Sierra Nevada, Italian Dolomites, and Scottish Highlands. The risk of getting bitten varies geographically, seasonally, and diurnally. Seek specific advice.

- Sensible clothing should be as ample and protective as comfort allows.
- Long sleeves and long trousers should be worn after dusk.
- Light colours are less attractive to mosquitoes than dark ones. Blue colour attracts African tsetse flies (see Sleeping sickness 📖 p. 483).
- Hats and face veils may protect against assaults on face and scalp by swarms of Scottish midges (*Culicoides*), or tropical black flies (*Simulium*) and sand flies (*Phlebotomus, Lutzomyia*).
- Effective repellents include diethyl-toluamide (DEET) and *p*-methane-diol (Mosiguard)-containing preparations applied to exposed skin or impregnated into cotton clothing or ankle bands.
- Clothes can be impregnated with pyrethroid insecticides at the expense of waterproofing.
- Protect sleeping quarters. Mosquito proofing of sleeping quarters and insecticide spraying at dusk reduces the risk. Night bites by mosquitoes that transmit malaria (📖 p. 470), cone-nosed (triatomine) 'kissing' bugs (Central and South America) that transmit Chagas' disease (📖 p. 484), bed bugs, ticks that transmit tick-borne encephalitis and tick-borne relapsing fever (📖 p. 268), and even vampire bats that transmit rabies (📖 p. 459) can be prevented by sleeping under a pyrethroid-impregnated mosquito net. Burn pyrethroid releasing mosquito coils or, if there is electricity, plug-in insecticide vaporizers. Ceiling fans deter mosquitoes from biting.

Ectoparasitic infestations

Fleas, lice, mites, ticks, invasive flies (myiasis), and leeches

Some blood-feeding invertebrates take up temporary or long-term residence on the surface of humans' bodies or clothing. Tropical climate and poor socioeconomic conditions increase the risk of acquiring ectoparasites from other humans or from the environment. The very presence of these creatures, visible or palpable, is irritating, distressing, and embarrassing, but it is only in the past century that westerners have grown less accustomed to being flea-ridden and lousy. For example, Marie Curie was awoken by a myriad of bed bugs falling off her back as she rolled over in her poor Paris attic bedroom.

The biting and burrowing of these ectoparasites causes pain and irritation, and may lead to hypersensitivity, secondary local infection, or transmission of systemic diseases such as:

- Rickettsioses and plague by fleas.
- Viral encephalitides and haemorrhagic fevers, spirochaetoses, rickettsioses, and bartonelloses by ticks.
- Spirochaetoses and rickettsioses by lice.
- Scrub typhus by trombiculid mites.
- Local *Streptococcal* infection leading to acute glomerulonephritis by scabies mites.

Fleas

Humans can be infested and bitten by human fleas (*Pulex irritans*) and by dog, cat, rat, pigeon, and other animal fleas. Direct contact with an infested person or animal is not necessary. Tropical rodent fleas (*Xenopsylla* species) transmit plague and murine typhus. The first evidence of fleas is the appearance of small groups of intensely itchy bites (red macule with a central punctum), often in a line a few centimetres apart, especially on the trunk or buttocks. Fleas may not remain on the body after feeding but retreat to bedding or crevices and cracks in the bed or room. Examination of underclothing or turning back the bedclothes may reveal the jumping fleas.

Treatment: itching bites are treated with counter-irritants, topical corticosteroid, or systemic antihistamines (see Insect bites above). Domestic animals and the infested environment should be kept as clean as is practicable and treated with pyrethroid or other pesticides.

Lice

Human head lice (*Pediculus capitis*), body (clothing) lice (*P. humanus*), and pubic lice (*Pthirus pubis*) are obligate human parasitic insects that spread through close physical contact.

- *Head lice*: flourish in the human scalp even in hygienic, affluent conditions, especially among teenage school girls. Eggs ('nits') stuck to head hairs are recovered using a fine comb. Itching and scratching may cause secondary infection with occipital lymphadenopathy.
  - *Treatment*: repeated application of insecticide lotion (pyrethroid, organophosphate, or carbamate) and combing.
  - *Prevention*: avoid head-to-head contact.

- *Body lice*: infestation is promoted by poor hygiene (unwashed clothes and bodies) and crowding, common accompaniments of disasters, wars, forced immigration, and cold, wet seasons as in the highlands of Ethiopia. Lice and their eggs may be discovered on skin, body hair, or in clothing, especially in the seams. More than 21 500 lice have been found on one person. Individual bites look like flea bites but there is no linearity and only mild local irritation.
  - *Treatment*: burn clothing or heat-sterilize and impregnate with pyrethroids. Bathe infested people with soap and 1% lysol.
- *Pubic (crab) lice*: sexually transmitted infestation of the pubic hair and also body hair, eyebrows, and eyelashes. Provoke itching, scratching, secondary infection, and curious bluish staining (maculae caeruliae). Eggs are stuck to the hairs.
  - *Treatment*: apply insecticides (see above) to affected areas and leave on for 1–2 days then repeat after a week. Treat sexual contacts.

Mites

- *Scabies mites* (*Sarcoptes scabei*): burrow under the skin, creating linear papulovesicular tracks, typically in the interdigital clefts and skin creases. There is intense itching, especially at night, provoking scratching, excoriation, and secondary infection. Transmitted by close physical contact. Exuberant crusting **(Norwegian scabies)** develops in immunocompromised patients.
  - *Treatment:* two treatments a week apart of aqueous lotion—0.5% malathion or 5% permethrin. Apply lotion to the whole body surface of all affected people and leave on for 24 h before being washing off. Itching may persist for several weeks and requires topical counter-irritant and corticosteroid (e.g. crotamiton and hydrocortisone) and sedating antihistamine (chlorphenamine at night). Ivermectin (200 mcg/kg single dose) is used for Norwegian scabies and in patients whose severe excoriations make topical treatment intolerably irritating and painful.
- *Trombiculid (harvest) mites:* sometimes known very misleadingly as 'chiggers' (see Tungosis 📖 p. 270), can infest in large numbers, especially under tight underpants, causing multiple, persisting, painful, itchy, blistering bites.
  - *Prevention:* use DEET-containing repellents, tuck trousers into boots, and avoid notorious 'mite islands' densely infested with trombiculids in cleared areas of jungle.

Bed bugs (Cimex)

At night, bed bugs emerge from cracks and crevices in the bedroom to bite sleeping humans. Insomnia and painful, red papules result.

Prevention

Discourage bites by keeping the light on all night, by sleeping under a permethrin-impregnated mosquito net, and putting newspaper under the under-sheet. Eradication is by thorough cleaning of the environment and application of the usual residual insecticides. Sleeping bags should be exposed to the sun (including both outside and inside) and treated with insecticide. However, insecticide-resistance has developed and bed bugs are becoming more abundant.

Ticks

- *Soft (argasid) ticks:* live in animal burrows and human dwellings. They attach briefly at night, engorge rapidly with blood, and then drop off and hide in cracks and crevices. Ticks of the genus *Ornithodoros* transmit relapsing fever.
- *Hard (ixodid) ticks* or their tiny nymphs may be picked up from vegetation or brought into gardens by deer or indoors by the dog. They find a secluded area (groin, perineum, waist, umbilicus, axilla, scalp, even external auditory meatus) and feed for days until they are spherical and engorged. Some species transmit Lyme disease (📖 p. 467), Rocky Mountain spotted fever (📖 p. 471), African tick fevers (📖 p. 471), European tick-borne encephalitis (📖 p. 458), Crimean–Congo haemorrhagic fever (📖 p. 464), Colorado tick fever, louping ill, babesiosis, ehrlichiosis, and other human infections. Some ticks in North America and Australia inject a neurotoxin (📖 p. 540).

Prevention of tick-transmitted infections

- Examine yourself at likely tick attachment sites (see above and use a mirror or a friend) when undressing at night while on the expedition.
- Avoid contact with tick-infested domestic animals.
- Wear light-coloured trousers against which ticks are more visible.
- Tuck trouser bottoms into boots.
- Apply DEET-containing repellents.
- Specific antibiotic chemoprophylaxis against tick-transmitted infections is not justified.

Removing ticks

Grasp the tick as close to your skin as possible with fine curved (iris) forceps (avoid squeezing the engorged body) and pull it out gently without twisting (Fig. 8.5). If the mouth parts break off, remove them separately with forceps or a needle. The aim is not to leave the barbed hypostome in the wound as it may provoke inflammation and granuloma formation. Keep the tick for later expert examination in case you become ill.

Invasive fly larvae (myiasis) and fleas (tungiasis)

Larvae (maggots) of some tropical flies hatch from eggs contaminating human skin and burrow into tissues, creating an uncomfortable, inflamed boil which seems to wriggle, exudes blood-stained pus, and has a definite head through which the larval spiracles may protrude ('myiasis'). Secondary infection may cause fever and lymphadenopathy.

The **human bot fly** (*Dermatobia hominis*) of Central and South America is also known as ver macaque, berne, el torsalo, or beefworm. Eggs are laid on mosquitoes which deposit them on human skin. The larvae grow for 10 weeks.

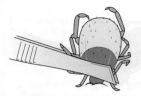

Fig. 8.5 Tick removal using forceps.

The **tumbu fly** (*Cordylobia anthropophaga*) of sub-Saharan Africa and southern Spain is also known as putsi fly or ver du cayor. Eggs are laid on sand, stick to clothes (e.g. washing laid out on the ground to dry), and hatch on the skin. Larvae penetrate and grow for 10 days.

• *Treatment:* folk remedies such as raw steak or bacon fat, and occlusion of the maggot's breathing hole in the skin with paraffin, petroleum gel, and candle wax occlusion sometimes work. However, attempts to squeeze them out like giant blackheads make matters worse. Injecting local anaesthetic into the base of the lesion may force the maggot out. The final solution is removal through a small scalpel incision.

• *Prevention:* hang washing to dry on a clothes line in strong sunlight; do not lay clothing on the ground. Iron washing to kill the tumbu fly ova.

Congo floor maggots, larvae of the fly *Auchmeromyia luteola*, live in earthen floors of huts throughout tropical Africa between latitudes 18°N and 26°S. They suck blood from those sleeping on the ground, causing local swelling and itching. Fumigate the hut and treat the bites symptomatically, making sure that no secondary infection is introduced (wipe the skin with tincture of iodine, and give systemic antimicrobials if there are signs of infection).

• *Prevention:* if possible, don't sleep on the ground (there are several other good reasons for this advice—see snake bites!).

Invasive myiasis, involving wounds, body orifices, and cavities: aggressive larvae of screw worm flies, such as *Cochliomyia (Callitroga) hominivorax* in Latin America and *Chrysomyia bessania* in eastern Europe, Africa, and Asia, hatch from eggs laid on wounds or on healthy mucosae (especially of the eye, orbit, nasal cavity, or external auditory meatus), and invade body cavities, orifices, and living tissue, causing life-threatening destruction and secondary infection.

- *Clinical:* there is pain, irritation, a feeling of wriggling movement, discharge of serosanguineous matter and maggots, obstruction (e.g. of the external auditory meatus causing deafness), and symptoms of secondary bacterial infection.
- *Treatment:* irrigation with sterile saline solution and dilute antiseptic is a first aid measure but eventually, thorough surgical debridement is essential.
- *Prevention:* protect wounds from flies.

Tungosis ('chigger', 'jigger' or 'chigoe' flea) (*Tunga penetrans*) occurs in Latin America and Africa. After fertilization the female flea jumps (feebly) and burrows alongside the nail fold or into the skin of the groin, loses its legs, and produces eggs each night. A painful swelling develops on the foot, typically under a toe nail, and there is a risk of secondary bacterial infection and ulceration.

- *Treatment:* the encapsulated flea must be curetted out (excised, ideally with a small surgical spoon with sharpened edge) and iodine applied. Complete enucleation is required.
- *Prevention:* wear proper shoes; do not walk around bare-footed.

'Creeping eruption' (cutaneous larva migrans): arthropod infestations must be distinguished from creeping eruption (**Coloured Plate 1**) which occurs in tropical countries worldwide. It is caused by larvae of cat and dog hookworms, such as *Ancylostoma braziliense, Uncinaria stenocephala,* and *Ancylostoma caninum*. Contact with contaminated ground (especially from sleeping rough on beaches in Central/Southern America) allows filariform larvae to penetrate the skin. They crawl under the skin a few millimetres each day, causing excruciating itching. Feet, buttocks, knees, hands, and back are commonly affected, sometimes by dozens of worms. The best treatment is 10–15% thiabendazole applied topically in paraffin ointment under occlusion for 1 week or, if that fails, oral albendazole 400 mg daily for 3 days or a single 200 mcg/kg dose of ivermectin (adult doses).

Leeches

Leeches are blood-sucking ectoparasites that live in the water or on moist land surfaces. Usually those encountered are small, 7–40 mm, but the largest ones are 45 cm long.

Aquatic leeches cause bleeding after entering the nose, mouth, nostrils, ears, eyes, vulva, urethra, or anus of swimmers or being swallowed in water from natural sources. They tend to remain attached for longer than terrestrial leeches.

Land leeches inhabit moist vegetation and may drop onto upper limbs from trees or vegetation, or rapidly climb up from the ground, fastening onto the legs. Usually, they are far more upsetting than harmful.

Attachment is via a three- or two-jaw bite giving a Y- or V-shaped incision.
There may be a tickling sensation or sharpness as they bite but, as they
inject local anaesthetic as well as anticoagulants, bites often go undetected
until bleeding is noticed. This may ooze for hours, but blood loss from a
single bite is insignificant.

- *Prevention:* leeches can squeeze through small gaps such as
  shoelace holes, and so boots, socks, or trousers offer little protection.
  Application of DEET to boots, socks, and skin or coarse tobacco
  rolled into the top of socks and kept moist is repellent. Take care
  when swimming and drink only filtered sterilized water. British
  troops in Malaya wore condoms at night for fear of urethral
  invasion by leeches while they slept.
- *Treatment:* if detected before attachment flick or pull off.

Once attached: ripping off can leave the mouth parts behind and predispose to infection. Apply salt (kept dry in a screwtop plastic container or
film canister), iodine tincture, alcohol, lighted cigarette, tobacco, or other
irritant to persuade them to release. This may precipitate regurgitation of
ingested blood into the wound and, to avoid secondary infection, treat as
an open wound; clean, apply antiseptic, and compression dressing.

If animal has attached inside the mouth, gargle with strong salt solution
but don't swallow as it may induce vomiting.

Leeches will spontaneously release after feeding. They harbour in their
gut symbiotic *Aeromonas hydrophila* which are potentially pathogenic.

Tropical ulcers

Tropical (phagedenic) ulcer

In tropical climates, even trivial wounds seem to heal slowly or persist. Classical tropical ulcers usually affect the shins and affect 30% of some indigenous communities. They start as minor abrasions (thorn prick, scratch, insect bite, existing skin lesion, pressure blister) that become infected with saprophytic bacteria (e.g. *Fusobacterium ulcerans*, *Borrelia vincentii*) in mud or stagnant water.

Clinical

A pustule appears and after 5–6 days discharges foul-smelling pus. Over the next few weeks a painful, circular ulcer develops with a defined, raised, undermined edge and floor of granulation tissue covered with purulent discharge. Over subsequent months and years the ulcer becomes painless but the infection penetrates to deeper tissue, tendon sheaths, periosteum and bone, becomes gangrenous and may show malignant transformation.

Treatment

In the early stages, high dose penicillin or erythromycin, preferably parenteral, may promote healing. Later, surgical debridement and recon-struction or even amputation may be needed.

Prevention

In tropical environments, especially in wet conditions, protect legs and ankles from scratches and pricks, and treat any new injury, however trivial, by washing with sterile (drinking) water, applying antiseptic or topical antibacterial (e.g. mupirocin), and protecting with a dry dressing.

Other types of tropical ulcer

(For Genital ulcers see p. 395)

Ulcerating skin lesions can be caused by many different tropical pathogens:

- Pyogenic bacteria (*Staphylococcus*, *Streptococcus*, *Berkholderia pseudomallei*—melioidosis).
- Cutaneous diphtheria ('desert' or 'veldt' sore).
- Spirochaetes (yaws).
- Mycobacteria (tuberculosis, *M. ulcerans*, 'Buruli ulcer').
- Protozoa (leishmaniasis).
- Fungi (histoplasmosis, cryptococcosis, and deep fungal infections).
- Non-infectious diseases such as sickle cell disease, varicose veins, and other vascular problems.

Other infective skin lesions

Other infective skin lesions

Pustules, furuncles, boils, styes, abscesses, paronychias, whitlows, cellulitis, erysipelas, ecthyma, and other painful, inflamed, and obviously infected skin and soft tissue lesions should be treated promptly. Depending on their stage of development and severity, they may require only topical antiseptic or antibiotic treatment, but systemic antibiotics are often needed.

Marine wound infections

Swimmers, scuba divers, fishermen, sailors, other boat people, and anyone in contact with marine or brackish water or sea animals are susceptible to wound infections and otitis externa caused by unusual pathogens acquired from salt water. Heatwaves associated with higher sea temperatures, even in the Baltic and North Seas, increase the risk. Infections complicate injuries such as coral cuts (📖 p. 545), skin penetration by fish or sea urchin spines and stings (📖 p. 542–6), and fish hooks, merely handling fish (erysipeloid) and other traumas associated with fishing and boating.

Marine pathogens

- Vibrios: *Vibrio vulnificus* infection starts with local erythema round the wound, followed by swelling, haemorrhagic blisters, necrotic ulceration, and severe systemic symptoms (fever, rigors, septic shock). Case fatality is high, especially in people with chronic debility (immunocompromise, chronic alcoholism, diabetes mellitus). *Vibrio parahaemolyticus* (see also Travellers' diarrhoea 📖 p. 380), *V. cholera*, and *V. alginolyticus* can also cause inflammation, sometimes within 8 h of injury, with the risk of deep, severe wound infections and bacteraemia in immunocompromised people.
- *Aeromonas hydrophila*: (brackish and fresh water) can cause myonecrosis and pyomyositis.
- *Erysipelothrix rhusiopathiae* (erysipeloid, 'seal finger', 'whale finger'): demarcated red/violaceous plaques appear on the hands after handling fish. The rash spreads proximally and may be associated with arthritis.
- *Plesiomonas shigelloides*, *Acinetobacter* spp., *Chromobacterium violaceum*, *Flavobacterium* spp. and *Pseudomonas aeruginosa* are commonly cultured from marine wounds.
- *Mycobacterium marinum* causes chronic granulomatous lesions in aquarium keepers and others who are exposed to sea water.
- *Staphylococcus aureus*, pyogenic *Streptococcus*, and enteric pathogens derived from the patient rather than the marine environment. However, the sea water near some popular beaches (e.g. Waikiki Beach, Honolulu) is heavily contaminated with *Staph. aureus*, including MRSA.
- Achlorous algae (*Prototheca* spp.): causes a chronic papule, plaque or ulcer, or olecranon bursitis, and may become disseminated in immunocompromised people.
- Free-living amoebae (*Acanthamoeba*, *Naegleria*, *Balamuthia mandrillaris*): a hazard of tropical ponds, swimming pools, saunas or spas can cause keratitis in contact lens wearers and encephalitis.

Diagnosis

Clinical suspicion based on history of marine exposure and underlying illness is crucial for early antibiotic treatment. Expert microbiology involves special cultures in 3% saline media. Biopsy and histopathology may yield the diagnosis.

Treatment

Urgent surgical debridement is needed if there is any suggestion of necrotizing fasciitis or myositis

Blind antibiotic treatment:
- For mild lesions: oral doxycycline or co-trimoxazole
- For severe lesions with systemic illness: combination treatment— tetracycline + aminoglycoside (e.g. gentamicin) + cefotaxime *or* tetracycline + aminoglycoside + a fluoroquinolone.

Specific treatment:
- Marine vibrios: doxycycline, co-trimoxazole, fluoroquinolone, gentamicin, cefotaxime, or co-amoxiclav (Augmentin).
- *Aeromonas hydrophila:* doxycycline, fluoroquinolone, gentamicin, or cefotaxime.
- Erysipeloid: penicillin or erythromycin or tetracycline.
- *M. marinum*: doxycycline or co-trimoxazole for trivial lesions; rifampicin and ethambutol for destructive lesions.

Others: as directed by laboratory sensitivities.

Prevention

Sensible behaviour, acquisition of technical skills, and appropriate protective clothing may reduce the risk of marine injuries. Beachcombers should not expose open wounds to sea water and should avoid eating undercooked or raw shellfish. Wounds contaminated by sea water should be cleaned immediately with drinking water (not rinsed in the brine). Foreign bodies should be removed and the wound watched carefully for early signs of infection. Start blind antibiotic treatment at the first hint of infection. For those at high risk of invasive marine vibrio infection (see above), prophylaxis with doxycycline or co-trimoxazole is recommended.

Minor skin conditions

Superficial fungal infections (dermatophytosis, ringworm, tinea)

Infection of the skin by *Trichophyton, Microsporum,* and *Epidermophyton* species is spread by direct contact with infected humans or animals or from soil saprophytes. It is common in tropical climates.

- *Clinical:* the classic lesion is a circumscribed round or oval scaly patch with vesicles around its border and central clearing (Colour Plate 2). Scalp, face, body, beard area, hands, nails (📖 p. 280), intertriginous areas (groins, axillae, 'dhobie's itch') and feet ('athletes foot' 📖 p. 280) may be affected. Hyperkeratotosis caused by scratching, and follicular and granulomatous lesions may be present.
- *Diagnosis:* direct microscopic examination of scrapings incubated for 20 min in 5–20% potassium hydroxide may reveal hyphae and spores. *Microsporium* spp. fluoresce green with Wood's lamp.
- *Treatment:* topical creams or ointments containing imidazoles or terbinafine are usually effective (see Athlete's foot 📖 p. 280), but nail and scalp infections require systemic treatment with imidazoles (e.g. ketoconazole 200 mg each day), triazoles (e.g. itraconazole 200 mg each day), or terbinafine (250 mg each day) for many months (adult doses).

http://www.bad.org.uk/healthcare/guidelines/Tinea_Capitis.pdf

Tinea (Pityriasis) versicolor

Skin infection with the yeast *Pitysporium orbiculare (Malassezia furfur)* spreads by direct contact, affecting half the population in some tropical communities. Scaly macular rashes coalesce over large areas usually of the trunk. They appear hyperpigmented or hypopigmented, or yellowish or brownish. Fine scales can be scraped off these lesions.

- *Treatment:* topical imidazoles, 20% sodium thiosulphate solution, Whitfield's ointment, or selenium sulphide, or ketoconazole shampoos are applied overnight repeatedly. Relapses are common.

Skin conditions of the hands and feet

Ingrowing toenails

An edge of a big toe nail is forced into the nail fold either by pressure of tight footwear or abnormal growth. This causes trauma, pain, bleeding, or serosanguineous discharge and infection of the nail fold (inflammation, swelling, pus formation; paronychia see below) that can make walking very painful.

- *Treatment:* soak in saline, clean with antiseptic, apply antiseptic cream, and relieve compressing footwear. Trimming the nail may make matters worse. Curative treatment of intractable ingrowing toenails: under digital block (📖 p. 566) incise the side of the nail back to and including the nail bed (Fig. 8.6).
- *Prevention:* cut toe nails straight across and avoid wearing tight footwear, especially brand new boots that have not been worn and thoroughly broken in before the expedition.

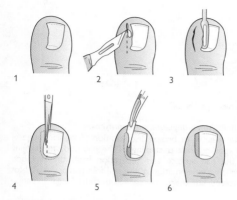

Fig. 8.6 Relief of paronychia or ingrowing toenail.

Paronychia

Frequent immersion of the hands in infected water may result in chronic *Candida* and acute staphylococcal nail fold infections. There is painful redness and swelling of the nail fold. Pus may be trapped under the nail. *Pseudomonas aeruginosa* infection causes greenish discoloration of the nail and foul-smelling greenish pus.

- Treatment: initially, warm saline soaks, topical antiseptic or antibacterial cream, and drainage of abscesses may be curative. Otherwise, consider systemic antibiotics or removal of the nail edge(s) under digital block (📖 p. 566) as for ingrowing toe nails.

Whitlow (felon)

Acute swelling, redness, inflammation, and throbbing pain of the pulp space of finger or toe is usually caused by *Staphylococcus* or *Streptococcus* from a splinter or spread from paronychia. Contact with Herpes simplex causes a whitlow with painful vesicles. Orf, a sheep virus, causes pustular whitlow. Inflammatory swelling in the pulp space may compress the digital artery, causing necrosis. The terminal phalanx may be infected. Nail biters, especially diabetics, may self-inoculate oral *Eikenella corrodens*.

- Treatment: initially try warm saline soaks and antibiotics for suspected pyogenic infection (flucloxacillin or erythromycin) and aciclovir for herpetic whitlow. If tense, painful swelling persists, a relieving incision (Fig. 8.7) may be needed under digital block (📖 p. 566). Herpetic whitlows should not be incised as this may spread the infection.

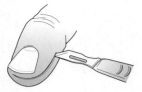

Fig. 8.7 Incision for relieving a whitlow.

Fungal infection of nails (tinea unguium, onychomycosis)
Initially there is white, yellow, or brown discoloration of the free edge of the nail and later hyperkeratotic thickening of the nail bed, and ridging and crumbling of the nail surface and separation from the nail bed (onycholysis). There is no inflammation of the nail fold (paronychia). Not all the nails are involved but there is usually superficial fungal infection elsewhere.

- *Treatment:* early infection responds to topical amorolfine (Loceryl) nail lacquer or tioconazole (Trosyl) cutaneous solution. Established infection requires systemic terbinafine 250 mg or itraconazole 200 mg each day for 3 months.

http://www.bad.org.uk/healthcare/guidelines/onychomycosis.pdf

Athlete's foot (tinea pedis)
In shoe and sock wearers, skin of the interdigital spaces between the toes, especially the third and fourth, may become greyish white, moist, macerated, fissured, dehiscent, itchy, and sore. An associated vesicular eruption is common. Lesions may become secondarily infected, causing cellulitis of the lower leg.

- Treatment: wear sandals at least in camp and keep the interdigital spaces dry and clean. Terbinafine (Lamisil) cream applied twice daily for 1 week is the most effective antifungal, but a wide range of cheaper preparations is also effective such as compound benzoic acid (Whitfield's) ointment and -azole creams (e.g. clo-trimazole).

Head and neck

Section editor
Chris Johnson

Contributors
Stephen Hearns, Annabel Nickol, Paul Cooper,
Daniel Morris, and David Geddes

Anatomy

The skull is a complex structure, initially comprising 29 bones, but these fuse during childhood, leaving mobile only the lower jaw and three pairs of tiny bones within the middle ears. Eight bones form the cranium that protects the brain, while another fourteen provide the supporting structure for the eyes, nose, and facial muscles. Areas of the head are described according to their underlying bony parts (Fig. 9.1). The eyes lie protected within the orbit, while the prominent nose is susceptible to injury.

The breathing and digestive passages cross in the oropharynx, requiring complex mechanisms to ensure correct routing (Fig. 9.2). The nose and upper airway form a humidification and filtering mechanism. The opening to the lower airway is the larynx, a complex cartilaginous structure hung from the hyoid bone, which in turn is slung from the base of the skull. When foods or fluids are swallowed, the epiglottis, a roof-like flap, closes over the glottis and protects the trachea. Inside the lower end of the larynx are the vocal cords, used both to provide a watertight seal to the airways and to phonate. These are fixed in the midline anteriorly, but attached to the arytenoid cartilages posteriorly. Movement of the arytenoids permits alterations both to the position and the tension of the vocal cords. The two prominent thyroid cartilages form the anterior border, the 'Adam's apple' of the larynx. Just below these cartilages is an obvious groove, the cricothyroid membrane—the safest location of emergency surgical access to the airway.

The swallowing mechanism primarily involves the tongue and oropharynx. Movement of a food or fluid bolus to the back of the mouth causes reflex closure of the larynx and a peristaltic wave to pass down the oesophagus. Tongue swelling or a sore throat will disrupt swallowing.

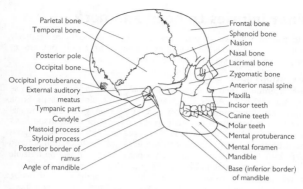

Fig. 9.1 Bony structures of head.

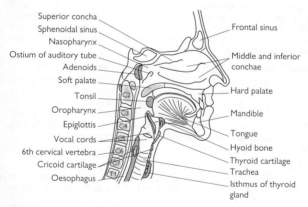

Fig. 9.2 Anatomy of the airway.

Minor injuries to head and neck

Head injuries such as bruises, black eyes, or lacerations are relatively common; more serious head injuries are fortunately rare, but are an ever-present risk during outdoor activities.

Lacerations (📖 p. 252)

Scalp lacerations tend to bleed a lot initially and can look a lot worse than they really are. Apply firm pressure until the bleeding stops. Small wounds can be closed using cyanoacrylate tissue glue. Conventional superglue has been used for this purpose, but can provoke tissue reactions and is not recommended[1]. The area around larger lacerations should be shaved and cleaned, and the edges of the laceration sutured (📖 p. 254). If appropriate medical kit is not available, it may be possible to approximate the wound by tying the patient's hair across it.

Facial lacerations usually heal well, but it is important to minimize scarring. Clean the wounds and, where possible, use glue or skin fixers (Steri-Strips™, etc.) to bring the edges together. If wounds are deep, try to remove tension from the surface by placing subcutaneous sutures to approximate the edges and then suture the skin itself using as fine a suture material as possible (ideally '6/0') to finish the job. Ensure that tension is even throughout the wound and that the edges are aligned. When a lip has been cut, make every effort to realign the vermilion edges, as even small deviations are very obvious and may require subsequent corrective plastic surgery.

Nasal injuries (see Nasal fractures 📖 p. 287 and Epistaxis 📖 p. 320)

Injured noses tend to bleed a lot. If a nose is broken and deformed it may be possible to straighten it soon after the injury, although the casualty may be reluctant to permit this. Apply cool compresses and pressure to areas of bruising. Pressure over the soft tissues of the nose will control almost all nose bleeds, although rarely it may be necessary to pack a nostril using either a nasal tampon or ribbon gauze lubricated with paraffin ointment or a suitable antibiotic ointment.

Tongue

Bitten tongues and burnt tongues are usually made worse by attempting surgical treatment. Provide pain relief, rest, and keep the patient head-up if there is significant airway swelling.

1 Cascarini L and Kumar A. Case of the month: Honey I glued the kids: tissue adhesives are not the same as "superglue". *Emerg Med J* (2007) **24**: 228–31.

Fractured facial bones

Detailed diagnosis of facial bone fractures is impossible and irrelevant in a remote environment. Fractures to both the mandible and maxilla will cause pain and swelling, limit diet, and may threaten the airway. The best advice is to arrange early evacuation to the nearest specialist care. However, this may take time and in the interim the following can help, assuming there are no other life-threatening injuries:

- Reduce and stabilize the fracture.
- Apply comfortable and supportive bandaging.
- Arrange for a soft food or liquid diet if the upper and lower teeth have been splinted together.
- Provide details of the circumstances of the accident, treatment to date, and medication.
- Arrange for a carer to accompany the patient to specialist care.

Mandibular fractures

There are two common fracture sites. Both are seen following a fall or blow to the chin.

- *Condylar fracture*: a horizontal fracture through the base of the condyle about 2 cm below the temporomandibular joint (TMJ).
- *Vertical fracture*: in the premolar region, often associated with the mental foramen, which is positioned between the root apices of the lower premolar teeth. The nerve exiting this hole provides sensation to the lower lip.

Treatment of a condylar fracture

A *condylar fracture* is beyond your ability to reduce in the field. It will typically present as an inability to open and close the mouth, and pain in and below the TMJ. The upper face may be very swollen. Treat as follows:

- Make casualty comfortable with padded vertical bandaging to immobilize the mandible.
- If there are no contraindications, give NSAIDs (ibuprofen or diclofenac) to reduce swelling. If swallowing tablets proves difficult, persuade the casualty that suppositories are a good idea.
- Arrange soft food diet.
- Evacuate.

Treatment of a vertical fracture

In a very remote area, you may be able to reduce and splint a **vertical fracture** through the mental region of the mandible using figure-of-eight wiring (Fig. 10.2) around the teeth. The location of the fracture will often be obvious, as there may be a step between the fractured segments. The muscles of the neck will have the effect of pulling the most mobile fractured element downwards. The objective is to identify teeth that are not mobile on either side of the fracture line and reduce the fracture by splinting using wire in lengths of about 20 cm. Once the fracture is reduced, it can be located by applying a figure-of-eight wire to the opposing upper teeth and then connecting the two sets of wires. That is the theory. This is a fussy procedure that is possible in the field if you have good light, an accurately placed mandibular local anaesthetic block, wire, strong tweezers, and wire-cutting thin-nosed pliers. The patient will need to be stoical.

- Decide whether to attempt wire splinting.
- Apply padded vertical bandaging.
- If no contraindication, give NSAIDs (ibuprofen or diclofenac) to reduce swelling. If swallowing is difficult, persuade the casualty that suppositories are a good idea.
- Arrange soft food diet.
- Evacuate.

Maxillary fracture

There are many categories. Fractures will most commonly occur to the zygomatic arch where the chewing muscles attach. Difficulty in opening and closing the jaw will be typical, with pain in the region of the temporalis muscle. Fractures of the middle third of the face may be suspected if there is evidence of periorbital bruising and swelling. This can look quite dramatic. Make the casualty as comfortable as possible with vertical padded bandaging (Fig. 9.3) and evacuate immediately.

Nasal fracture

- Examine for signs of significant head injury in patients with nasal injuries.
- The diagnosis of a nasal fracture is a clinical one. X-rays are not routinely required. Swelling, tenderness, and possibly deformity of the bridge of the nose are visible.
- It is essential to look for and exclude a septal haematoma—a smooth swelling of the midline of the nose that can develop into septal necrosis. In the wilderness a septal haematoma should be incised under local anaesthetic, and then the nostrils packed to prevent recurrence.

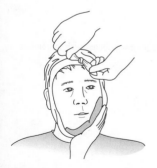

Fig. 9.3 Vertical padded bandage. If the casualty is conscious and not seriously injured, sit them up with head well forward to allow secretions to drain. Support jaw with soft pad. Ask casualty to hold in place and tie bandage around the casualty's head, tying it with knot on top of head. Additional padding is required for maxillary fractures.

- Swelling often prevents an early assessment of the degree of nasal deformity. Between 5 and 7 days after injury, the nose should be re-examined; if there is evidence of deformity or septal deviation, the patient requires evacuation for specialist ENT assessment and management. Deformities should be corrected operatively within 10 days of injury.
- Open fractures of the nose require prophylactic antibiotics such as co-amoxiclav or erythromycin.

Blow-out fracture of orbit following blunt trauma

Blunt trauma to the globe of the eye, perhaps from a fall or a punch, can cause the bony orbit to fracture (Fig. 9.4). The weakest point is the orbital floor and a blow-out fracture inferiorly often causes prolapse of orbital fat into the maxillary sinus below. There can also be tethering of the inferior rectus eye muscle, causing double vision, particularly when the patient looks up.

Diagnosis is made of the basis of:
- History
- Pain on eye movement
- Double vision (diplopia)
- Sunken eye (enophthalmos).

If you suspect this injury:
- Check visual acuity
- Assess globe integrity
- If the double vision is intolerable, cover the damaged eye with a patch (see Fig. 9.6).

Injuries of this type may also lead to:
- Corneal abrasion
- Hyphaema (blood in the anterior chamber of the eye)
- Subluxed lens
- Vitreous haemorrhage
- Retinal detachment
- Posterior globe rupture.

If visual acuity is reduced following blunt trauma, evacuation is imperative.

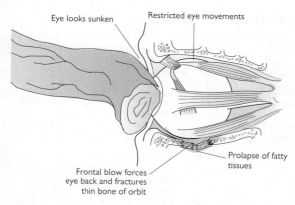

Fig. 9.4 Mechanism of injury in an orbital blow-out fracture.

Cervical spine injuries

Neck injuries occurring in remote areas are challenging as they are accompanied by a fear of missing an unstable injury that could lead to neurological impairment. In an urban environment it is relatively straightforward to immobilize patients with neck injuries for short periods en route to hospital where significant injuries can be excluded by an experienced emergency physician or radiological imaging. Such practice in remote areas may not be as appropriate, as prolonged immobilization during evacuation is potentially harmful to the patient and to rescuers. Therefore thorough examination techniques and appropriate experience are required in assessing and managing cervical spine injuries in the expedition environment.

Anyone who has had a significant force applied to their head or neck, especially if they are now unconscious, should be considered to have a neck injury and should have their neck initially immobilized until it can be fully assessed. The history taken should include the mechanism of injury, location of pain, and the presence of any neurological symptoms. Examination should identify areas of localized tenderness, swelling, or bruising. Sensation, tone, and power should also be examined and documented for all four limbs. Active range of cervical spine movement should only be assessed if the medic is sure that the presence of any significant underlying injury is unlikely.

Spinal immobilization

When initially assessing a patient with a potential neck injury, the patient's head should be gently supported on either side. Avoid covering the patient's ears as this makes communication difficult. The head and spine should be held in a neutral position. Careful manual in-line stabilization is a satisfactory method of preventing further injury.

If a neck injury cannot be excluded in the field then the patient will require immobilization for transfer. Complete spinal immobilization is only possible if a properly fitted cervical collar is used, together with sandbags on each side of the head, and tapes to fix position relative to the two sides of the stretcher. Cervical collars used without bags or tape provide insufficient immobilization. Cervical collars come in a variety of sizes. In the expedition setting it is appropriate to carry one adult multi-size collar such as the Stifnek select™. This cuts down on weight and cost.

Patients transferred on stretchers are prone to pressure area necrosis; this is more common in the presence of a sensory deficit. For this reason, spinal boards, whether commercially manufactured or improvised, should be used for extrication only, and should not be used for evacuation. Best practice for prolonged transfer of spinally-injured patients is a vacuum mattress, but only very large expeditions would be likely to take such a piece of equipment. It would be advisable to place a Thermarest™ or Karrimat™ type sleeping mattress under the patient if carried on a hard surface during evacuation.

Assessing and managing neck injuries

Most but not all spinal injuries will result from one of the following three causes:

- A fall from a height
- Being struck by a falling object
- A high speed road traffic collision (RTC).

The neck should always be fully immobilized if there has been a dangerous mechanism of injury, such as:

- Fall >1 m or five stairs
- After diving
- A high speed road traffic collision (>65 mph), a rollover, or ejection from a vehicle.
- If the patient is over 65 years of age, the risk of injury increases and immobilization is recommended.

Provided that:

- The casualty is fully alert (GCS score 15)
- The casualty is not under the influence of drugs or alcohol
- There is no distracting painful injury such as a chest, abdominal, or thigh fracture
- There are no neurological signs or symptoms such as tingling
- There is no midline bony tenderness of the neck bones

and if any of the following apply:

- The neck pain has a delayed onset
- The patient is sitting or has walked since the injury
- The neck injury followed a rear-end vehicle collision.

then it should be safe to let the patient move their head 45° to the left and right slowly. If this is possible then the neck collar can be removed and investigations are not required. Stop and reapply the collar if tingling develops in the extremities. These rules follow the principles of NICE guidelines and the Canadian rules for radiography of cervical spines following injury[2].

Acute neck sprains

These most commonly result from low velocity rear-end road traffic collisions. The trapezius and sternomastoid muscles may be injured. Neck sprains are managed with analgesia and encouragement to mobilize. Immobilization with neck collars causes stiffness and should be avoided.

Fractures and dislocations of the neck

These are indicated by the mechanism of injury, usually severe pain, and localized midline tenderness of the cervical spine. Assessment and exclusion without the aid of X-rays is difficult, especially for the inexperienced. If in doubt, immobilize and evacuate for specialist assessment.

2 Eyre A (2006). Overview and comparison of NEXUS and Canadian C-spine rules. *Am J Clin Med* **3**: 12–16.

Head injury

A person should be considered to have a head injury if they have suffered any trauma to the head, apart from superficial lacerations to the face. Head injuries can be:
- Direct or indirect
- Closed or open

and may result in:
- Primary or secondary brain damage.

Epidemiology

It is best to avoid a head injury! About 60% of adults with moderate head injuries and 85% with severe head injuries remain disabled 1 year after their accident. Even a minor head injury can ruin a trip: 3 months later 80% have persistent headaches and 60% have memory problems.

Causes

- Direct head injuries are caused by a blow to the head of some form; this can result in a closed injury, without penetration of the skull, or an open injury, where the skull is penetrated.
- Indirect injury is caused by a 'whiplash' effect of the brain moving within the skull, though without a direct blow to the head; this can result in brief concussion, but in a young adult is unlikely to cause significant damage.

History and examination

- Ask about amnesia for events before or after the injury. Brief amnesia, of less than 1 min, is common with even mild concussion, but any significant amnesia should be a cause for concern. Significant head injuries are usually associated with amnesia of 30 min or more.
- Care is particularly needed for high energy injuries, for example a pedestrian struck by a vehicle, any high speed road traffic collision or any accident involving motorized off-road vehicles such as snowmobiles, jet skis, or quad bikes. High-energy injuries also include any significant fall from a height, or any rock fall.
- Assess *level of consciousness*, using the Glasgow Coma Scale (📖 p. 192). This is easily and reliably administered with minimal experience and is particularly useful to monitor progress. Failure of the GCS to improve and, in particular, a fall in GCS is of significant concern. The scale has a range of 3–15. A score of 8 or less indicates a very severe head injury, one that, if it were available, would prompt immediate critical care. A score of 12 or less at any point after a closed head injury indicates possible significant injury, but secondary intracranial bleeding can develop even in someone fully conscious initially.
- Carry out *careful inspection* of the head, looking particularly for signs of any skull fracture. Classically basal skull fracture may be associated with:
  - Cerebrospinal fluid leaking from ear (otorrhoea) or nose (rhinorrhoea).
  - Blood behind tympanic membrane ('haemotympanum').

- 'Battle sign' (bruising and tenderness over mastoid).
- 'Panda eyes' (black eye(s) without orbital injury).
- However, these signs are often absent.
- Carry out and document a **simple neurological examination**. As a minimum this should include:
  - Examination of pupil size and reaction.
  - Check of visual acuity.
  - Eye movements.
  - Examine tympanic membranes if possible.
  - Always assess hearing.
  - Gag reflex if not fully conscious.
  - Examine for any focal motor deficit, including plantar responses.
  - Check for any sensory loss.
  - Ask about paraesthesia.
  - Check for ataxia.
- Look out for irritability and/or altered behaviour, persistent headaches, or vomiting. An apparent convulsion at the moment of impact is a well recognized feature of concussion, often seen in contact sports, and need not be of great significance. Any subsequent seizure is of great concern.
- Do not attribute a depressed conscious level and/or altered behaviour to intoxication with alcohol or drugs unless you are sure that there has been no significant brain injury. Any intoxicated person with a suspected head injury needs close observation.
- Always carefully examine the spine, especially the cervical spine in any significant head injury, particularly those with a dangerous mechanism of injury. Around 10–15% of those knocked out with a head injury have an associated neck injury (📖 p. 290).
- Document any findings and repeat examination; judgement is needed to determine the frequency and extent of repeat examination, but if you are concerned about a possible significant head injury it would be reasonable to repeat GCS every 15 min for 2 h; by then the GCS should be 13 or better. Continue to repeat regularly until the GCS is normal, and do not leave the person alone for 24 h.

Avoiding head injury

Wear a helmet! Even a minor head injury from a falling stone, or standing up too quickly in a confined space such as a cave, can result in persistent dizziness, headaches, and poor concentration.

Clinical features

Closed head injury:
- Results from falls, RTCs, etc.
- Typically high energy injury.
- No penetration of the skull.
- *Primary* damage tends to be diffuse:
  - Diffuse axonal injury.
  - Some focal damage, particularly to vulnerable areas such as frontal lobes, anterior temporal, and posterior occipital poles.

Open head injury:
- Results from bullet wounds, etc. with penetration of the skull.
- *Primary* damage is largely focal but the effects can be just as serious.

Secondary deterioration is usually due to:
- *Oedema* (swelling) of damaged tissue, resulting in increased intracranial pressure and possible brain herniation.
- Intracranial haemorrhage (bleeding) from torn vessels, which can be:
  - *Subdural*: between the dura and the brain.
  - *Extradural*: outside the dura, beneath the skull vault.

Swelling inside the closed cranium interferes with blood flow into the brain. Cerebral perfusion pressure (CPP) is the balance of mean arterial pressure (MAP) less intracranial pressure (ICP):

$$CPP = MAP - ICP$$

It is therefore important to maintain blood pressure, with fluid replacement, and minimize ICP. Factors that increase ICP that can be correctable in the wilderness include pain and hypoxia due to altitude.

Management

Management options for a significant head injury in a remote environment are limited.
- Maintain airway and breathing, and replace fluids when possible.
- Assess and manage cervical spine.
- Give adequate analgesia to control pain, and try to be calm and provide reassurance. Opiates, if available, may be needed to control severe pain, but can mask signs of deteriorating cerebral function. Tramadol is best avoided unless nothing else is available as it can increase the risk of seizures and can cause confusion.
- Elevation of the head to 20° improves venous outflow from the brain and may reduce ICP, therefore increasing CPP. This should only be attempted after any hypovolaemia has been corrected. If a patient is hypovolaemic, elevating the head will reduce MAP.
- If the casualty is at altitude sufficient to cause hypoxia then, if possible, bring them down, and give oxygen when available.
- Steroids should not be given; they have been shown to increase mortality rates.
- Secondary deterioration owing to cerebral oedema may respond to diuretics. Mannitol is preferred because it causes less electrolyte disturbance than loop diuretics, but it is unlikely to be available. Furosemide and other diuretics should be used with care; give sufficient to induce diuresis, but ensure that blood pressure is maintained.
- Deterioration caused by intracranial bleeding is usually untreatable in the wilderness, though a doctor familiar with the technique might in desperation attempt a burr hole to relieve a developing extradural haematoma.

- The major issue is whether to arrange evacuation. This decision depends on the situation and the severity of the injury. Most head injuries do not require neurosurgery, but there are many factors following any significant injury that are better managed in hospital, and secondary deterioration because of intracranial bleeding is potentially correctable. If evacuation is realistically possible, following anything other than a minor head injury it should be arranged.

Complications

- *Infection*: meningitis is a recognized complication of any skull fracture where the integrity of the blood–brain barrier may be breached. If transfer to hospital may be delayed it is appropriate to give a broad spectrum antibiotic. There is particular risk if there is a CSF leak, a common presentation of which is the loss of clear, slightly salty, watery fluid coming from the nose or ear.
- *Seizures*: epileptic seizures can occur early or late. Early seizures, within 24 h, may not require long-term treatment, but in the wilderness any seizure is best treated until definitive care is available. A seizure should be considered a sign of possible intracranial deterioration. Medication available is likely to be limited to a benzodiazepine such as lorazepam or diazepam. The risk of sedation is outweighed by the need to control seizures.
- *Neurological symptoms*: these can be divided into minor symptoms that can follow any concussion, and more significant deficits. Headaches, disequilibrium, and poor concentration are common after minor head injury; they are likely to last for up to 3 months and possibly longer. Benign positional vertigo can follow any blow to the head; it results in intense vertigo with a sensation of spinning precipitated by movement of the head. Give prochlorperazine or cyclizine and arrange an ENT assessment.

Severe head injuries have protean consequences, and may require long-term rehabilitation.

Website

http://www.nice.org.uk/guidance/CG56

Blackouts, syncope, and epilepsy

Blackouts

An episode of transient loss of consciousness is often referred to as a 'blackout'. This is a useful colloquialism, because it makes no inference as to the mechanism of transient loss of consciousness, or the underlying pathophysiology.

Blackouts commonly result from:-

• A disorder of the circulation—e.g. syncope (fainting).
• A disorder of the brain—e.g. epilepsy.
• A disorder of the psyche—e.g. psychogenic blackouts.

It may prove difficult, if not impossible, to determine the cause of some blackouts in the wilderness. Misdiagnosis is common, with rates exceeding 25% even if diagnostic facilities exist. Any previous diagnosis in an expedition member should be treated with caution, particularly if there are unusual features about the new attack.

Epidemiology

Blackouts are universal, although the possible causes vary between populations owing to various factors, including endemic diseases and cultural factors. Various neurological infections such as neurocysticercosis may present with seizures; many conditions associated with HIV, particularly toxoplasmosis, may cause epilepsy, and there are a number of well recognized culturally determined causes of psychogenic attacks, such as Latah in Malaysia. Latah occurs in certain cultural groups, where a minor fright leads to a prolonged and vigorous physical display of fear or anger over which the victim has little or no control. These factors may influence the likely causes of blackouts seen in local populations.

Incidence

Doctors often assume that a blackout is neurological, due to epilepsy. In fact, cardiac syncope accounts for most blackouts, and of these the majority are cases of reflex syncope, with up to 30% of people suffering reflex syncope during their lives. In contrast, epilepsy only affects about 0.5% of the population at any one time, with a lifetime incidence of 2%, although many of these will develop at one or other extreme of age. Blackouts are also often seen in the absence of organic physical disease; these attacks may be accompanied by apparent convulsive movements, and the possibility that an episode may be psychological should be considered, particularly in the context of stressful situations.

Syncope

Syncope is a cardiovascular disorder. Causes can therefore be divided into *cardiac* and *vascular*:

• *Cardiac causes* are either underlying structural heart disease or an arrhythmia. Sudden death in young people is occasionally associated with a structural cardiomyopathy. An arrhythmia in the wilderness is likely to be a marker of myocardial infarction. Syncope *during* (as opposed to *after*) exercise is potentially serious and may presage sudden cardiac death owing to a familial arrhythmia syndrome such as long QT.

- *Vascular causes* are more likely, and include:
  - Reflex causes, such as vasovagal syncope.
  - Situational causes, such as cough and micturition syncope.
  - Postural causes, such as orthostatic hypotension which may reflect dehydration.
- In hot environments, consider heatstroke.
- Pulmonary embolism.

Clinical diagnosis

Diagnosis is made from the history, particularly the circumstances around the blackout. Syncope results in transient self-limited loss of consciousness owing to transient global cerebral hypoperfusion, typically leading to collapse; most attacks, particularly those with vascular causes, therefore occur when patient is upright, although fainting can occur while sitting.

- The patient may recall a brief prodrome of lightheadedness, when voices sounded distant, and vision faded.
- Onset is rapid; recovery is spontaneous, complete, and usually prompt.
- During the episode the pulse may be slow and blood pressure low, but often the episode is too brief and the bystanders too panicked for either to be reliably measured.
- The patient characteristically appears limp and white.
- Myoclonic limb jerks commonly occur. These are usually brief, but complex movements resembling epilepsy can be seen. This 'convulsive syncope' often results in panic in bystanders and may be reported as an 'epileptic fit' by even medically trained observers unfamiliar with the phenomenon.
- The profound pallor of syncope often results in witnesses saying afterwards that they thought that the person had died.
- During recovery there may be brief bewilderment, but prolonged confusion is rare.
- If the person gets up too quickly they may collapse again.
- Victim may be sweaty, and complain of thirst.

Epilepsy

Broadly, epilepsy, as a disorder, can be classified as *idiopathic*, a condition in isolation, or *symptomatic*, resulting from some underlying disease. The resulting seizures are either *generalized*, involving the whole brain from onset, or *focal*, starting in one area but then maybe generalizing.

- *Idiopathic epilepsy* usually starts in childhood, and is therefore unlikely to be a diagnostic issue in the wilderness; however, there are some syndromes that may first appear during adolescence, and may therefore affect youth groups (see below). Idiopathic epilepsies usually cause generalized seizures, tonic–clonic convulsions, myoclonus, and absences.
- *Symptomatic epilepsy*, particularly in the context of wilderness medicine, is more likely to result in focal or secondarily generalized seizures. The fit may indicate an underlying localized brain disorder, and in these circumstances concern should be raised about infection, including cerebral malaria.

A separate classification describes the resultant seizures: these are *partial* or *generalized*.

Partial (or 'focal') seizures
- More likely to be caused by a symptomatic epilepsy; that is, where pathology has developed in part of the brain, causing the seizures—this is potentially of more concern in the wilderness.
- Start in one area, and spread; this is reflected in the associated symptoms and behaviour, which may or may not result in loss of awareness, and which may or may not result in collapse.
- An essential component of any witness's account, to determine that the episode is a partial seizure, is therefore a detailed description of the onset of the attack, which may include automatic behaviour, asymmetrical limb jerking, or a forced turn of the head.
- The patient may afterwards recall a strong unpleasant smell, or a brief but intense sense of déjà-vu.

Generalized seizures
- Involve the whole of the brain.
- Best recognized form is a tonic–clonic convulsion.
- Onset is sudden with an initial tonic phase; all muscles stiffen, the limbs are rigid, and there may be a strangled cry; the person falls to the ground. Victim may become cyanosed.
- The subsequent clonic phase involves rhythmic jerking of the limbs; initially this may be vigorous, but the movements slow and become irregular.
- Victim is then usually unconscious for a period.
- When they come round they may be confused, which can be prolonged, muscles may ache, and they will usually complain of headache.
- They may have bitten the tongue (usually the side).
- The tonic–clonic seizure itself rarely lasts more than 1–2 min, but post-ictal drowsiness and confusion can be prolonged, with general malaise occasionally lasting 24 h or more.
- A generalized tonic–clonic convulsion can also develop from an initial partial seizure, the seizure activity starting focally and then spreading to the whole brain; these are secondarily generalized convulsions.

The other types of generalized seizures are unlikely to be an issue in the wilderness. These include collapse, rigid (*tonic seizure*) or without loss of muscle tone (*atonic seizure*); these usually only occur in the context of a complex epilepsy associated with learning disability. Generalized seizures also include *absences*, with preserved posture, and *daytime myoclonus*, both of which may be seen in idiopathic childhood and juvenile epilepsies which will usually have been previously diagnosed.

Psychogenic blackouts and disturbances

These range from simple panic attacks with hyperventilation, which rarely cause blackout and are usually readily recognized, to a wide spectrum of non-epileptic seizures. Patients are usually adolescents or young adult women[3] and may have very frequent episodes, sometimes occurring many times a day. Attacks are non-stereotypical and unresponsive to medication, without obvious cause for apparent intractable epilepsy. The assessment of psychogenic blackouts is likely to be very difficult in the wilderness, requires specialist advice, and, although the circumstances of an expedition may well predispose to such attacks, the diagnosis should only be made with extreme caution.

Differential diagnosis of blackouts and seizures

If you consider that the blackout is due to syncope, then check for any systemic illness, which may have predisposed to this:

- Anaemia is a common factor, particularly in young women who faint; check for blood loss—acute or chronic.
- Dehydration or heat exhaustion.
- Salt deficiency.
- Excess alcohol can predispose to fainting, possibly due to dehydration, and excess alcohol can also be a factor in epileptic seizures.
- Hypoxia and high altitude cerebral oedema (HACE 🕮 p. 626) may cause fitting.
- An initial epileptic seizure may be an indication of an underlying neurological disease presenting for the first time. This is especially likely if the seizures are focal in onset. There are several possible causes:
  - *Neurocysticercosis* is the most common cause of new adult onset epilepsy in rural, developing countries with poor hygiene, where pigs are allowed to roam freely. It results from human ingestion of the eggs from the pork tape worm. Visitors are vulnerable, the condition usually presenting some months after exposure. Other parasitic diseases, including *schistosomiasis*, may also present with epilepsy.
  - *Bacterial meningitis* can cause seizures, but the individual is likely to be unwell with fever, photophobia, and a stiff neck at this stage. Likewise, *cerebral malaria* can present with seizures, and should always be considered in malarial zones.
  - There is a specific epilepsy syndrome, *juvenile myoclonic epilepsy* (JME), which commonly starts in adolescence, and in which seizures typically occur in the morning, precipitated by sleep deprivation with or without excess alcohol. JME presents with generalized convulsions and is often accompanied by myoclonic jerks. It may be a consideration in youth groups; there is often but not always a family history.

3 Reuber M, Elger CE (2003). Psychogenic nonepileptic seizures: review and update. *Epilepsy & Behavior* **4(3)**: 205–16.

Investigations

Few investigations are possible in the wilderness. Check pulse and temperature to check for systemic illness, and check blood glucose if possible. If you consider syncope and have access to ECG then this is worthwhile. Measure oxygen saturation if a pulse oximeter is available.

Management

- Assess whether the diagnosis is likely to be epilepsy, or if the episode might be convulsive syncope.
- Question the patient carefully for any prior history that they may have concealed to secure a place on the trip. If they are confused, or you doubt their medical history, consider contacting their family or GP if communications are available.
- Carry out as comprehensive a neurological examination as you are able to, looking carefully for papilloedema if possible, and checking for any persisting focal neurological deficit.
- If you assess this to be a first seizure, particularly if the patient is unwell, if there are any focal features to the seizure, or focal neurological deficit, then evacuate if at all possible.
- Consider cerebral malaria (📖 p. 474) and give therapeutic doses of antimalarials if in doubt.
- Seizures can rarely complicate HACE (📖 p. 626); if this is the case then intensify treatment for the HACE and hasten descent.
- If you believe that a team member has developed epilepsy for the first time in a wilderness environment, particularly in the tropics, then seek expert advice or evacuate if possible.

Treatment

- During the seizure, move the patient only if essential to protect from injury. Take the pulse; it is quicker and easier to compare the patient's pulse to your own, rather than to try and count it. If the pulse is weak, thready, and particularly if slow then consider convulsive syncope.
- Turn patient on their side into the recovery position.
- Give oxygen if available, particularly if the seizure is prolonged.
- Do not attempt to force anything into their mouth.
- Your choice of available anti-epileptic drugs is likely to be limited. Most seizures are self-limiting, and a single seizure does not require treatment unless the situation is such that a further seizure could be catastrophic.
- If the seizure is prolonged, with a convulsion lasting more than 2 min, then give any available benzodiazepine intravenously, intramuscularly or rectally at a dose equivalent to 20 mg of diazepam (30 mg if rectal).

- If you wish to give continuing preventive treatment, either following repeated seizures or if any further seizures might be particularly hazardous, then give the equivalent of oral diazepam dose 10 mg twice daily, and increase to 20 mg twice daily if seizures occur despite this. There may be a compromise between anti-epileptic treatment and sedation; individual circumstances must be considered, but if possible avoid sedation following any significant head injury. In many parts of the developing world the locally available anti-epileptic is likely to be phenobarbitone, or maybe phenytoin. If either is available then, to prevent further seizures, give 60 mg of phenobarbitone initially, then 30 mg daily thereafter, or 1000 mg phenytoin initially, then 300 mg daily thereafter.
- An alcoholic binge-induced seizure may be complicated by hypoglycaemia; in chronic alcoholics there may well be thiamine deficiency, and correcting the hypoglycaemia without supplementing thiamine can precipitate Wernicke's encephalopathy. Therefore, if alcohol may be a factor, glucose should be accompanied by thiamine.

Migraine

Migraine is a disorder characterized by recurrent, usually unilateral, moderate to severe headaches that may be accompanied by dizziness, nausea, vomiting, or extreme sensitivity to light and sound. Migraine is common in young adults. Most migraine sufferers will be aware of their liability to headache, so a first attack would be unusual but could be precipitated by, for instance, altitude. The cause of migraine is unknown; the two main hypotheses focus on either a primary vascular instability, or on an imbalance of central neurotransmitters.

Risk factors

Women may be more prone to migraine if on the oral contraceptive pill.

Focal migraine is a contraindication to the use of the oral contraceptive pill—it may increase risk of stroke, so the Pill should be stopped if focal migraines develop. Stress, tiredness, exertion, and menstruation may precipitate migraine in susceptible individuals. There are a number of well recognized dietary precipitants:

- Alcohol, especially red wine.
- Citrus fruits.
- Cheese.
- Chocolate.
- Caffeine.

History and examination

Migraine usually produces a fairly stereotypical progression of symptoms.

- *Prodromal:* many notice a change in mood, or other biological functions that may predate the headache by more than a day. These symptoms include negative or positive features; for instance, depression or restlessness, tiredness or listlessness.
- *Aura:* the aura is characterized by visual abnormalities, including flashes, shimmering, and other hallucinations.
- *Headache* phase. The headache itself is typically one-sided but may affect both sides of the head. It is usually gradual in onset, moderate to severe in pain intensity, throbbing, and worse with physical exertion, and it can last anywhere from 2 h to 2 days in children and 4 h to 3 days in adults. The headache stage is often accompanied by loss of appetite, nausea, vomiting, sensitivity to light and sound, blurred vision, tenderness of the scalp or neck, lightheadedness, sweating, and pallor. In severe cases there may be visual field defects and lateralizing limb weakness; these are very frightening symptoms which should be treated seriously unless the patient knows that they are regularly associated with their migraines.

Differential diagnosis

Diagnosis of migraine at low altitude is usually straightforward, particularly if the individual has a prior history.

The main issue at high altitude is distinguishing migrainous headache from acute mountain sickness (AMS). AMS commonly produces a throbbing headache with nausea, and may be indistinguishable from migraine. Any headache developing at altitude should be assumed to be AMS and treated as such, including adequate hydration and descent if severe.

Treatment

- Rest, hydration, and adequate analgesia.
- If the individual is known to have migraine they may have brought their medication with them. Otherwise, give 900 mg soluble aspirin with available antiemetic, which should be given with a glass of milk, if available, to protect the stomach. Metoclopramide or domperidone are particularly useful as they promote gastric emptying, but avoid metoclopramide in adolescents and young adults, as it can precipitate an extrapyramidal reaction. Prochlorperazine is a suitable alternative.

Complications

Complications are unlikely. Migraine can occasionally result in stroke. If migraine develops for first time in women on oral contraception then this should be stopped, particularly if migraine has focal features.

If features suggestive of stroke develop at altitude, assume AMS with likely high altitude cerebral oedema (HACE 📖 p. 626).

Sleep disturbances

On an expedition, many factors may disturb sleep, including time zone shifts, unfamiliar harsh living conditions, physical discomfort, environmental extremes, sport-specific disturbances (night watches sailing/dawn starts climbing), and psychological factors such as anxiety about the venture ahead or homesickness. Few things erode team morale and daytime performance as much as disturbed sleep; however, forward planning and simple measures can improve things considerably.

General measures to improve sleep

- Comfortable bed—careful choice of tent site, padded sleeping mat, under-tent lumps shifted before night fall.
- Temperature control—fan, hot water bottle (e.g. tomorrow's boiled drinking water wrapped in a fleece), appropriate sleeping bag and mat.
- Mosquito deterrents—nets and repellents.
- Ear plugs.
- Safe environment—away from rock fall, avalanche run out zones, flood pathways, or marauding animals.
- Secure valuables if necessary.

Jet lag

Many body functions are under circadian control, including hormone secretion, body temperature, cellular and enzymatic function, and sleep. The natural circadian rhythm approximates 24 h. Rapid travel across time zones is associated with desynchronization between the body's circadian clock and the actual local time, resulting in jet lag. This is experienced as difficulty getting to sleep following an eastward flight, wakening early following a westward flight, disturbed sleep, daytime sleepiness, difficulty concentrating, irritability, depressed mood, anorexia, and nocturia. These symptoms usually only pose a minor inconvenience for travelers; however, performance, including decision-making, may be impaired in the first few days following arrival in a new time zone, and this should be allowed for in the travel schedule.

Decreasing jet lag

- Obtain adequate sleep. Use daytime flights in preference or sleep as much as possible during overnight flights. Use short naps terminated by an alarm clock to improve daytime alertness and concentration. Avoid napping late in the day as this will decrease the drive to sleep at night.
- Adopt the new time frame in the country you are leaving and in transit, including bed and get up times and meal times. Adhere strictly to the new time zone on arrival.
- Optimize light exposure. The light–dark cycle is the principle time cue for resetting human circadian rhythms. Bright light exposure during the daytime for the new time zone and avoidance of bright light at other times of day may have a beneficial effect on the circadian clock and jet lag. This usually means maximizing the exposure to light early in the day after flying eastwards and late in the day after flying westwards.

- Take exercise. Exercise both improves sleep quality and has a minor effect on entraining circadian rhythms, with night-time exercise delaying the circadian clock.
- Avoid excess caffeine and alcohol as these can have a deleterious effect on sleep quality.
- Short-acting hypnotic drugs used on overnight flights and for a few nights after arrival may help. Drug-induced sleepiness carrying over into the next day must be taken into account, particularly after short flights followed by driving.
- Melatonin is a hormone that is secreted by the pineal gland and linked to the circadian rhythm; it has soporific and temperature lowering effects. However, there is no consistent evidence that it has a beneficial effect upon jet lag.

Altitude

- The high altitude environment is often associated with harsh living conditions and cold that may disrupt sleep. In addition, hypoxia directly disturbs sleep by leading to waxing and waning of breathing, known as periodic breathing.
- Pathophysiology of sleep disordered breathing at altitude:
  - Reduced oxygen tension or hypoxia stimulates breathing at high altitude. This lowers carbon dioxide below the critical level required to stimulate breathing, known as the apnoeic threshold. During wakefulness, cortical drives to breathe are maintained; however, during sleep the relative importance of chemical drives to breathe increase, and an apnoea, or pause in breathing, may ensue. Central apnoeas are frequently followed by arousals consisting of increases in heart rate, respiratory rate, and awakening or lightening of sleep, which lower carbon dioxide, thereby helping to sustain periodic breathing. A brisk hypoxic ventilatory response (HVR) produces a greater overshoot in ventilation, so leading the cycle to repeat itself. Periodic breathing results. Recurrent awakenings or lightening of sleep impair sleep quality, and if the sleep duration period cannot be extended may lead to fatigue the next day.

Prevalence

Periodic breathing and central apnoeas are nearly universal in native lowlanders at high altitude. This is in contrast to Sherpa natives who are longstanding high altitude dwellers, and is attributed to their blunted HVR. With increasing altitudes, the proportion of the night spent in periodic breathing increases, and periodic breathing hyperpnoea/hypopnoea cycle time decreases.

Implications of sleep-disordered breathing at altitude

- It is likely that poor sleep and sleep disruption reported by climbers act synergistically with hypoxaemia to impair judgement, vigilance, and safety at extreme altitude.
- Sleep disturbance at altitude is a feature of AMS and high altitude pulmonary oedema (HAPE) (📖 p. 622). Vigilance amongst group members must be maintained to recognize these conditions, and to take rapid action in the event of severe AMS or onset of HAPE.

- Periodic breathing is increased by a brisk HVR. It may be argued that this is a 'good' thing (the brisker HVR is associated with reduced oxygen desaturations during exercise at altitude), or a 'bad' thing (at extreme altitudes ventilation is greater during exercise, and therefore the trekker has less ventilatory reserve between their actual ventilation and maximum voluntary ventilation).

Treatment of periodic breathing

- Periodic breathing and nocturnal hypoxaemia diminish with acclimatization. Graduated, slow ascent, allowing time for acclimatization (📖 p. 618), will improve sleep quality. When severe, descent should be considered.
- Increased sleep duration may compensate in part for reduced sleep quality. This is often impractical during climbing expeditions!
- At extreme altitudes, oxygen supplementation during sleep improves sleep quality.
- Acetazolamide significantly reduces periodic breathing at altitude. It also helps to prevent and treat altitude-related illness (📖 p. 628).
- Temazepam has been shown to reduce periodic breathing at altitude without any impairment of next day vigilance, reaction time, or cognition.

The eye

Ophthalmology is viewed by the general physician with anything from mild boredom to abject fear. Unfortunately, these fears may have to be faced in the wilderness and this section is designed to equip you with the tools you need to assess and treat an eye problem in the field.

Ocular anatomy

It is important to have a basic understanding of ocular anatomy to assess the severity of an injury. Figure 9.5 shows an external and internal view of the eye; note that the cornea is continuous with the sclera and also that the conjunctiva lines the inside of the eyelids and covers the sclera up to the cornea.

Pre-expedition ocular history

Relevant ocular information can be obtained from the pre-departure health questionnaire (📖 Box and also pp. 21, 58).

- Do you wear contact lenses?
  - If yes, what type are they? (e.g. hard/soft, monthlies/dailies)
- Have you ever been treated by a doctor for an eye problem?
- Have you ever had laser eye surgery or any other operation on your eyes?
  - If yes, what kind and when?
- Does anyone in your family suffer from glaucoma or any other eye disease?
- Are you diabetic?

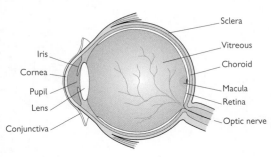

Fig. 9.5 Anatomy of the eye.

Examination of the eye

- *Visual acuity* is the single most important sign when examining the eye and you do not need a Snellen chart to test it; either compare it with the other eye or simply ask the patient if their vision has changed.
- Do not be afraid to *dilate* the pupil to obtain a reasonable view of the retina. If tropicamide alone is used, it can be easily reversed with pilocarpine in the extremely unlikely event of an acute rise in intraocular pressure owing to angle closure.
- Measurement of *intraocular pressure* does not require specialist equipment. Ask the patient to close their eyes and, with your thumbs, simply press gently on the globe, comparing one eye with the other. This will easily reveal the 'marble' of high pressure from the 'avocado' of normal pressure.
- *Fluorescein* is useful to assess the integrity of the corneal epithelium and the globe. It should only be administered after topical anaesthetic (e.g. amethocaine). It is best viewed with a blue light in the dark.

Drops or ointment?

- Drops are easy to administer but are shortlived. Ointment has a soothing, lubricating effect but blurs the vision. It is therefore worth having antibiotics in both preparations depending on the patient's needs.
- Acute eye problems are often very painful, and the patient may require systemic analgesia.

Refractive surgery and high altitude

Refractive surgery is becoming increasingly popular amongst outdoor enthusiasts. However, high altitude can affect the surgical results, causing blurred vision which resolves upon descent. During this type of surgery, the refractive power of the cornea is changed either through surgical incisions or laser ablation. Radial keratotomy (RK) has now been super-seded by laser *in situ* keratomileusis (LASIK), laser epithelial keratomileusis (LASEK), and photorefractive keratectomy (PRK).

RK tends to cause long-sightedness (hypermetropia) at altitude whereas LASIK, LASEK, and PRK may cause short-sightedness (myopia) at altitude. This phenomenon is not predictable and can severely affect vision.

Any decreased vision, redness or pain in the eyes of someone who has had refractive surgery should be taken seriously, as they are more vulnerable to infection. If necessary, consider descent and evacuation.

Patients should be advised not to have refractive surgery within 3 months of an expedition as refraction can be unstable and the eye is at risk of infection.

Contact lenses

Contact lens users are vulnerable to dry eyes and serious corneal infection in the wilderness setting, so they should be advised on sensible contact lens use (no more than 8 h a day) and strict hygiene when handling lenses. They should also be reminded to take their spectacles as well as plenty of spare contact lenses.

Any potential infection, even what appears to be a simple conjunctivitis, should be taken very seriously. Contact lens wear should be stopped and intensive broad spectrum antibiotic drops should be started (e.g. ofloxacin hourly). If there is no improvement within 5 days, the patient should be evacuated.

Case study

A 29 year old short-sighted man took daily disposable soft contact lenses for his attempt on Mount Everest (8848 m) from the north side. However during his summit bid he forgot to remove or change his lenses for four days. As the sun rose on summit day he removed his goggles and put on his designer sunglasses. After the 'Second Step' his vision started to become blurred so that as he reached the summit he was unable to appreciate the view and more importantly navigate. He was helped back down the mountain by two Sherpas on what was luckily a fine day. He was diagnosed with snow blindness and bacterial keratitis; a doctor was able to peel the contact lenses from his eyes with difficulty but the subsequent corneal scarring has left his visual acuity permanently reduced.

Lesson: This mountaineer made two mistakes, one was to not change his contact lenses daily and the other was to dispense with his goggles on summit day and use sunglasses, leaving his eyes vulnerable to snow blindness and dryness. This could have cost him his life.

Dry eyes

- Dry eyes can be exacerbated by the dry, windy, bright conditions found at high altitude or in polar regions. Contact lens wearers are particularly vulnerable.
- Eyes are red, painful, and gritty. Symptoms are relieved by topical anaesthetic; subsequent fluorescein reveals punctuate staining.
- Use an ocular lubricant frequently.
- Minimize contact lens wear.
- Goggles can decrease tear evaporation.
- Although usually just a nuisance, severely dry eyes are very painful, can significantly blur vision, and leave the eyes open to infection.

Conjunctivitis

Conjunctivitis is the most common eye problem that is likely to be encountered in the wilderness setting.

Symptoms and signs

Unilateral or bilateral red, painful eyes with pus (bacterial), profuse watering (viral), or itch (allergic) depending on aetiology. Usually there is no decrease in visual acuity and, while the conjunctiva is red and inflamed, the cornea is clear.

Treatment

Bacterial conjunctivitis should respond rapidly to topical antibiotics, whereas viral conjunctivitis can persist for many days but is eventually self-limiting. If the patient is a contact lens wearer then follow the specific advice earlier in the chapter. Allergic conjunctivitis may respond to sodium cromoglicate.

Bacterial and especially viral conjunctivitis are extremely contagious so strict hygiene measures should be enforced.

Corneal abrasion

A corneal abrasion is a tear in the corneal epithelium, usually through mild trauma such as removing a contact lens or perhaps even whilst asleep.

Symptoms and signs

An acute and exquisitely painful eye. Topical anaesthetic will provide immediate relief, but should not be used as a treatment. Fluorescein will confirm the diagnosis.

Treatment

* Antibiotic ointment
* An eye pad is not usually necessary and can encourage infection.

Snow blindness

Snow blindness is caused by unprotected exposure of the cornea and conjunctiva to ultraviolet light (UV-B). Like sunburn, by the time you realize there is a problem, it is too late, and it can be extremely painful.

Prevention and treatment are discussed on 📖 p. 604.

Corneal foreign body

Occasionally the protective blink reflex fails and allows a foreign body to embed itself into the cornea. This can be metallic or organic; a metallic foreign body will often leave a rust ring.

Symptoms and signs

Red, painful, gritty eye, and foreign body sensation. The foreign body is usually very small, but fluorescein and a magnifying loupe can assist identification and removal.

* Don't forget to evert the eyelid to exclude a subtarsal foreign body.

Treatment

* The foreign body should be removed either with a cotton bud or a 25 G needle. Irrigation with sterile saline may also assist removal.
* Antibiotic ointment.
* An eye pad is not usually necessary and can encourage infection.
* Remember to ask about the mechanism of injury, as a high velocity foreign body, such as a shard of metal from an ice-axe, is more likely to penetrate the globe.

Chemical eye injury

Immediately irrigate a chemical injury before any further assessment.

A chemical splash can be sight-threatening. It is important to identify the chemical because alkali penetrates the ocular tissues much faster than acid and therefore has a worse prognosis.

Symptoms and signs
- A red irritable eye following chemical splash.
- Visual acuity may be impaired.
- If severe, there may be blepharospasm.

Treatment
- Immediate profuse irrigation, preferably with sterile normal saline and a giving set. If unavailable, use the cleanest water at hand.
- Check the pH with litmus paper and continue irrigation until pH is 7.
- If unsure of pH, irrigate for a minimum of 30 min.
- Antibiotic ointment (e.g. chloramphenicol tds).
- Ocular lubrication (e.g. artificial tears hourly).
- Cycloplegic drops for pain relief (e.g. cyclopentolate tds).
- If there is any concern regarding a chemical injury, especially if visual acuity is impaired or if there was any delay initiating irrigation, evacuation for specialist treatment is indicated.
- Remember that a white eye following chemical injury could indicate severe ischaemia.

Eyelid laceration

The eyelids play an important role in protecting the eye and preventing corneal desiccation. If they are damaged, the eye can be rendered vulnerable.

Assessment
- Firm pressure to stop bleeding.
- Check visual acuity.
- Assess globe integrity.
- Examine the eyelid carefully for any embedded foreign body.
- Decide whether the eyelid margin is interrupted.

Management
- Remove any foreign body from the eyelid.
- Clean the wound thoroughly.
- Consider primary repair using a 6/0 non-absorbable suture if the eyelid margin is interrupted and the ends are not opposed. This is especially important with the upper eyelid.
- Antibiotic ointment.
- Broad spectrum oral antibiotics to prevent orbital cellulitis.
- Patch the eye if there is concern about corneal exposure.

Complications
- Corneal exposure is a problem, especially after upper eyelid laceration. This can affect visual acuity and encourage infection.
- Lacerations near the medial canthus may involve the tear duct and, if left unrepaired, may cause a permanent watery eye (epiphora).
- A patient with an eyelid laceration with the eyelid margin severed should be evacuated—a primary repair needs to be done properly by an ophthalmic surgeon under magnification. A poor repair performed in the field is likely to result in a permanent defect in the lid margin, which will require revision at a later date.
- Always check that there is no underlying penetrating injury to the globe, especially if the mechanism of eyelid injury was high velocity.

Penetrating eye injury
A penetrating eye injury involves disruption of the globe integrity and is a serious, sight-threatening problem. The mechanism of injury is important in determining whether there could be an intraocular foreign body or a perforating injury (entry and exit).

Symptoms and signs
- Pain.
- Decreased vision.
- Soft watery eye.
- Peaked pupil.
- Expulsion of ocular contents.

Siedel's test involves a drop of fluorescein (after topical anaesthetic) on a suspected corneal penetrating injury. The leak of aqueous fluid out of the wound will dilute the dye, showing up easily with a blue light and loupe. Beware of false negatives, however, as some wounds will seal themselves quickly, potentially leaving an undiscovered intraocular foreign body.

Management
- A casualty with a suspected penetrating eye injury should be evacuated as soon as practical.
- Do not touch any expulsed ocular contents.
- If available, use a topical antibiotic eye ointment.
- Start broad spectrum systemic antibiotics.
- Both eyes should move as little as possible.
- Protect the injured eye using a double pad and eye shield (Fig. 9.6).
- An increased suspicion of penetrating injury should be maintained in any high velocity eye injury, such as those involving firearms or hammering.

Orbital cellulitis
Orbital cellulitis is a sight-threatening condition that can also be life-threatening if it spreads to form a brain abscess. The infection often arises from an adjacent ethmoid sinus or from mild trauma to the orbital region.

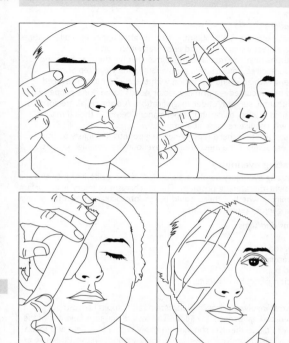

Fig. 9.6 The correct technique to pad an eye.

Symptoms and signs
- Pain.
- Reduced and painful eye movements.
- Conjunctival redness.
- Possible visual loss.
- General malaise.
- Pyrexia.

Treatment
- Broad spectrum antibiotics, preferably intravenous.
- Optic nerve function should be closely monitored (see below).
- Immediate evacuation for hospitalization.

Complications
- Decreased vision owing to optic nerve compression. This can be permanent without rapid orbital decompression.
- Orbital abscess requiring surgical drainage.
- Brain abscess which can be fatal.

Preseptal cellulitis

Preseptal cellulitis involves only the eyelid. There is periorbital inflammation and swelling but none of the other features mentioned above. However, preseptal cellulitis can progress to orbital cellulitis so should be treated with broad spectrum oral antibiotics and closely watched.

Painful loss of vision

Painful loss of vision should be of great concern to the expedition doctor, especially if no obvious cause can be found, such as snow blindness. Always consider evacuation for specialist evaluation.

- Take a full history.
- Optic nerve function (see box).
- Digital intraocular pressure (as described on 📖 p. 309).
- Eye movements.
- Ophthalmoscopy.

> ### Tests of optic nerve function in the wild
>
> - Visual acuity: compare with the other eye.
> - Colour vision: 'How red is my hat compared with the other eye?'
> - Visual fields: simple confrontational fields.
> - Pupils: check for a relative afferent pupillary defect.
> - Ophthalmoscopy: look for optic disc pallor compared to the other eye.

Differential diagnosis

- Snow blindness.
- Orbital cellulitis.
- Bacterial keratitis.
- Acute angle closure glaucoma.
- Optic neuritis.
- Giant cell arteritis.
- Endophthalmitis.

Painless loss of vision

Painless loss of vision in one or both eyes, even transiently, should be taken very seriously. Follow the list of investigations as above, especially the tests of optic nerve function. If there is any doubt the patient should be evacuated for specialist assessment.

Differential diagnosis

- Migraine.
- Amaurosis fugax (transient ischaemic loss of vision).
- Cerebral hypoxia.
- High altitude retinopathy (HAR).
- Hypertensive retinopathy.
- Ischaemic optic neuropathy.
- Retinal artery occlusion.
- Retinal vein occlusion.
- Vitreous haemorrhage.
- Retinal detachment.

High altitude retinopathy

HAR is defined as 'one or more haemorrhages in either eye of a person ascending above 2500 m'. It is normally asymptomatic but affects around 30% of lowlanders ascending to 5000 m.

Signs
- Retinal haemorrhages (flame, pre-retinal, dot and blot).
- Cotton wool spots.
- Optic disc hyperaemia.
- Decreased visual acuity (only if the macula is affected).

Aetiology
Retinal vascular tortuosity and engorgement are part of the normal physiological retinal response to the hypoxia of high altitude. However, a combination of factors, including exertion and speed of ascent, cause HAR. It is confusing to include papilloedema in the definition of HAR as this implies raised intracranial pressure; the relationship between HAR and the potentially fatal high altitude cerebral oedema (HACE) is not yet known.

Any visual disturbance at altitude is an indication for descent.

Ocular first aid kit

The first aid kit listed below is lightweight and will fit into a small pouch. However, as an expedition doctor you should have some experience of using a magnifying loupe and ophthalmoscope as well as administering eye drops and applying a double eye pad.

Case study

A 36-year-old man was diagnosed with hypertension several months before a trekking expedition to climb Mera Peak (6476 m) in Nepal. He was prescribed a beta-blocker which had controlled his blood pressure, but he regularly forgot to take his medication during the trek into base camp. At 4200 m a doctor was summoned as he had gone suddenly blind in both eyes and was feeling unwell. Dilated fundoscopy revealed multiple haemorrhages and cotton wool spots consistent with HAR. However, his blood pressure was 220/110 and a diagnosis of hypertensive retinopathy was made. He was re-started on his medication and evacuated by helicopter whereupon he made a full recovery.

Lesson: People often forget to take their regular medication during an expedition. There are other causes of haemorrhages at altitude than HAR; for example, central retinal vein occlusion has also been reported at altitude. It is always worth measuring blood pressure if possible.

Equipment
- Pentorch ± blue filter.
- Pocket ophthalmoscope.
- Magnifying loupe.
- Eye pads.
- Eye shield.
- Surgical tape.
- pH paper.
- Minor operations kit.
- Single use drops ('Minims'™):
  - Tetracaine (amethocaine)/Benoxinate (topical anaesthetic).
  - Fluorescein 1% (use only after topical anaesthetic for corneal staining).
  - Cyclopentolate 1% (pupil dilation and pain relief).
  - Artificial tears (dry eyes and snow blindness).
  - Tropicamide 1% (for pupil dilation).
  - Pilocarpine 2% (for reversal of pupil dilation by tropicamide).

Other topical medication:
- Antibiotic ointment and drops (e.g. chloramphenicol) (conjunctivitis, any minor infection, or snow blindness).
- Ofloxacin (reserve for more serious corneal infection and all contact lens-related infection).
- Sodium cromoglycate (allergic conjunctivitis).
- Fluorometholone (mild steroid; use cautiously in snow blindness).

These drops are given four times daily except ofloxacin, which can be given hourly for serious corneal infection.
- Remember oral analgesia is required for a painful eye.

Ear problems

Ear problems are relatively common, particularly on diving expeditions owing to pressure changes and prolonged exposure to salt water.

Otitis externa

This is an infection of the outer ear usually associated with constant moisture due to diving or living in tropical environments. The ear is itchy, painful, and a discharge may occur. In severe cases, hearing loss develops if the external canal is blocked by debris and swelling. Movement of the pinna elicits pain. Severe cases result in systemic upset with lymphadenopathy. The external canal looks swollen and red debris is usually obvious.

Otitis externa should be treated by gentle cleaning of the external canal with saline or clean water. A combination preparation of antibiotic and steroid such as Gentisone HC™ should be used four times a day. Severe cases merit oral antibiotics such as co-amoxiclav. Avoid further exposure to water until the condition has resolved.

Otitis media

This is a viral or bacterial infection of the middle ear. It presents as pain and decreased hearing. The pain is made worse by changes in pressure. It may be associated with an upper respiratory tract infection.

Through an otoscope, the eardrum will usually appear red. If there is pus collected behind the drum it can appear yellow. In some cases the drum will perforate, with hearing loss, relief of pain, and a pus discharge.

Prescribe painkillers such as co-codamol and a non-steroidal drug such as ibuprofen or diclofenac for pain. In the expedition environment you should prescribe a basic antibiotic such as amoxicillin or erythromycin.

A decongestant such as oral pseudoephedrine or nasal drops may help to relieve Eustachian tube obstruction.

Very occasionally, severe cases of otitis media can be complicated by *mastoiditis* which causes pain, tenderness, and inflammation over the mastoid process, the bony prominence immediately behind and below the pinna. High dose oral or, ideally, intravenous antibiotics should be commenced and the patient must be evacuated for specialist care because there is a small risk that meningitis or cerebral abscess could develop.

Tympanic membrane rupture due to trauma

This may be caused by direct trauma or associated with a base of skull fracture. Most eardrum perforations heal spontaneously and do not require specific management. Avoid swimming until the hole has healed.

Barotrauma

This results from changes in pressure during diving, usually due to failure to equalize adequately or in the presence of a blocked Eustachian tube.

Middle ear barotrauma or 'squeeze' causes pain, and the tympanic membrane will appear inflamed or blood may be visible behind it. In severe cases the drum may rupture, with bleeding from the ear. In simple cases treatment is symptomatic, with analgesia and decongestants. In the presence of tympanic rupture, amoxicillin or erythromycin should be prescribed. Do not dive until fully resolved.

Inner ear barotrauma is unpleasant. It results from inner ear haemorrhage or a rupture of the oval window. Patients experience vertigo, hearing loss, and tinnitus. Evacuation and examination by an ENT surgeon is advised.

Foreign bodies in the ear

On expeditions, these are most commonly insects that have crawled into the external canal. Insects should be drowned in oil and will usually float out. Other foreign bodies may require removal with suitable hooks.

If difficulty is experienced in foreign body removal, do not persist at the expense of damage to the tympanic membrane or external canal.

Nasal problems

Epistaxis (nose bleed)

Nose bleeds are quite common in expedition situations, and may be precipitated by the low humidity found at altitude, in cold climates, or aircraft cabin atmospheres. Other associations include direct trauma to the nose and upper respiratory tract infections. Ninety per cent are anterior and 10% are posterior.

First aid measures are usually effective in controlling haemorrhage. Press on the soft part of the nose with a finger for 15 min. If simple pressure is unsuccessful, try cauterizing off any identified anterior bleeding points with a silver nitrate stick. Before cauterizing the vessel you should apply a topical local anaesthetic such as lidocaine and adrenaline. Look up the nose using a head torch and apply the cauterization stick to the bleeding point for no longer than 5 s.

If cautery is not possible or is unsuccessful, then insert a commercially available nasal tampon. Such tampons should be lubricated before insertion. Once correctly positioned, expand the device by dropping saline from a syringe. Often both nostrils have to be packed. They are uncomfortable so prescribe painkillers. If nasal tampons are unavailable, then the nose can be packed with lubricated gauze or a small vaginal tampon.

Nasal packs can precipitate sinusitis and in the expedition setting amoxicillin should be prescribed. Leave the packs in place for 48 h and then remove them.

If bleeding continues despite insertion of a nasal tampon, it is probable that the bleeding point is in the posterior part of the nose. Remove the tampon and insert a deflated urinary catheter along the floor of the nose. Gently inflate the balloon with air and pull the catheter forward until resistance is felt. The pack or tampon should then be re-inserted.

A patient with a persistent nose bleed that does not respond to the measures described will have to be evacuated for further treatment and investigation which must include a blood count and clotting studies. Rarely, transfusion is required.

Nasal fracture (📖 p. 287)

Nasal foreign bodies

Foreign bodies in the nose need to be removed as they may lead to infection or aspiration. Anterior foreign bodies can be removed with hooked implements or forceps using a head torch to look up the nose.

Upper respiratory tract

Coryza (common cold)

Upper respiratory tract infections are very common and infection has often originated before departure. The condition is usually self-limiting and requires only symptomatic treatment. Catarrh may block sinus openings and Eustachian tubes. Pressure differences may cause ear or sinus pain, which may be severe. Nasal decongestants such as phenylephrine taken before travel can help. Antibiotics are worthwhile if persistent sinus pain and tenderness suggests secondary bacterial infection.

Pharyngitis/tonsillitis

Sore throats with painful swallowing are common in travellers, especially following air travel. The throat infection may be associated with fever and systemic upset. Most are viral in origin. Pus around the tonsils suggests bacterial infection but it is not usually possible to differentiate the two clinically.

Most cases of tonsillitis settle with time and analgesia. In the remote setting, if symptoms fail to improve after a few days then antibiotics should be prescribed. The antibiotic of choice for the most common bacterial pathogen, beta haemolytic streptococcus, is penicillin V 500 mg for 7 days. Erythromycin is an alternative in penicillin-allergic patients.

Peritonsillar abscess (quinsy)

Quinsy causes severe unilateral throat pain and dysphagia, with associated pyrexia and systemic upset. Trismus (an inability to open the mouth due to pain) and drooling occur. The tonsil is swollen, inflamed, and deviated medially; the uvula is usually displaced away from the affected side. Intravenous antibiotics are required. In the remote setting the abscess should be drained by needle aspiration rather than incision and drainage.

Throat foreign bodies

These are most commonly fish or chicken bones. The patient complains of pain, especially on swallowing. Foreign bodies stuck in the tonsil or base of the tongue can usually be seen and removed with forceps. If no foreign body is visible it is possible that it may simply have scratched the pharyngeal mucosa on passing. A foreign body stuck out-of-sight in the pharynx may become infected and abscesses can develop, so if symptoms persist the patient must be evacuated for further treatment.

Useful equipment and drugs for ENT problems

- Head torch.
- Forceps.
- Nasal tampons.
- Gentisone HC™ ointment.
- Amoxicillin.
- Silver nitrate sticks.

Remote emergency dentistry for doctors

Section editor
Chris Johnson

Contributor
David Geddes

Preparation for remote dentistry

Most doctors receive little education in the management of dental problems during their training, but dental problems are common, especially on longer expeditions, and it is worthwhile learning to recognize and treat them. This chapter offers advice on treating dental and orofacial problems in the field, and indicates those conditions that should lead to evacuation for expert care. Ideally, doctors visiting a remote area should obtain practical instruction before departure.

Dental pain in its chronic phase can be as continual, intense, and as disabling as renal colic. Table 10.1 gives a guide to the likely cause and required treatment.

Avoiding dental problems

It is essential that all expedition members should have a full dental examination with full mouth radiographs at least 3 months before departure. This enables third molar extractions or root treatments to be arranged. All previous dental work of a dubious quality should be electively replaced; this is a lesser risk than leaving it in place and trusting to fate.

Atraumatic restorative technique

This technique involves the removal of decay using a chelating chemistry, the placing of a silver diamine solution to recrystallize damaged dentine, and the placement of a glass ionomer cement as a filling which could be expected to serve many months and perhaps years even when placed in the field. Atraumatic restorative technique may be worth learning for a physician on a long term and remote deployment without recourse to evacuation. A full description of the technique is beyond the remit of this chapter.

Mixing materials

Most modern dental materials are no longer mixed but are command set by the use of a blue light at a wavelength of approximately 480 angstrom. Suitable light sources are now made in pen size and are mains-rechargeable, the charge lasting for many applications. The chemical preparation of the tooth for such materials is also much easier, with a combined preparatory solution that etches the tooth and then provides a chemical bond. This eliminates the need to wash and dry the teeth involved. There are some definite benefits in being able to apply blue light-activated materials for certain forms of filling work, and definitely for splinting that would avoid the need for wiring splints.

If you do not have blue light technology in the field you will be limited to traditional materials that are mixed and set through a chemical reaction. You should practice the mixing technique. There are two distinct timings. The first is the mixing time, during which the material is workable and will not set, and must be placed in the mouth. The second is the setting time, during which the material needs to be undisturbed, and maintained in a dry location, and adjusted so that it does not interfere with other teeth or the chewing function. Given that you may be working using a mirror with copious volumes of saliva, a little practice is merited.

A comfortable working position with visibility

The mouth is full of nervous tissue and attached to a conscious nervous patient. It is dark, and full of saliva. You need to work with a patient who is comfortable enough to relax and give you good visibility. A good light with a wide beam and the means to control saliva flow are both essential. An ergonomic position that can be sustained comfortably for many minutes and sometimes hours will be required. These all need some practice.

Appropriate skills, especially for extractions

The section on extractions instructs that considerable experience of tooth removal is essential if this service is considered an appropriate one for the risks to which your patients are to be exposed. Teaching may be arranged in a teaching dental hospital or general hospital oral surgery department, although most work may be carried out in this environment using general anaesthetics. Seeking experience in a walk-in emergency clinic or busy general practice where extractions are common may be preferable. There is a very considerable advantage in obtaining supervised learning for placement of dental local anaesthetic, extractions, placing temporary fillings into a dry location using a mirror for visibility, and differential diagnosis. Observing in general practice may be a start but is insufficient on its own.

Cross-border manifests

When transporting pharmaceuticals and materials across international boundaries, one should be in possession of a manifest in triplicate, for each new country visited, covering all the materials for which you are responsible.

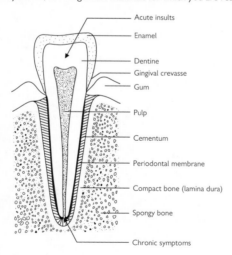

Fig. 10.1 Dental anatomy.

Toothache and dental swellings

In any attempt to treat dental pain it helps to understand one fact. Dental pain is caused by swelling and pressure around the profuse dental pressure proprioceptors, blood vessels, and surrounding tissues. The guiding principle of treatment of dental pain in an expeditionary environment is to reduce this pressure swiftly, whether it originates from tooth, gingival, or third molar infections. In pragmatic terms, the remote doctor will be treating the effect of dental disease and not the cause.

Diagnostic advice

Many serious dental procedures are indelibly etched on the patient's memory. Treatment may have been difficult, highly skilled, took a long time, and was preceded by significant symptoms and pain. Your patient, given time, will relate almost all the information you need, albeit in lay terms. Please use the following chart to refine your differential diagnosis to the point at which you can follow the progression of previous events and decide upon expedient and correct treatment.

Table 10.1

Patient complains of	What is likely to be happening	Likely recent history	Plausible previous history	What to do?
Brief twinges from hot, cold, or sweet stimuli, becoming increasingly uncomfortable	Dental nerve within the visible tooth is being insulted by hot, cold, and sweet stimuli. Pulp is not insulated	Broken or lost filling Cracked enamel Undiagnosed decay	Known damaged tooth Recent minor trauma No recent dental care	Avoid the stimuli Attempt temporary filling to achieve insulation
Twinges from hot, cold, and sweet developing into aching pain of few minutes duration	Dental nerve within the tooth is being insulted and becoming oedematous, but is capable of recovery	Long-term history of reaction to hot, cold, and sweet becoming worse	Known untreated dental damage	Essential to seal the damaged area with an effective temporary filling+NSAIDs
Twinges gradually lessen and replaced by continual aching toothache	Dental nerve is damaged to the point it cannot recover	Long-term history of reaction to hot, cold, and sweet	Known untreated dental damage and history of increasing symptoms	Essential to seal with effective temporary filling, give NSAIDs and consider antibiotics and advise unavoidable need for root canal therapy or extraction

Table 10.1 (Contd.)

Patient complains of	What is likely to be happening	Likely recent history	Plausible previous history	What to do?
Recent continual toothache from hot, cold, and sweet stimuli; now subsiding to no symptoms	Dental nerve is becoming necrotic but not yet with any abcess symptoms	Long-term history of reaction to hot, cold, and sweet	Known untreated dental damage or history of heavily treated tooth without root treatment	Leave open as blocking with temporary filling will seal in oedematous pressure. Give NSAIDs and antibiotics
Pulsing continual toothache, with little respite, worse on lying down	Dental nerve is necrotic and infected with infection spreading beyond tooth structure and into the peri-odontal membrane, bone, and main dental neurovascular bundles. Tooth starting to become tender to percussion	Dental symptoms at some time previously, recent upset to immune system	Previous serious restorative dental work close to the dental nerve without root treatment	Leave open as blocking with temporary filling will seal in oedematous and infective pressure Give NSAIDs and antibiotics and advise extraction is most probably outcome
Pulsing continual toothache, lessening as swelling appears	Dental nerve is necrotic and infected, visible periapical abscess is forming Tooth is very tender to percussion	Recent continual aching toothache	Previous serious restorative dental work close to the dental nerve without root treatment	Leave open as blocking with temporary filling will seal in oedematous and infective pressure Give NSAIDs and antibiotics and advise extraction is most probably outcome Attempt to lance swelling if it has started to point

Pulsing continual toothache, lessening as swelling points and discharges pus	Dental nerve is necrotic and infected, periapical abscess is well formed. Tooth is very tender to percussion	Recent continual aching toothache and swelling	Previous serious restorative dental work close to the dental nerve without root treatment. Various occasional nagging symptoms	Seriously infected tooth and bone structure spreading anaerobes systemically. Heavy dosage NSAIDs and antibiotics and advise extraction inevitable on return. Try to maintain discharge from pointing sinus
Rapid onset aching toothache with little previous warning plus radiating face ache, typically involving ear ache for lower molars, temporal ache for upper molars, and lower border of the eye/edge of nose for upper canines or upper premolars. Worse when sleeping prone	Long-term well formed granulomatous chronic abscess in long-term necrotic tooth, with or without previous root treatment	History of serious dental trauma or treatment in long-term past	Can relate to accident in childhood, or teens, with little intervening symptoms. Patient unlikely to have had regular comprehensive dental care with radiographs	Seriously infected tooth and bone structure spreading anaerobes systemically. Heavy dosage NSAIDs and antibiotics and advise extraction inevitable on return. Try to maintain discharge from pointing sinus. Advise sleeping in a seated position

Treatments for dental pain

Painkillers

When pain is severe use a non-steroidal anti-inflammatory drug (NSAID) such as ibuprofen 400 mg up to six times per day. This high dose should be reduced after 36–48 h as symptoms decrease. (Avoid NSAIDs if the patient has contraindications to their use such as asthma, history of peptic problems, bleeding tendency, or renal problems.) Codeine and paracetamol, singly or in combination, are an alternative, and all three may be used in combination in very severe pain. Opiate painkillers and tramadol are not very effective in dentistry other than for the relief of pain from an unreduced facial or mandibular fracture.

Antibiotics

Dental infections are typically caused by anaerobic bacteria and require treatment with a broad spectrum antibiotic. In remote situations, use penicillins, cephalosporins, or erythromycin in that order of preference, the dose being 500 mg tds for 1 week. For severe infections, add metronidazole 400 mg tds for 1 week. Metronidazole interacts with alcohol, which must be avoided. If alcohol cannot be avoided, Augmentin® 500 mg tds for 1 week is a reasonable alternative. There is an element of 'making sure' with these dosages for remote locations that one might not routinely use in general practice. Antibiotics will generally reduce swelling and associated pain in 2–3 days. At this point anti-inflammatories can be reduced drastically in dosage.

Mouthwashes

Infections of the gum structure occur with poor oral hygiene around buried or partly erupted third molars. Gums will appear swollen, reddish purple in colour, will bleed spontaneously on touch with an instrument, and may smell foul. When an infection appears to be located in the gingival tissues rather than related to a tooth (for instance, acute ulcerative gingivitis, periodontitis, or third molar infections), the control of anaerobes between teeth and under gingival margins is essential.

- Encourage improved oral hygiene immediately after all meals to remove food substrates from breeding bacteria plus the vigorous use of mouthwash for at least 3 min.
- Give an antibiotic such as metronidazole 200 mg tds for 5 days.
- Encourage the use of mouthwashes such as those which liberate oxygen (e.g. 'Peroxyl'), or use chlorhexidine in high concentration (2%+), (eg 'Corsodyl').
- In the absence of these, use hot concentrated salty mouthwash.
- The patient will need to be encouraged to brush a painful area vigorously for some minutes. It's a case of being cruel to be kind.

Fillings

Temporary filling materials are used to insulate the pulp from temperature, hypertonic solutions, chemicals or irritating foods. If a tooth is damaged during an expedition—whether through a lost or broken filling, decayed dentine, or cracked or broken enamel—but is not giving symptoms, then a temporary filling is probably unnecessary.

Temporary filling materials suitable for placement when in a remote location fall into two categories:

• Premixed in a sealed tube; squeeze out and apply.
  • The premixed materials (e.g.'Cavit') are easier to use but have less structural strength.
  • They will erode and may require replacing as often as every few days.
  • Their chemistry is usually a variation on zinc oxide powder and versions of oil of cloves.
  • The cavity can be damp but not wet.
  • They will soothe reversibly damaged dentine and dental pulp.
  • Require powder and fluid to be mixed before application.
• Materials that require mixing (e.g. IRM—intermediate restorative material—or any glass ionomer cement/filling) are fussy. Consider the following before starting:
  • The exact ratio of powder to liquid is critical.
  • The mixing time is about 1 min and the setting time is similar.
  • Mix on a glass slab with a flat spatula into a dough-like consistency.
  • Apply and compress into a dry cavity, immediately removing all excess material from the biting surface.
  • A small aerosol used to clean the inside of cameras is a handy way of drying the cavity.
  • The cavity must be protected on either side with absorbent pads or cotton wool until the filling has set. Working from above and behind the patient will establish this control.
  • IRM can be colour-coded: white for a clean cavity, blue for decay present, red for pulpal symptoms. This code is used to avoid clinical notes by the military of many nations and is universally understood.
  • Both IRM and glass ionomers are soothing to reversibly damaged dentine and dental pulp.
  • The same glass ionomer filling materials, if mixed into a 'double cream-like' consistency, are excellent for reseating and cementing crowns. For greater effectiveness, after removing excess cement, seal the margins of the cement around the crown, whilst setting, with petroleum gel to protect from saliva erosion.

Dislodged crowns and bridges

Crowns (commonly known in lay terms as 'caps') are made of porcelain, sometimes with an inner metal core, and usually restore all the outer structure of a badly damaged tooth. Bridges are a series of joined crowns used to support and replace a missing tooth. Normal crowns rarely dislodge.

Two common and two rare categories of crowns typically dislodge:

- The crown retained by a metal post which inserts into an existing prepared root. This tooth will have already been root-treated (the root tip sealed to prevent bacterial colonization).
- The crown where the cementation has failed or been removed by trauma. In the case of trauma the crown may hold original tooth structure that has fractured.
- The implant-retained crown; this is such a specialist field that you should avoid offering any treatment that tampers with implant-retained prosthetics. Implants are osseo-integrated titanium replacement roots placed surgically.
- The adhesive bridge located to the hidden surfaces of teeth by metal wings and strong adhesives—this instead of crowns for support; there is nothing you can do for this. The chemistry, tooth preparation, and moisture control needed for restoration are impossible in the field.

Re-cementing a crown with post

Check by flexing the root with a long probe to ensure that the root is not vertically split. If it is, then do not re-cement the crown as a gingival abscess may ensue. If the root is intact then:

- Clean the inside of the root with an aerosol camera cleaner until clean and totally dry.
- Maintain this moisture control.
- Test, by rehearsing the positioning, the ease or difficulty placing of the post.
- Have someone else mix the glass ionomer cement into a thick creamy consistency.
- Apply a little inside the root and most to the clean post.
- Reposition and hold in the correct place until set (2–3 min).
- Remove excess when still soft with the probe, and seal the cement margins with petroleum gel.

Re-cementing a crown with broken core

A problem arises if the core of the tooth required for accurate fixation of the crown breaks off inside the crown. If the tooth is already root-treated, no harm will be done if the crown is left out as the nerves have already been removed. The root treatment can typically be seen as a pink rubbery material running up the long axis of the centre of the root. Root-treated teeth are brittle and damage of this type is quite common.

However, if the stump has not been root-treated and the exposed nervous tissue is very sensitive, you are duty-bound to try to cover the sensitive area. If there is no core inside the dislodged crown, re-cement the crown using a glass ionomer mixed into cement consistency. The steps are the same as for the post crown. If there is bleeding from the core of the tooth, prescribe antibiotics and NSAIDs to reduce nerve and blood vessel inflammation which will lead to dental pain.

If the tooth is not root-treated and has the original remaining tooth structure fractured and remaining inside the crown then attempt the following technique:

- Remove the core and fractured tooth substance as best you can.
- Clean and dry the fitting surface.
- Clean and dry the remains of the tooth.
- Have someone else mix a glass ionomer cement into a wet dough-like consistency.
- Place a slight surfeit of cement into the crown.
- Press home onto the remaining tooth, seating it down fully.
- Check the patient can bite correctly and is not propped open by the crown.
- Hold in this position for 2–3 min until setting is established.
- Remove any excess with the probe, and seal the margins with petroleum gel.
- Alternatively, preserve the root for future treatment options by sealing the post hole with a temporary filling material. Make sure the patient retains the crown for possible re-use.

It is possible mistakenly to place some crowns back to front. Check the orientation before cementation. A porcelain crown made on a metal base will usually have a shiny metal margin on the inner aspect of the tooth.

Dental injuries

Reduction of tooth luxation after trauma

Repositioning a tooth that has been moved by trauma involves the reduction of fractured alveolar bone (the bone immediately surrounding the roots). This is not difficult and is not normally too uncomfortable for the patient. It must be done as soon as possible after an accident to stand much chance of success—certainly within an hour and preferably within 20 min of the injury. One of three situations can occur:

- Tooth or teeth and bone have been moved a short distance but are reasonably solid. There is a good chance the teeth may have retained a patent blood supply and will survive. The patient, with encouragement, may be able to bite these teeth the short distance back into the correct relationship.
- Tooth or teeth are very loose, independent of what has happened to the bone structure. If the blood supply has been severed—and there is no way of being sure other than speculating on the looseness—then root treatment will be required soon, and splinting will be required now. Reduce all malpositioned teeth, support the teeth by wire and/or glass ionomer cement splinting if you can, and consider evacuation to specialist care.
- Tooth or teeth may be mobile because of fractured roots. You are advised to remove the fractured teeth and leave the roots to be removed by an expert; consider evacuation to specialist care.

In all cases prescribe antibiotics and NSAIDs.

Teeth that have been loosened in bone that has been fractured can be moved quite easily. Typically, upper incisors will have been moved towards the palate by frontal trauma. They will be in cross-bite with the lower incisors in any attempt to bite together naturally. To reduce the cross-bite, with or without local anaesthetic:

- Place yourself above and behind the patient.
- Exert slow but very firm forward pressure from your thumb placed on the palatal aspect of the pre-maxilla and palatal aspect of the loose teeth.
- Maintain the firm pressure until the bone and teeth move back into a normal occlusion.
- The patient will tell you when they can bite together naturally.
- You now need to consider whether the reduction will hold naturally or will need a wire splint, for which you will have been wise to practice before leaving home!
- It's fussy the first time, but easier than it looks on all subsequent occasions, but it is vital to secure the luxed teeth.
- Failure to try to reduce such impact damage early may mean that the patient will face bills of up to £2500 per tooth for surgical bone augmentation, implant and crown placement, so field treatment is worth attempting.

Tooth avulsion after trauma

The repositioning and fixation by splinting of any totally avulsed tooth is getting into the realms of dental heroics, especially in the field. Consider:

- Are there bigger clinical issues that take precedence for triage?
- If the patient requires or is likely to require airway intubation then do not reposition.
- If the root is fractured then do not attempt repositioning.
- Repositioning may just work if the accident was less than 40 min ago.
- Repositioning stands a worthwhile chance of success if the accident was less than 20 min ago.
- The tooth and root needs to be clean.
- The best way to carry the tooth after avulsion is in the mouth—saliva is reasonably isotonic, is at body temperature, and the presence of friendly commensal bacteria and protein matrices will help control the risk of infection.
- Never handle the avulsed tooth by touching the root; always handle using the enamel.
- Are you equipped for wire splinting?
- If so, are the teeth adjacent to the avulsed tooth sound enough to provide adequate splinting support?

(a)

(b)

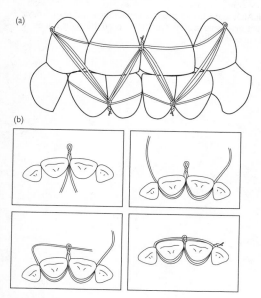

Fig. 10.2 Dental support wiring for avulsed tooth.

Replantation of an avulsed tooth

Normal haemostasis in the tooth socket will occur within 8 min. This blood clot will have to be removed to make way for the root to be firmly embedded full depth into the socket. In removing the clot, it will be necessary gently to stimulate bleeding again from the periodontum with a sterile instrument to improve the chances of healing. Use the following technique:

• The tooth should be taken from the saliva.
• Rinse the tooth in sterile water at 37°C.
• Re-insert full depth into the socket so that it stands confluent with the adjacent teeth and no longer or shorter than their height.
• Hold in position until haemostasis is re-achieved—typically 4–8 min.
• Splint to adjacent supporting teeth using figure-of-eight wire ligatures. You may use one or two teeth on either side of the recently avulsed tooth.
• If possible, enhance the splinting by placing a strong temporary filling material over the meticulously dry outer (labially facing) surfaces of the splinted tooth and its supporting teeth; squeeze when soft between the teeth for increased rigidity.
• Once set, cover the materials with petroleum gel to avoid softening from moisture contamination.
• Prescribe NSAIDs and a broad spectrum antibiotic for at least 5 days.
• Ensure diligent oral hygiene after every meal even though it will be difficult and uncomfortable.

Dental local anaesthesia

Being able to apply local anaesthetic (LA) accurately is a great boon in many circumstances. Upper and lower jaw blocks differ significantly. Local anaesthesia is useful:

• To enable treatment for painful teeth.
• To give immediate relief from intractable chronic toothache and allow sleep.
• To enable reduction of fractures and splinting.
• To permit dental extractions.

There are three main styles of dental LA delivery:

• Block
• Infiltration
• Intraligamentary.

Almost all dental LAs are premixed in cartridges and include a vasoconstrictor. The vasoconstrictor aids the retention of the LA in the locality of the symptoms. A well placed block to the mandible will give pain relief for up to 3 h. Premixed dental anaesthetics come in either 1.8 ml or 2.2 ml cartridges. Check that the syringes you take match the cartridges! The needle gauge will be either 27 or 30, and the length needs to be at least 3 cm.

Metal dental syringes are heavy. Disposable syringes offer an option. Use 1–2 ml of 2% lidocaine with, typically for minor injury, 1/100 000 epinephrine as a vasoconstrictor. Serious injury may require a greater percentage of vasoconstrictor.

Mandibular (inferior dental) nerve block

The mandibular branch of the trigeminal nerve runs down the inside of the mandible. Halfway down the bone the nerve divides into two, with the inferior dental nerve entering a canal within the mandible, and the long buccal nerve continuing outside the bone (Fig. 10.3). The bony cortex of the mandible is so dense that infiltration of LA will not work. Place the LA just above the canal entrance (lingula):

• Open the patient's mouth as wide as possible.
• For a left-sided block, approach needle insertion with the syringe barrel lying over the right premolars, and vice versa (Fig. 10.4).
• Insert the needle tip at mid-height in the muscular pillar that connects the lower third molar region to the upper third molar region.
• Angle the needle backwards towards and just above the lingula.
• The needle should touch bone at 3 cm deep. A more shallow touch indicates you are in front of the lingula and in the wrong place. No touch on bone when 3 cm of needle are inserted indicates you are incorrectly angled and probably deep to the lingula.
• Aspirate the syringe to check you are not in a blood vessel and reposition as necessary.
• Deliver a full cartridge slowly.
• Wait for a clear indication of anaesthetic effect to the midline of the mandible and full length on the side of the tongue. This may take seconds or minutes. Work should commence only when there is a clear sensory distinction across the mandibular midline.

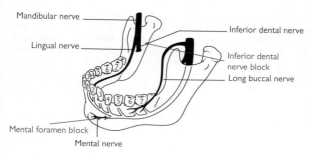

Fig. 10.3 Lower jaw anatomy and nerve supply.

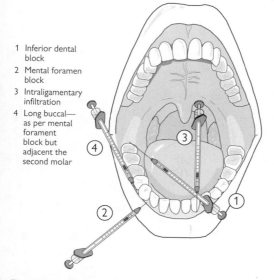

1 Inferior dental block
2 Mental foramen block
3 Intraligamentary infiltration
4 Long buccal— as per mental foramrent block but adjacent the second molar

Fig. 10.4 Mandibular dental blocks.

Maxillary nerve infiltrations

Infiltrating local anaesthetic into the gingival tissues below the roots of mandibular teeth, rather than using block anaesthesia, is notoriously ineffective.

Maxillary dental nerves appear from three locations (Fig. 10.5). They interconnect widely rather like lots of minor roads on a map. Block anaesthesia is therefore difficult. It is preferable to use a number of infiltrations above the buccal/labial sulcus both forward and behind the tooth in question. The infiltration is delivered slightly above the apices of the tooth roots. Most roots can be considered to be about 20 mm from the occlusal surface of the tooth. Upper canines can occasionally be up to 30 mm long.

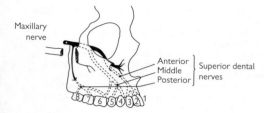

Fig. 10.5 Maxillary division of trigeminal nerve.

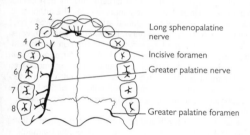

Fig. 10.6 Palatal nerves.

1 Buccal/labial
  infiltration

2 As per no 1 but go to
  the level of the lower
  orbit—suborbital
  block

3 Sphenopalatine
  block

4 Incisal papilla block

5 Intraligamentary
  infiltration

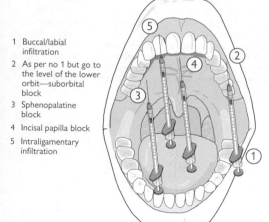

Fig. 10.7 Maxillary dental nerve blocks.

- Insert the needle into the buccal or labial sulcus and slightly angled towards the facial bone structure.
- Place the needle tip above the level of the root apices.
- Deliver a full cartridge.
- When delivering LA for incisors and canines, place the needle slowly and inject very slowly. The tissue is tight and the nerve plexus considerable. This is a very painful injection if rushed.
- If attempting an extraction, a very small infiltration must also be placed on the palatal side of the tooth until visible blanching is seen. This is also an unpopular injection site.

Buccal/labial infiltration (Fig. 10.8)

The objective is to place a small amount of LA directly into the periodontal ligament with a very fine gauge and preferably short needle. The intention is to use the vascularity of the narrow periodontal attachment between root and bone to deliver the LA to the apical nerve fibres. This approach, when in practised hands, is sufficient even for extractions. In the context of field-work it should be considered as an adjuvant to block or infiltration to gain profound local anaesthesia. It is particularly useful when attempting to anaesthetize a locality that has been heavily infected or luxed. When infection has been present for some time there is often buffering of the LA. The intraligamentary approach is sufficiently direct to overcome this problem.

- Select a fine short needle.
- Place the needle tip between tooth and bone by sliding the needle along the tooth surface and inserting 2–3 mm into the periodontal ligament.
- The needle will always follow the long axis of the root of the tooth.
- Using considerable pressure, place about 0.2 ml of LA.
- Repeat for each root—molars have three roots, premolars can be considered to have two, while incisors and canines have one root.

If, after your best efforts, there is insufficient anaesthetic effect, then repeat all stages again and again. Seven or eight full cartridges might be considered a maximum dose for a fit young person. Then wait, and wait. It once took 3 h for a very badly infected lower wisdom tooth to anaesthetize. The tooth then came out painlessly and the climber subsequently summited Lhotse Shar when otherwise his expedition was over.

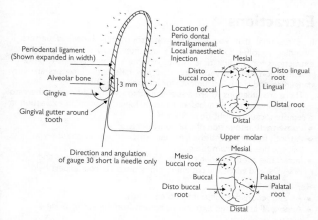

Fig. 10.8 Intraligamentary dental nerve block.

Extractions

It is essential that you seek appropriate training before departure if intending to offer extractions as a treatment. Do not attempt dental extractions for the first time in the wilderness. There are many patterns of extraction forceps, each applied slightly differently. Luxators are very dangerous and sharp instruments for inexperienced hands.

There are situations where a successful extraction might mean otherwise inevitable evacuation is avoided. Reasons for attempting an extraction in a remote location might be as follows:

• Loose teeth either side of a bone fracture.
• A tooth fractured with the live neurovascular pulp exposed—you will see bleeding from the pulp.
• Intractable toothache which does not respond to antibiotics and NSAIDs, and when the patient is a long distance from expert help.

Remember:

• All extractions are difficult to do efficiently.
• Almost all attempted extractions benefit from loosening using a luxator or elevator.
• Each tooth requires a specific style of forceps.
• Forceps are gripped in a very specific manner.
• The tooth root is gripped by the forceps as far below the gum level as possible.
• A great deal of very focussed force is slowly and relentlessly applied up or down the long axis of the root.
• One never pulls a tooth—they are all pushed and slowly rotated out using a figure of eight movement and following the line of least resistance, which can be increasingly sensed.
• Upper teeth are extracted standing in front of the patient.
• Lower teeth are extracted from a stance behind the patient.
• The jaw and head both need to be immobilized to avoid the extraction force being dissipated. This may necessitate the help of a colleague.
• Force is never applied in any other way than very precisely along the long axis of the roots. Failure to do this—force applied tangentially to the root long axis—will cause tooth breakage. This makes the situation very much worse and perhaps irretrievable.

Extraction aftercare

Once the tooth is out, a surgically created gap remains that is open to bone and periosteum. This can be very prone to painful infection lasting 14 days. The main responsibility is to establish complete coverage of bone by a solid blood clot. A small firm pack of cotton wool roll or absorbent paper can be placed over the socket and the patient invited to bite hard onto this. Continual pressure will almost always achieve haemostasis within 5 min. The pack should be rotated out to avoid lifting the clot with the pack. Antibiotics are seldom required unless the previous infection was considerable. NSAIDs or paracetamol may be required for the first 12 h. Suturing is occasionally necessary to close the surgical wound. Black silk or vicryl 3/0 sutures on a small curved needle should be used while LA is still working. Black silk sutures can be removed after a minimum of 5 days. Thorough oral hygiene must be advised even though this is uncomfortable.

Advice to patient after extractions

The objective is to avoid further bleeding, return for further treatment, and infection. The patient should be advised as follows.

• No hot drinks, smoking, alcohol, or heavy lifting for 4 h.
• Use a pressure pack to control any subsequent bleeding. Bite hard on this for 8 min and then gently rotate out.
• Red-coloured saliva is not a bleed and can be expected; a bleed looks like a substantial mass of 'jelly-like' blood clot.
• Mouth washing and gentle brushing after every meal is essential to limit the food source of damaging bacteria which will cause infection.

One last word of advice concerning extractions

A tooth, once extracted, cannot be used for any fixed dental prosthesis. Fixed prosthetics are considered best practice. The eventual replacement of an extracted tooth may involve the placement of a titanium implant, connector, and crown. This might commit the patient to thousands of pounds or dollars of treatment. So avoid dental extractions if at all possible.

Further reading

Atraumatic Restorative Techniques—'ART'—Internet search recommended for variety of helpful. pdf files

Andreasen JO, Andreasen FM (1990). *Essentials of Traumatic Injuries to the Teeth*. Munksgaard.

Wray D, Stonehouse D, Lee D, Clark AJE (2003). *Textbook of General and Oral Surgery*. Churchill Livingstone.

Remote dentistry kit list

For supply contact: The Dental Directory, 6 Perry Way, Wiltham, Essex CM8 3SX. Tel: 0800 585 586. http://www.dental-directory.co.uk

- Sterile surgical gloves
- Cotton wool rolls
- Sealed alcohol swabs
- Sachets of surgical instrument sterilization solution
- 2 dental mirrors
- 1 sickle probe
- 1 locking tweezer
- 1 flat-bladed filling plugger
- 1 spatula to mix filling material
- 1 glazed paper mixing pad
- 1 Spencer Wells fine suturing forceps
- Black suture silk on fine semilunar needle
- 1 fine curved surgical scissors
- Disposable scalpels
- Extraction forceps of your choice—upper molar left and right, lower molar, upper single root, lower single root provide a minimum capability
- Extraction elevators or luxators depending on preference
- Aspirating LA syringe, 3 cm/gauge 30 or 27 needles, LA cartridges to match syringe size
- Antibiotics and NSAIDs
- Sachets of hydrogen peroxide mouthwash
- Table salt to make hot mouthwash
- Petroleum gel
- Temporary filling materials—Cavit, glass ionomer powder/water-filling material, IRM (intermediate restorative material)—colour-coded
- Stainless steel wire for eyelet wiring or electrical cord for harvesting copper wire
- Gas aerosol suitable for camera cleaning for moisture control in the mouth (unsuitable for export by airline)
- Petzl Tikka LED head torch x 2
- Disposable plastic instrument trays
- Secure DIY toolbox to carry all equipment.

Optional equipment
- Blue light (led) as curing source for materials (mains re-chargeable)
- Light-cured filling materials for splint construction and temporary fillings.

Chest

Section editor
Annabel Nickol

Contributors
Andrew Drain, Jonathan Ferguson, Jonathan Leach, Julian Thompson, Andy Thurgood, and David Warrell

Introduction

The chest is the region of the body between the neck and the abdomen, along with its internal organs and other contents. It is mostly protected and supported by the ribcage, spine, and shoulder girdle. The chest contains:
- Heart and major blood vessels
- Trachea, lungs, and pleura
- Diaphragm
- Oesophagus.

Also protected by the lower ribs are:
- Liver and gallbladder
- Spleen
- Upper part of stomach
- Upper poles of kidneys.

Injuries to the ribcage may damage the underlying organs. Chest pain may originate from thoracic or intra-abdominal organs.

Chest pain

Chest pain is a relatively common complaint on expeditions. Most chest pain is musculoskeletal in origin and may be treated by analgesics and, where possible, rest. However, severe central chest pains and pleuritic pain made worse by deep inspiration may signal more serious conditions that might require urgent treatment or evacuation. Diagnosis of these conditions is covered on p. 224 and the algorithm on Fig. 7.8, p. 225.

Myocardial infarction

A myocardial infarction or 'heart attack' results from sudden blockage of a coronary artery that distributes blood to the heart muscle. Although this may, especially in the elderly, go almost unnoticed, the symptoms and signs are usually obvious and the victim may collapse. The vascular obstruction can result in failure of the heart to pump properly (cardiac failure) or irregular heart rhythms that can be fatal. Myocardial infarction is most likely to develop in middle-aged men and post-menopausal women, but occasionally affects adults in their twenties.

Symptoms
- Central, crushing retrosternal pain
- Pain may radiate to shoulder and neck
- May mimic severe heartburn, but discomfort not relieved by antacids
- Palpitations
- Breathlessness.

Differential diagnosis
Causes of chest pain are discussed in Chapter 7.

Signs
Patient is anxious, distressed, and often pale, cold, and clammy.

Monitoring
If facilities are available, monitor blood pressure and pulse (by palpation or oximeter). Portable fully automated defibrillators are becoming cheaper and more widely available; they are located in many transport terminals and large stores. Apply electrode pads and listen to instructions. Medics covering charity treks and major endurance sporting challenges should consider whether obtaining an automated defibrillator would be practical and worthwhile.

Management
Options are limited in the wilderness:
- Give supplementary oxygen if available
- Obtain iv access
- Give analgesia—opiates are valuable both for treating pain and relieving breathlessness. Use tramadol if opiates not carried
- Give aspirin 300 mg if no contraindication
- Consider use of glyceryl trinitrate (GTN) as spray or skin patch
- Inform rescue services of possible diagnosis; in remote areas many paramedics are permitted to administer thrombolytic ('clot-busting') drugs
- Evacuate as soon as possible to tertiary care hospital.

Rib fractures

Most rib fractures are not dangerous in themselves, but are extremely painful. The pain will probably prevent further participation in the expedition as sleep will be disturbed and carrying a rucksack impossible. Morbidity correlates with the degree of injury to underlying structures. Average blood loss per fractured rib is 100–150 ml.

The pain from a fractured rib can severely restrict breathing and can predispose to reduced movement and infection of the underlying lung. Basic treatment involves managing the pain and monitoring for more serious injuries. When there is evidence of significant injury (as opposed to just chest wall bruising), the patient should be evacuated to definitive medical care as soon as possible.

Signs and symptoms

Suspect a simple fractured rib if any of the following are present:
- Chest wall bruising
- Tenderness over a specific bony point on the chest
- Sharp pain when coughing or breathing
- Deformity of the chest.

Treatment

- If possible, stop all activity, reassure, and try to keep the patient calm to reduce effort of breathing. Assess ABCD (see Chapter 6). Deal with the identified rib fractures once you are sure there are no other life-threatening problems such as an obstructed airway or bleeding.
- If available, give patient high flow oxygen using a non-rebreathing oxygen mask.
- Administer ibuprofen 400 mg to 800 mg stat (with food) then 400 mg qds for pain. If additional pain relief is required add paracetamol 1 g qds.
- Encourage the injured person to cough frequently, breathe deeply every hour at least, despite the pain, in order to prevent secretions from pooling in the lung, which could cause chest infection.

Serious fractures

Look for signs that may suggest injury to the lungs:
- Rapid and shallow breathing
- Elevated heart rate
- Increased difficulty breathing
- Coughing up blood.

The mechanism of injury may indicate serious underlying chest injury; for instance, fall from height, crushing forces, or rapid deceleration injuries in a road traffic collision.
- Place one hand on each side of the injured person's chest and observe the way in which the chest moves with inhalations. If one side of the chest rises during inhalation while the other falls, at least three ribs have been broken on the falling side of the chest—a 'flail chest.' This is best visualized by looking from the patient's feet along the patient's body towards their head, meanwhile watching the chest rise and fall—the 'sunset view' of the chest wall.

- If the casualty is having severe difficulty breathing, or if the chest is rising and falling asymmetrically during breathing, roll them onto the injured side. This makes breathing less painful. If the patient does not improve try another position.
- Keep the casualty on their side and continually monitor for breathing difficulties. Consider the possibility of a tension pneumothorax (see below).
- Evacuate immediately to a hospital for even the simplest of rib fractures. The injured person must be flown or carried out if there are any signs of respiratory distress (consider chest drain if risk of pneumothorax), but may be able to walk out with simple fractures.
- Morphine or other analgesics: the pain of the fractures may hinder breathing sufficiently for it to be necessary to administer small amounts of an opiate painkiller to enable more effective breathing. Morphine should be administered, ideally intravenously. Give 1 mg doses every 1–2 min and monitor closely the effects of the analgesia. A fit adult may require 20–30 mg and sometimes more of morphine in total to relieve severe pain, but be careful not to give so much that respiration is depressed. Any dose of opiate can cause nausea, reduced awareness and confusion, and can make evacuation more difficult. Tramadol 10–20 mg doses may be similarly titrated to relieve pain. Up to 300 mg may be required. Tramadol is less likely than an opiate to cause respiratory depression, but may cause light-headedness, nausea, and vomiting.
- Traditional firm (not tight) strapping may help pain but, by restricting expansion, encourages infection.

Tips and warnings

- Examine the patient's left and right, front, back, and sides for hidden rib injuries.
- Serious rib fractures will very likely have underlying lung bruising accompanying the condition and this injured lung reduces lung function. The patient must be monitored closely for deterioration and evacuated as soon as possible.
- Older persons are more prone to rib fractures than younger adults owing to weaker bones.
- Position of the fractured rib in the thorax helps identify potential injury to specific underlying organs. Fracture of the lower ribs is usually associated with injury to abdominal organs rather than to lung tissue.
- Fracture of the left lower ribs is associated with splenic injuries.
- Fracture of the right lower ribs is associated with liver injuries.
- Fracture of the floating ribs (ribs 11, 12) is often associated with kidney injuries.

Spontaneous pneumothorax

A pneumothorax is a collection of air or gas within the pleural cavity. (See also traumatic pneumothorax, 📖 p. 182) They typically occur in tall, thin, young males but may occur during scuba diving or during acute asthma attacks.

Symptoms and signs
• Shortness of breath
• Increased respiratory rate
• Lateral sharp chest pain on breathing in
• Central cyanosis (blue lips)
• Reduced chest movement and air entry on the affected side
• Hyper-resonant to percussion on the affected side.

Treatment
• Oxygen, if available
• Pain relief
• All patients with a pneumothorax require hospital assessment
• Regularly reassess the patient for the development of a tension pneumothorax
• Unless the patient is compromised or must be evacuated by aircraft, avoid insertion of needles or drains into the chest. Note that the pneumothorax will expand with gain in altitude. See also Heimlich valve and chest drainage (📖 p. 184).

Acute chest infections

Respiratory infections are a common medical problem on expeditions. Chest infections often follow an initial upper respiratory tract infection (URTI). URTIs, including coryza, sore throat, tonsillitis, quinsy, and sinusitis, are covered in Chapter 9 Head and neck (📖 p. 322).

Acute lower respiratory tract infections (ARI) can be caused by a wide range of pathogens. Those likely to affect members of expeditions include:
- Viruses
  - Influenza viruses
  - Measles—rare if immunized
  - Respiratory syncytial virus (RSV)
  - SARS Corona Virus—epidemics only!
- Bacteria
  - *Streptococcus pneumoniae*
  - *Haemophilus influenzae*
  - *Mycoplasma pneumoniae*
  - *Chlamydia* spp.
  - Q fever—*Coxiella burnettii*
  - *Legionella*
  - Tuberculosis—especially in local populations
- Fungi
  - *Pneumocystis (carinii) jirovecii*
  - *Histoplasma capsulatum*
  - *Cryptococcus neoformans*.

Immunocompromise and underlying chronic illness determines special vulnerabilities, for example to *P. jirovecii* pneumonia in HIV-positive patients, to *Strep. pneumoniae* in alcoholics, and to a range of pathogens in smokers and chronic bronchitics.

Transmission is usually by inhaled aerosol from infected people, including asymptomatic carriers and, in the case of some pathogens, from animals (e.g. *Chlamydia psittaci*) and from the environment (e.g. Q fever, fungal pneumonias). Crowded and enclosed areas such as buses, hostels, travel terminals, aircraft, and underground trains increase the risk of transmission.

Symptoms
- Cough with or without sputum production developing after URTI or influenza
- Fever (sometimes with rigors)
- Breathlessness
- Exacerbation of underlying asthma
- Pleuritic chest pain
- Myalgia
- Other 'flu-like' symptoms.

Examination

- Temperature
- Cold sores
- Upper respiratory tract—catarrh and post-nasal drip from sinusitis
- Rashes (e.g. measles, *Mycoplasma pneumoniae*)
- Displaced mediastinum
- Auscultation:
  - added sounds
- Evidence of lobar or patchy consolidation
- Lobar collapse
- Pleural effusion
- Pleural friction rub.

Lower lobe pneumonia can cause misleading upper abdominal tenderness. Look at the sputum! Yellowish, greenish purulent sputum, sometimes 'rusty' or streaked with frank blood is a typical sign of infection.

Complications include: respiratory failure, septicaemic shock, metastatic infection such as meningitis and infective endocarditis, pericarditis and pericardial effusion, pneumothorax, pneumomediastinum, empyema, and lung abscess.

Diagnosis

In the field, diagnosis is made on clinical grounds and can be confirmed later by chest radiography, sputum microscopy, blood cultures, leucocyte count, serology, and antigen detection in urine (*Legionella*).

Treatment

Antibiotics

Clinically convincing ARI during an expedition in a remote location deserves immediate antibiotic treatment.

If classic pneumococcal lobar pneumonia is suspected, treatment with oral amoxicillin 500 mg three times a day for 5–7 days (or erythromycin 500 mg four times a day for penicillin-hypersensitive patients). In severe cases, or if oral treatment is impossible, start ceftriaxone iv or im, 2 g once a day.

For broader spectrum blind treatment (also covering *H. influenzae*, *Legionella* spp., *Mycoplasma*, *Chlamydia*, Q fever), use oral doxycycline 100 mg twice each day, or clarithromycin 250 mg bd.

Supportive treatment

Cough suppressants (cough mixture, linctus) have limited effect but can be soothing, especially if sleep is disturbed. Codeine or pholcodine linctus or sedating antihistamines such as chlorphenamine (Piriton®) may be helpful provided they do not cause respiratory depression.

Asthma exacerbations should be treated with bronchodilators and, in some cases, a short course of oral corticosteroid (see asthma 📖 p. 362).

Severe pleuritic pain warrants strong analgesia. Start with regular full dose paracetamol. Non-steroidal anti-inflammatory drugs, tramadol, or opioids may be needed (beware of respiratory depression).

Oxygen (if available, for example, on climbing expeditions) may relieve severe dyspnoea and hypoxaemia. Affected mountaineers should be moved to lower altitudes. Oxygen may be needed for air evacuation of patients with ARI.

Prevention

Vaccination against *Strep. pneumoniae* and influenza viruses (📖 p. 492) is appropriate if a high risk of exposure is anticipated; this depends on the expedition's programme, the influenza epidemic status, and the medical history of the expedition member.

Provision of antiviral treatment or prophylaxis (ribavirin for RSV; amantidine for influenza A, zanamivir or oseltamivir for influenza B) would be appropriate only in exceptional circumstances such as unavoidable travel to an area where an epidemic was predicted.

References

http://www.brit-thoracic.org.uk/c2/uploads/MACAPrevisedApr04.pdf
http://www.cdc.gov/ncidod/diseases/submenus/sub_pneumonia.htm
http://www.cdc.gov/mmwr/preview/mmwrhtml/rr5315a1.htm

Asthma

Asthma affects 10–15% of the population and is becoming increasingly common, especially in the young. It is characterized by recurrent episodes of shortness of breath, cough, and wheeze caused by reversible airway obstruction. Up to 2000 deaths/year in the UK are caused by asthma, with most occurring outside hospital. Risk factors for death include chronic severe disease, inadequate medical treatment, and those with adverse behavioural and psychosocial factors.

Asthma on expeditions

A person with well controlled asthma should be able to participate in most expeditions, although any obstructive airways condition except very mild asthma is a contraindication to diving (📖 p. 656). Remote environments restrict the treatment available for severe asthma attacks. Severe or unstable asthma may preclude an individual from joining a trip to a remote area (see Chapter 2, Pre-existing disease, 📖 p. 59). Any new environment can alter symptoms, either worsening or improving the condition. Emphasis must be placed on the prevention of asthma attacks, and plans made for early evacuation if symptoms develop.

Asthmatics should be identified at the pre-expedition planning stage and efforts made to optimize the condition, assess medication requirements, formulate a plan for an exacerbation, and, if necessary, modify CASEVAC plans. If space permits they should bring a peak flow meter.

During an expedition, an asthmatic person should note symptoms and, if worsening, record their peak flows regularly. This will identify exacerbations early and prompt the use of prearranged medication increases. Spares of essential medications should be packed separately from regular supplies and a β_2 bronchodilator included in the expedition medical kit.

Altitude: symptoms may improve in some people at altitude owing to reduced airway resistance and fewer allergens. In others, cold air and exercise may exacerbate it. Peak flow meters may marginally under-read at altitude because of reduced air density.

Prevention of acute asthma attacks

Provoking factors

Cold air, exercise, emotion, allergens (house dust mite, pollen, animal fur), infection, drugs (aspirin, NSAIDs, β-blockers).

Ensure:
- Medication compliance and good inhaler technique
- Written asthma action plan for deteriorating symptoms and reduced peak expiratory flow.

Avoid:
- Triggering allergens
- Smoking
- Acute asthma.

Symptoms

- Shortness of breath, wheeze, cough and sputum, especially at night or first thing in the morning.

Signs
- Rapid respiratory rate
- Widespread, polyphonic wheeze
- Hyperinflated and hyper-resonant chest
- Diminished air entry
- Severe life-threatening asthma may have no wheeze and a silent chest.

Assess and record
- Peak expiratory flow rate
- Symptoms and response to self-treatment
- Heart and respiratory rates
- Oxygen saturation (by pulse oximetry if available).

Severity of acute asthma
Moderate asthma
- Peak expiratory flow >50% best or predicted
- Speech normal
- Respiration <25 breaths/min
- Pulse <110 beats/min.

Acute severe asthma
- Peak expiratory flow 33–50% best or predicted
- Unable to complete sentences
- Respiration >25 breaths/min
- Pulse >110 beats/min.

Life-threatening asthma
- Peak expiratory flow <33% best or predicted
- SpO_2 <92% (caution: saturation may be maintained in severe disease, particularly when supplementary oxygen administered)
- Silent chest, cyanosis, or feeble respiratory effort
- Bradycardia, dysrhythmia, or hypotension
- Exhaustion, confusion, or coma.

Differential diagnosis
- Upper airway obstruction
- Pneumonia/lower respiratory tract infection
- Hyperventilation
- Anaphylaxis (📖 p. 222)
- Pulmonary oedema
- Congestive cardiac failure
- High altitude pulmonary oedema (📖 p. 620)
- Chronic obstructive pulmonary disease
- Pneumothorax.

Immediate management
- High flow oxygen (if available)
- $β_2$ bronchodilator—e.g. salbutamol
- 4–6 puffs repeated at intervals of 10–20 min (via spacer or nebulizer if available)
- Hydrocortisone 100–200 mg iv
- Prednisolone 40–50 mg orally.

If there is acute severe asthma, life-threatening asthma, or a poor response to initial treatment, CASEVAC to hospital.

If moderate asthma and good response to initial treatment (reduced symptoms, respiratory rate, and heart rate, PEF >75%), consider increasing usual treatment and continue oral prednisolone 30 mg for 5 days. CASEVAC if any further deterioration.

Life-threatening asthma in remote environment

- Fatality is caused by cardiac arrest secondary to hypoxia and acidosis. Give high flow oxygen if available.
- Consider tension pneumothorax (📖 p. 182).
- Epinephrine (adrenaline) 1:1000 solution 0.5 ml im may be used to relieve brochospasm if peri-arrest.
- In a resource-poor environment: a paper bag or empty water bottle can be used as an improvised spacer for inhalers. Caffeine, a methylxanthine in coffee, tea, and chocolate, is a bronchodilator. Caffeine is readily absorbed from the buccal mucosa and instant coffee granules may be administered in this way.

Reference

The British Thoracic Society publishes comprehensive guidelines for the assessment and management of asthma: http://www.brit-thoracic.org.uk/guidelinessince%201997_asthma_html

Abdomen

Section editor
Sarah Anderson

Contributors
Tim Campbell-Smith, Claire Morgan,
and Jane Wilson-Howarth

Acute abdominal pain

Abdominal pain is a relatively common complaint when overseas and exposed to new cultures, diets, and living conditions. Acute abdominal pain can be a cause of great anxiety in a wilderness setting. Often the first thought is of appendicitis. Indeed, acute appendicitis gives rise to undue concern, historically so much so that, until relatively recently, those venturing to the Antarctic were offered a prophylactic appendicectomy. In reality, acute surgical emergencies account for only 0.7% of medical problems during an expedition.[1]

When a patient presents with acute abdominal pain in a remote location it is far more important to establish whether there is evidence of peritoneal inflammation, and hence the need for evacuation, rather than worrying about specific diagnoses. The hallmarks of peritoneal inflammation are tenderness with guarding. The presence of percussion tenderness (a more subtle form of 'rebound') adds further evidence of serious intra-abdominal pathology. Resuscitation, pain relief, and antibiotics (if appropriate) can be given whilst plans for evacuation are organized.

Abdominal pain is more common in women, but the incidence of surgical disease causing abdominal pain is more common in men.

Managing acute abdominal pain

History

- Age
- Sex, including menstrual history
- Pain:
  - Onset
  - Location, character, severity, and radiation
  - Exacerbating and relieving factors
- Associated symptoms, i.e. vomiting, diarrhoea, fever, melaena, etc.
- Past medical history.

Examination

- General
- Conscious level
- In pain or distress?
- Dehydrated?
- Lying still or rolling in pain?
- Flushed, cold, and clammy?
- Cardiovascular system
  - Tachycardia?
  - Hypotension?
- Respiratory system
  - Cyanosis
  - Respiratory rate
  - Breath sounds (pneumonia can mimic acute abdominal pain)

---

1 Anderson S.R., Johnson C.J.H. Expedition Health of Safety: a risk assessment. *Journal of the Royal Society of Medicine* 2000; **93**: 557–62.

- Abdomen
  - Note any scars, distension, or tenderness
  - Is there guarding (reflex contraction of the abdominal wall muscles on palpation)?
  - Is the guarding localized or generalized?
  - Is the guarding distractible (i.e. voluntary)?
  - Is there 'rebound tenderness'?
  - A more sensitive test is for 'percussion tenderness'. Percuss gently over the abdomen and watch the patient's face for signs of discomfort
  - Listen for bowel sounds
  - Signs of chronic liver disease.

Rectal and vaginal examinations are valuable if the situation allows. Always have a chaperone.

Always document consultation findings, differential diagnoses, and management plan. These are invaluable to look back on, and medicolegally important.

Management plan for patient with acute abdomen

- Good analgesia.
- *Opiates*, if possible intravenously, particularly if vomiting. (This will not mask the signs of peritonitis.)
- Antiemetic such as cyclizine.
- Oxygen, if available.
- Intravenous fluid resuscitation with normal saline (rectal fluids have been used successfully in the wilderness).
- Nasogastric tube if evidence of obstruction or persistent vomiting.
- Aspirate gastric contents or insufflate air and auscultate over the stomach to check position.
- Urinary catheter (if possible). This gives a good indication of adequate fluid resuscitation. Do not place if patient is to make an ambulatory evacuation.
- Check blood glucose (?diabetic ketoacidosis).
- Start broad spectrum antibiotics.
- Proton pump inhibitor (PPI) or H2 blocker if available (now available as sublingual preparations).
- If you have diagnosed a patient with signs of peritonitis, evacuate urgently.

Differential diagnosis

See Table 12.1.

Table 12.1 Table of differential diagnoses of acute abdominal pain

	Site of pain	Onset and character of pain	Associated symptoms	Examination findings
Perforated peptic ulcer	Epigastric. Previous history of ulcer disease	Sudden severe upper abdominal pain. Remains constant	Nausea, vomiting, anorexia (More common in smokers and NSAID takers)	Tachycardic, shocked, dehydrated. Initially upper abdominal tenderness and guarding then becomes generalized
Biliary colic	Epigastric or RUQ. Radiates to shoulder ip	Gradual. Constant pain until subsides	Nausea and vomiting. Pain may be precipitated by fatty foods	Mild RUQ tenderness. No guarding
Acute cholecystitis	Epigastric or RUQ. Radiates to shoulder tip	Gradual onset becomes constant	Nausea and vomiting	RUQ tenderness, localized guarding. Murphy's sign positive. Fever
Acute pancreatitis	Epigastric pain radiates through to back	Sudden onset. Severe, sharp pain	Nausea, vomiting, anorexia g jaundice	Epigastric or generalized tenderness with guarding. Can be shocked and hypoxic
Acute appendicitis	Periumbilical pain which migrates to & localizes in RIF	Gradual onset. Initially vague then sharp pain in RIF	Nausea, vomiting anorexia (common). Occasional diarrhoea	Flushed, fever 38°C, tachycardia. Localized tenderness and guarding RIF. Rovsing sign +ve
Intestinal obstruction	Vague central pain	Gradual onset, colicky abdominal pain	Vomiting, absolute constipation	Dehydration. Tachycardia, abdominal distension, vague tenderness. High pitched bowel sounds
Acute diverticulitis	LIF pain	Gradual onset, constant or colicky	Diarrhoea	Tenderness in LIF ± localized guarding. Occasional mass. Fever
Renal colic	Flank pain radiates around the groin to the penis/labia	sudden onset, colicky	Nausea and vomiting common. Haematuria (on diostick)	Rolling around in pain. Mild flank tenderness
Acute salpingitis	Bilateral adnexae, suprapubic or iliac fossae	Gradual onset, becoming worse	Nausea and vomiting occasionally	Fever. Vaginal discharge. Cervical tenderness, adnexal mass
Ectopic pregnancy	Unilateral low groin pain early on ± shoulder tip pain	Sudden or intermittent, sharp	Often none	Adnexal mass tenderness

Upper abdominal pain

Common causes of severe upper abdominal pain
- Peptic ulcer disease
- Indigestion and gastro-oesophageal reflux disease (GORD)
- Gallstone disease.

Peptic ulcer disease
Risk factors for peptic ulcer disease include smoking, stress, NSAIDs, steroids, and alcohol. Presentation can be insidious, with aching upper abdominal discomfort and irritability to severe abdominal pain, bleeding, or perforation.

Symptoms
- Gnawing upper abdominal pain
- Occurs 1–4 h after eating
- Relieved by bland foods such as milk and yoghurts which buffer stomach acids.

Examination findings
- None
- Mild epigastric tenderness.

Management
- Avoidance of risk factors
- Antacids
- H2 antagonists: ranitidine or cimetidine
- PPI, e.g. omeprazole, lansoprazole, etc.

Indigestion and gastro-oesophageal reflux disease
Symptoms
- Vague upper abdominal fullness
- Belching
- Regurgitation of food or stomach acid
- 'Heart burn'—usually worse after eating
- Improves about an hour or so later
- If intermittent, think of gallstones.

Examination findings
- Often overweight
- Usually none.

Management
- Avoid smoking
- Eat smaller meals
- Antacids ± PPI
- Try low fat meals (to minimize gallstone colic).

Gallstone disease
Gallstones are common, more so in women, and are found in up to 40% over the age of 40 years. Symptomatic stones are increasingly seen in younger people. Gallstones are often asymptomatic, but once symptoms

develop are usually recurrent. Conditions caused by gallstones range from 'flatulent' dyspepsia and fatty food intolerance to life-threatening acute pancreatitis and cholangitis. If a member of an expedition to a remote area has symptomatic gallstones, serious consideration should be given to having a cholecystectomy well in advance of departure.

Table 12.2 Differential diagnosis of gallstone disease

	Symptoms	Signs	Management
Biliary colic	Constant RUQ or epigastric pain Radiates to shoulders, some nausea or vomiting	Mild RUQ tenderness No guarding	Analgesia, rest Avoid fatty foods
Acute cholecystitis	RUQ pain, radiates to right shoulder tip Pain worse on deep breath Nausea and vomiting	RUQ tenderness, localized guarding, fever	Analgesia, antibiotics, co-amoxiclav 375–625 mg tds or ciprofloxacin 500–750 mg bd *Evacuate*
Acute pancreatitis	Epigastric or central abdominal pain, radiates through to the back Nausea and vomiting	Central or generalized tenderness and guarding Hypotension and tachycardia, sometimes fever, occasional jaundice	Analgesia, fluid resuscitation, catheter, omeprazole 40 mg and antibiotics (to treat other possible causes) *Evacuate*
Ascending cholangitis	RUQ or epigastric pain, rigors	RUQ tenderness, fever, jaundice	Analgesia, resuscitation, broad spectrum antibiotics (co-amoxiclav or ciprofloxacin) *Evacuate*
Obstructive jaundice	May be associated with any biliary condition, itching	Jaundice Pale stools Dark urine	Analgesia if required, broad spectrum antibiotics (if febrile) *Evacuate*

Acute pancreatitis: antibiotics are not usually part of the acute treatment of mild pancreatitis, but without the ability to confirm the diagnosis, treat as for a perforated viscus.

Lower abdominal pain

Differential diagnosis of lower abdominal pain

- Acute appendicitis
- Acute diverticulitis
- Gastrointestinal obstruction
- Hernias
- Obstetric and gynaecological problems.

Acute appendicitis

Acute appendicitis is a feared condition to diagnose in the wilderness, and often a cause of anxiety for those going even before the expedition leaves home shores. Appendicitis can occur at any age, but is more common in the young. The diagnosis, even in hospital, is essentially a clinical one, backed up with a white cell count and CRP. *A patient diagnosed with signs of peritonitis requires urgent evacuation.*

Pain begins as a vague central visceral aching pain. Over 12–48 h the pain migrates to settle in the right iliac fossa (RIF), becoming a more focal sharp pain, made worse by moving, coughing, or straining. Anorexia is common, and the most reliable associated symptom. Nausea is common, vomiting less so. Occasionally, patients have diarrhoea (pelvic appendicitis) but this is not profuse as in gastroenteritis. With children, watch them walk; if they limp or bend forward slightly, holding the RIF this is a good indicator of significant pain. Get patients to jump up and down; if they can do this without pain, it is unlikely that they have peritoneal inflammation. Examine them supine. Before even laying a hand, ask them to blow their abdomen up like a balloon and then suck it in. This will hurt if there is peritonitis.

Symptoms

- Central abdominal pain that migrates to the RIF **or** solely RIF pain
- Worse on movement, coughing
- Occasional loin pain (retrocaecal appendicitis)
- Anorexia (very common)
- Nausea and occasional vomiting
- Occasional loose stool.

Clinical findings

- Flushed, feverish, tachycardic
- Furred tongue, fetor oris
- Tenderness in the RIF with guarding
- Percussion tenderness
- Pain in RIF when palpating the left iliac fossa (LIF) (Rovsing's sign)
- Rectal or vaginal tenderness (pelvic appendicitis)
- Feel for cervical excitation (pelvic inflammatory disease—PID).

Management

- Analgesia
- Intravenous fluids (if available; if not, sip clear fluids slowly)
- Start broad spectrum antibiotics if >6 h from definitive medical care

- Cephalosporin and metronidazole (preferably iv, or PR metronidazole 1 g bd)
- Evacuation essential.

Differential diagnoses
- Mesenteric adenitis (children)
- Meckle's diverticulitis
- Mittleschmerz (mid-cycle ovulation pain)
- Ovarian cysts
- Ectopic pregnancy
- PID
- Sigmoid diverticulitis
- Crohn's ileitis
- Gastroenteritis
- Typhoid

If in doubt, treat as acute appendicitis and evacuate.

Acute diverticulitis

Diverticulosis is common in high income countries, and increases with age (rare under the age of 40 years), affecting 5% of 50-year-olds and up to 70% of 85-year-olds. Acute diverticulitis is caused by a microscopic perforation of a diverticulum with a resultant surrounding inflammation. This may cause mild systemic upset which resolves with antibiotics, or can progress to a pericolic abscess which, if it perforates, leads to generalized peritonitis.

Symptoms
- Lethargy and anorexia
- Lower abdominal pain, usually localized to LIF
- Diarrhoea
- Nausea, vomiting (occasional).

Examination findings
- Pyrexia
- Tachycardia
- Tenderness in the LIF ± localized guarding.

Management
- Analgesia
- Rest
- Fluid diet for 24–48 h
- Broad spectrum antibiotics
- If signs of peritonitis are present, *evacuate*.

Gastrointestinal obstruction

GI obstruction is a serious condition requiring fluid resuscitation, evacuation, and treatment of the underlying cause. The commonest causes in the UK are adhesional obstruction from previous surgery and strangulated hernias. In the wilderness, making a specific diagnosis is less important than recognizing the problem and initiating fluid resuscitation and evacuation. Fluid losses into the obstructed bowel can be considerable (several litres) and patients can rapidly become dehydrated and shocked.

Symptoms
- Abdominal pain (initially colicky then constant)
- Vomiting, maybe bile-stained (early with proximal obstructions)
- Absolute constipation (no passage of flatus or faeces)
- Abdominal distension
- Painful swelling (i.e. groin, umbilical).

Examination findings
- Dehydration
- Tachycardia
- Hypotension
- Oliguria
- Distended abdomen
- High-pitched (tinkling) bowel sounds
- Hernia
- Abdominal tenderness (a very worrying sign of possible perforation).

Management
- Analgesia
- Rest
- Intravenous fluids
- Nasogastric tube if vomiting
- *Evacuate*.

Hernias
Hernias should be diagnosed and repaired well before departure. The commonest sites are groin and umbilical. Most hernias will cause discomfort and limit activity, particularly heavy work. If strangulation occurs, urgent evacuation is required. If a hernia becomes apparent on an expedition but is not strangulated it does not require evacuation. Limit the patient to light activities which are comfortable to perform and avoid lifting (particularly rucksacks). Improvised trusses are of little or no value.

Symptoms
- Swelling
- Discomfort
- With strangulation:
  - Lump that 'won't go down'
  - Constant severe pain
  - Vomiting
  - Distension
  - Absolute constipation.

Examination findings
- Uncomplicated hernia:
  - Soft, non-tender swelling
    - *Groin (may extend in to the scrotum)*
    - *Umbilical*
    - *Femoral (higher risk of strangulation)*
    - *Associated with a surgical incision*
  - Reducible

- Strangulated hernia:
  - Tender swelling
  - Hot, erythematous overlying skin
  - Signs of obstruction.

Management
If uncomplicated:
- Avoid heavy lifting/work/carrying bags
- Simple pain relief

Strangulated:
- As for GI obstruction: *evacuate.*
- Intravenous antibiotics.

Acute ovarian conditions
Acute problems with the ovaries include haemorrhage, rupture of a cyst, and torsion. All these conditions are associated with pain. The time of pain can help distinguish the various diagnoses. Mittleschmerz pain is mid-cycle from ovulatory bleeding and is usually unilateral. Pain from a ruptured ovarian cyst can occur at any time in the cycle. There may be signs of peritonism or the patient may complain of shoulder tip pain if blood tracks up to the diaphragm. Torsion presents as sudden onset of unilateral severe lower abdominal pain and may be accompanied by nausea, vomiting, and diarrhoea. In hospital, these conditions are often thought initially to be appendicitis and are diagnosed at laparoscopy or appendicectomy. These patients, therefore, will commonly be evacuated.

Symptoms
- Lower abdominal/pelvic pain
- Nausea, vomiting, diarrhoea
- Shoulder tip pain
- Examination findings
  - Low iliac fossa tenderness ± guarding
  - Cervical tenderness and tender adnexae on vaginal examination
  - Tachycardia but apyrexial.

Management
- Check pregnancy test if possible
- Analgesia
- Rest
- Reassurance with Mittleschmerz
- If there are signs of peritonism: *evacuate.*

Ectopic pregnancy
All women of childbearing age with abdominal pain should have a pregnancy test performed. The site and onset of pain depends on site of implantation. Pain is usually preceded by a period of amenorrhoea for 6–8 weeks. Pain is usually unilateral. If there is enough blood, pain is more generalized or may give shoulder tip pain. Vaginal bleeding is scant and usually dark brown, and appears a few hours after the onset of the pain. Risk factors include intrauterine contraceptive devices (IUCD),

previous ectopic, progesterone only pill, IVF and previous pelvic sepsis, i.e. appendicitis or PID. Once suspected, evacuate urgently, as these patients can deteriorate rapidly.

Symptoms
- Amenorrhoea and breast tenderness
- Previous period atypical
- Lower abdominal pain
- Shoulder tip pain
- Vaginal bleeding (scant and often dark) in <50%.

Examination findings
- Lower abdominal tenderness ± guarding
- Signs of shock
- Vaginal bleeding
- Positive pregnancy test.

Management
- Analgesia
- Resuscitate
- Intavenous fluids
- *Evacuate.*

Pelvic inflammatory disease

PID is almost always caused by ascending infection from the genital tract. It is acquired as a sexually transmitted infection. The condition used to be commonly gonoccocal; now, up to half of cases are due to *Chlamydia*. Infection usually involves the endometrium and both fallopian tubes. Risk factors include age at first sexual intercourse, number of partners, and presence of an IUCD. The severity is variable, and it may be mistaken for appendicitis.

Symptoms
- Pelvic pain
- Fever
- Deep dyspareunia
- Dysmenorrhoea
- GI upset.

Examination findings
- Pyrexia
- Signs of systemic sepsis
- Bilateral iliac fossa tenderness ± guarding
- Cervical tenderness on vaginal examination
- Speculum examination may reveal pus from the external os
- Occasional pelvic mass.

Management
- Analgesia
- Combination antibiotics
- Co-amoxiclav or erythromycin + doxycycline
- Penicillin + metronidazole + doxycycline
- *Evacuate if there are signs of systemic sepsis.*

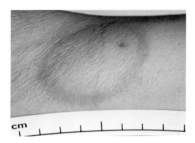

Plate 4 Lyme disease—erythema chronicum migrans.

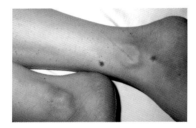

Plate 5 Meningococcal meningitis: early petechial rash.

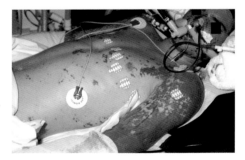

Plate 6 Meningococcal septicaemia: vasculitic/necrotic rash.

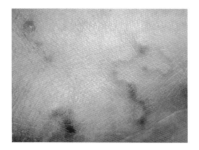

Plate 1 Cutaneous larva migrans (creeping eruption).

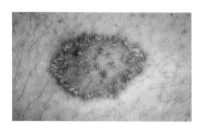

Plate 2 Superficial fungal infection (tinea).

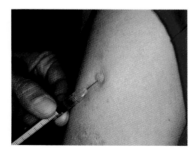

Plate 3 Intradermal injection technique.

Gastrointestinal bleeding

Upper gastrointestinal bleeding

This is a serious problem in remote areas.

Even in the hospital setting there is significant mortality.

With prolonged, effortful vomiting, minor streaks of blood may be seen in the vomitus. This is caused by small tears in the oesophageal mucosa (Mallory–Weiss tear), and is not serious.

If there is haematemesis (vomit of fresh blood), coffee ground vomiting, or the passage of melaena (black, sticky, offensive smelling, tar-like stools), then this is a true emergency requiring prompt treatment and evacuation.

If the expedition is in a very remote location, attempts to carry-out a casualty who is actively bleeding are not recommended. Evacuate by helicopter if possible.

If bleeding stops and the patient appears well, they should be evacuated urgently, as re-bleeding is common and carries a high mortality rate.

Symptoms
- Haematemesis
- 'Coffee grounds' vomiting
- Confusion
- Passage of malaena or dark blood per rectum
- History of peptic ulcer disease.

Examination findings
- Pale
- Tachycardia
- Hypotension (a very ominous sign in the young)
- Confusion and agitation
- Decreased urine output
- Concentrated urine
- Melaena on rectal examination
- Fresh blood per rectum; if from the stomach, indicates rapid haemorrhage.

Management
- Rest
- Place the patient supine with legs elevated
- Intravenous access and fluids if available
- PPI or H2 blockers (sublingual preparations are available, i.e. Fastabs®)
- Avoid NSAIDs, smoking, alcohol, caffeine
- Catheterize if possible or measure urine output
- *Evacuate.*

Lower gastrointestinal (rectal) bleeding

The passage of small amounts of fresh blood per rectum following defecation is common, and is usually due to haemorrhoids (piles). On expeditions, constipation can be a problem, particularly with dehydration, change in diet, and being confined to a tent in a storm.

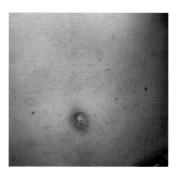

Plate 7 Typhoid rose spots.

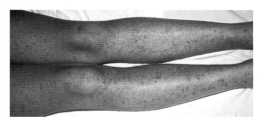

Plate 8 African tick typhus: generalised rash.

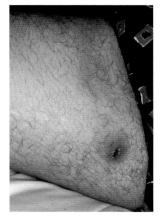

Plate 9 African tick fever: eschar and lymphangitic lines.

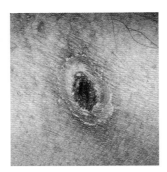

Plate 10 Scrub typhus: eschar.

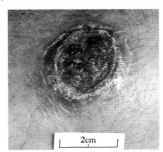

Plate 11 Cutaneous leishmaniasis.

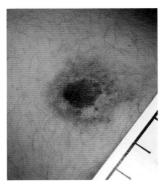

Plate 12 Recluse spider (Loxosceles) bite: red-white-and-blue sign 18 hr after the bite. Scale in cm.

Causes of lower gastrointestinal bleeding
- Haemorrhoids
- Anal fissure
- Diverticular disease (age generally >60 years; can be copious)
- Acute colitis (± pus and mucus; usually there is previous history)
- Dysentery (+ diarrhoea and fever) 📖 p. 385.

Haemorrhoids (piles)

Haemorrhoids are caused by abnormal swelling of anorectal tissue, which may become traumatized during defecation and bleed. They occasionally prolapse, strangulate, and thrombose. This requires pain relief and ice packs to reduce the swelling.

Symptoms
- Fresh red rectal bleeding following bowel motion (often painless and only seen on toilet paper)
- Perianal itching
- Prolapsing piles (very painful, if thrombosed).

Examination findings
- Unless prolapsed, haemorrhoids are impalpable.

Management
- Soften stools—high fibre diet and good hydration
- Avoid straining at stool
- Proctosedyl or Xyloproct ointment or suppositories can help
- Use baby wipes instead of toilet paper
- If thrombosed, use analgesia and ice packs (not directly on the skin).

Anal fissure

An acute, painful condition where there is a tear/split in the skin lining the anus. It is usually precipitated by an episode of constipation.

Symptoms
- Severe anal pain on defecation (like lemon juice on a cut)
- Small amount of fresh, red, rectal bleeding.

Examination findings
- Soft, non-tender abdomen
- Rectal examination is usually impossible due to pain and sphincter spasm (this gives the diagnosis).

Management
- Soften the stools—high fibre diet, good hydration, laxative (lactulose)
- Pain relief—local anaesthetic gel (Proctosedyl or Xyloproct ointment)
- Relax the sphincter spasm with Rectogesic® (0.4% GTN ointment—shelf-life 3 months). Use a pea size amount rubbed on to the perianal skin bd for 6 weeks. Can cause headache and postural hypotension.

Diarrhoea and vomiting

Up to a third of medical problems encountered on an expedition are related to gastrointestinal 'upset' or diarrhoea. Diarrhoeal illness world-wide causes over a billion episodes of illness a year, and in the developing world is a major cause of death in the young and the elderly. There are many reasons for developing diarrhoea whilst abroad: the change in water and diet, altered schedules, the stresses of foreign travel, and infection. If diarrhoea has continued for less than 3 weeks, then infection is the most likely cause.

The commonest route of infection is faecal–oral, i.e. poor hygiene or through contaminated water. Prevention with scrupulous hand hygiene and avoidance of untreated water are essential to minimize the risk of diarrhoeal illness affecting an expedition. Diarrhoea can be the cause of the expedition failing in its aims or just being a miserable experience, and is largely preventable.

- Diarrhoea = four or more loose or liquid stools per day
- Dysentery = acute diarrhoea with blood.

In taking the history ask about:
- Duration
- Stools: colour, consistency, frequency, blood or pus
- Vomiting
- Fever
- Abdominal pain
- Thirst? (a late symptom)
- Recent eating and drinking habits
- Others affected?

Examination
- General condition
- Signs of dehydration:
  - Reduced volume of concentrated urine
  - Dry mucous membranes
  - Skin turgor
  - Sunken eyes
  - Raised pulse (late sign)
  - Blood pressure—including postural drop (very late sign)
- Temperature.

Usually diarrhoeal illnesses will settle. Some will require specific treatments, but the most important factor in minimizing morbidity and mortality rates is hydration. Most patients can maintain their hydration with rest and oral rehydration, although occasionally intravenous fluids are necessary.

Table 12.3 Common causes of diarrhoea

Condition	Diarrhoea no blood	Diarrhoea with blood
No fever	Food poisoning (bacteria or toxins) Traveller's diarrhoea Viruses *Giardia*	Amoebic dysentery
Fever	*Salmonella*	*Shigella* *Campylobacter* *Salmonella*

General treatment guidelines and rehydration

- Rehydration is fundamental.
- Antibiotics are not first line treatment for diarrhoea. Most episodes are self-limiting and usually settle within 2 days.
- However, a single dose of ciprofloxacin (1 g) at the onset of diarrhoea may shorten the duration and, if symptoms persist, continue ciprofloxacin 500 mg bd for 3 days.
- Basic treatment is similar regardless of the cause.
  - *Rest.*
  - *Replace fluids, orally if possible, with oral rehydration fluids (Dioralyte)—frequent sips if vomiting.*
  - *Aim for good volumes (>0.5 ml/kg body weight/h) of clear urine.*
  - *Antiemetics may help (suppositories or im/iv injection).*
  - *Paracetamol if febrile or abdominal pain.*
  - *Avoid dairy products, but don't fast.*
  - *Avoid loperamide or lomotil unless absolutely necessary.*
  - *Loperamide (4 mg initially, then 2 mg after each loose stool) is useful to limit symptoms if travel is essential or tent-bound by a storm.*
  - *Intravenous fluids if unable to manage oral fluids (if iv fluids are required the patient should be evacuated).*
  - *(Anecdotally, rectal fluids via a Foley catheter have been used with success.)*
  - *If diarrhoea persists, it could be protozoal; give metronidazole or tinidazole.*

When to seek external medical attention:
- Temperature above 40°C
- Significant fever for over 48 h
- Diarrhoea lasting longer than 4 days
- Difficulty keeping fluid down
- Diarrhoea with blood.

Prevention of diarrhoeal illness

Prevention is better than treatment of diarrhoeal illness on an expedition which, once present, can spread rapidly through the group, disrupting plans, and at worst putting the group at risk. It is possible to prevent it entirely with education and care.

- Meticulous hand hygiene is essential.
- Ensure that there are facilities to wash hands at the latrine, whether soap and water or alcohol gel.
- Hands must be washed before entering a mess tent.
- Boil or sterilize water (📖 p. 106) before drinking, brushing teeth, or preparing salads
- Avoid ice in drinks
- Check seals on bottled water
- Avoid salads, unpeelable fruit, shellfish, and raw or undercooked meat (particularly chicken)
- Carefully clean mess tins and other cooking equipment.

Cholera

Infection is through contaminated water. Cholera can reach epidemic proportions where sanitation systems have broken down (natural disasters or in war). Profuse watery diarrhoea and rapid dehydration kill. Incubation is 1–3 days.

Symptoms and signs
- Mild diarrhoea initially
- Profuse watery diarrhoea ('rice water stools')
- Vomiting
- Prostration
- Fever
- Dehydration
- Signs of shock.

Treatment
- Rest
- Fluids +++
- Intravenous fluids
- Tetracycline 250–500 mg 6-hourly
- Evacuate.

Typhoid

This is a generalized infection, which later in its course can cause diarrhoea. Initially there may be constipation. Incubation is 7–14 days.

Symptoms and signs

- Fever
- Headache
- Abdominal pain
- Rash (rose spots—2 mm pink papules on torso which fade with pressure)
- After >7days:
  - General deterioration
  - High fever
  - Low pulse (= relative bradycardia)
- After 20 days:
  - Confusion
  - Gravely ill
  - 'Pea soup' diarrhea.

Treatment

- Rest
- Fluids—oral or intravenous
- Ciprofloxacin 500–750 mg bd
- *Evacuate*.

Table 12.4 Diagnosis and treatment of diarrhoea and vomitting

Category of diarrhoea	Organisms	Foods	Incubation	Symptoms	Treatment
Diarrhoea – no blood – no fever	*Staph aureus* (toxin)	Meat, poultry, diary produce, particularly, if eaten cold	Usual: 2–4 h Range:1–7 h	V, AP, (D) short-lived, Abrupt onset	Antibiotics infective, as due to toxins
	Bacillus cereus (toxin)	Fried rice, raw or dried foods particularly, if inadequate reheating	Usual: vomiting syndrome 1–6 h Usual: diarrohea syndrome 6–16 h	V and nausea—lasts <12 h D (short lived), AP—lasts <24 h	Antibiotics ineffective, as due to toxins
	E.coli (toxin) (known as travellers' diarrhoea)	Faecal contamination of water or food	Usual: 12–48 h	D (watery), AP(cramps) Duration: 2–5 days	Usually self-limiting but single dose ciprofloxacin 1 g or tetracycline 500 mg may shorten illness
	Clostridium perfringens	Cooked meat, poultry, particularly, if inadequate re-heating	Usual: 8–12 h Range: 4–24 h	D (watery, often violent), AP, V(racely)	Supportive only
	Cryptosporidium	Faecal contamination of food or water	Usual: 7–10 days Range:1–28 days	D (Watery), AP, bloating	Self-limiting but severe disease in immuno-compromised
	Viral Norovirus Rotavirus	Usually person–person or environmental contamination	Usual: 24–72 h Duration: 1–2 days	N—projectile vomiting, mild D, AP R—Watery D, V, fever	No antibiotics
	Giardia lamblia protozoal infection	Contamination water and mountain streams	Incubation: 7–10 days Duration:2–6 weeks	D (often pale and persistent AP (cramps), bloating Flatulence–'Eggy burps'	Metronidazole 400 mg tds for 5 days or tinidazole single dose 2 g

Table 12.4 (Contd.)

Category of diarrhoea	Organisms	Foods	Incubation	Symptoms	Treatment
Diarrhoea - no blood - FEVER	Salmonella	Undercooked or raw meat, poultry, dairy produce, eggs	Usual: 12–36 h Range: 6–72 h	D(± blood/mucus) V, AP (cramps), fever Duration: 2–5 days	Usually self-limiting ciprofloxacin 500 mg bd if needed
	Cholera	Contaminated water, shellfish or raw food	Incubation:1–3 days	D (profuse and watery = 'rice water') Rapid dehydration leading to shock	Fluids +++ (IV) Tetracycline 250–500 mg for 6 hourly. Evacuate
Diarrhoea - BLOOD - no fever	Entamoeba (amoebic dysentery; protozoal infection)	Raw or undercooked food Waterborne	Incubation: >7 days Duration: Until successfully treated	D (bloody/gradual onset) AP (cramps), Weight loss	Metronidazole 800 mg tds for 5 days Followed by Diloxanide 500 mg tds for 10 days
	E.Coli O157	Meat, poultry, dairy produce Contaminated water	Usual: 3–4 days Range: 1–9 days	D or D with blood, AP (severe) HUS (2–7%)	Antibiotics contra-indicated
Diarrhoea - BLOOD - AND FEVER	Shigella	Faecal contamination of water or food	Usual: 24–72 h Range: 1–7 days	D (Explosive and bloody) AP (cramps), fever, anorexia	Ciprofloxacin 500–750 mg td or trimethoprim 200 mg bd
	Campylobacter	Poultry, raw milk, eggs Contaminated water	Usual: 2–5 days Range: 1–10 days	D (often bloody and profuse), AP (severs cramps) ± fever Duration 2–7 days	Usually self-limiting, Ciprofloxacin 500–750 mg bd or erythromycin 500 mg qds or 1 g bd.

Symptom definitions: V, vomiting; D, diarrhoea; AP, abdominal pain.
Hawker J et al. (2005). Communicable Disease Control Handbook.

Other gastrointestinal problems

This short section deals with some less serious but more common problems. In themselves these are not major problems but in the wilderness can result in a very miserable time and/or the sufferer having to leave the expedition.

Constipation

Normal bowel habit varies enormously, from three stools per day to one stool every 3–4 days. Alterations of bowel habit are common on expeditions. Many people suffer diarrhoea with the change in environment and diet, but constipation can be equally disabling.

Dehydration, from exertion, high altitude, or confinement to a tent during a storm can predispose to constipation. Diets on expeditions can also lack fibre. Constipation is best avoided rather than treated. Ensure that the expedition food has adequate dietary fibre and encourage good hydration, aiming for the regular passing of dilute urine.

Symptoms
- Cramping abdominal pains
- Reduced stool frequency with passage of hard stools.

Examination findings
- Soft abdomen
- Mild tenderness occasionally
- May feel indentable stools in the LIF.

Management
- Good hydration
- High fibre diet
- Prophylactic laxatives are unhelpful
- Simple laxatives may be required (lactulose/senna).

Perianal haematoma

This is a painful small purple swelling at the anal verge, usually arising after having to strain at stool.

Management
- Anaesthetize the area (topical local anaesthetic or ice)
- Make a small stab incision
- Express the clot.

Perianal abscess

This is an acute painful condition of the anus, presenting with pain and swelling in the perianal skin. It comes on over a few days. If caught early and treated with antibiotics it may resolve.

Symptoms
- Perianal pain and swelling
- Fever
- Chills and rigors.

Examination findings
- Pyrexia
- Tender, erythematous perianal swelling.

Management
- Antibiotics (co-amoxiclav or erythromycin + metronidazole).
- Analgesia.
- If very remote some form of drainage will be required to enable ambulatory evacuation.
- An abscess will require surgical incision and drainage, but other abscesses (such as breast) are now treated with needle aspiration and antibiotics.
- It is reasonable to attempt to drain the abscess with a large needle through the most fluctuant area.
- Local anaesthetic does not work well in inflamed tissue—try oral analgesia, ice packs, and lidocaine to skin.
- Evacuate for formal drainage.

Pilonidal abscess
This is infection in the natal cleft, the area over the sacrum between the buttocks.

Symptoms
- Pain and swelling over the sacrum between the buttocks (there may be a previous history of this or even of previous surgery).
- Discharge (minimal serum to large amounts of pus).

Examination findings
- Swelling in the natal cleft (usually slightly to one side).
- The swelling maybe hot, red, and tender.
- On close inspection of the cleft, tiny black pits maybe visible in the midline (pilonidal pits).

Management
- Antibiotics (penicillin and flucloxacillin or erythromycin).
- If not settling, drain the abscess under local anaesthetic:
  - Infiltrate a wide area around the abscess with local anaesthetic (preferably non-inflamed tissue; local anaesthesia works better here).
  - Make a longitudinal linear incision off the midline into the most fluctuant part of the abscess.
  - Break down any loculations with a little finger and irrigate with sterile saline.
  - Cover with a dressing.
- If this then fails to settle: *evacuate*.
- If the situation makes draining the abscess inappropriate, *evacuate* for surgical drainage.

Urological problems

Urinary tract infection

This is a common problem, particularly among women. Symptoms include urinary frequency, a burning sensation during micturition (dysuria), which is maximal as flow stops. Fever is rare unless associated with pyelonephritis.

Examination
- Often clinically normal
- Blood, leukocytes, nitrites, and protein on urine dipstick.

Treatment
- Increase oral fluids
- Trimethoprim, amoxicillin, or ciprofloxacin.

Pyelonephritis

This is infection of one or both kidneys, usually as an ascending infection from the bladder or more rarely secondary to ureteric obstruction. Differential diagnosis: possible retrocaecal appendicitis

Symptoms
- Sudden onset of fever, sweats, rigors
- Flank and/or back pain
- Patient feels 'terrible'
- Dysuria, urinary frequency, and urgency.

Examination findings
- High fever
- Loin tenderness
- Blood, leukocytes, nitrites, and protein on urine dipstick.

Treatment
- Ensure good hydration
- Ciprofloxacin, co-amoxiclav, or a cephalosporin for 10 days

Indications for evacuation
- Failure to respond to treatment
- Systemic sepsis.

Acute urinary retention

This condition manifests as acute painful inability to void urine despite the intense desire to do so. It almost invariably affects men (middle age onwards). The symptoms are incapacitating and require prompt relief.

Symptoms
- Lower abdominal/suprapubic pain
- Intense desire to void
- Dribbling of urine
- Suprapubic distension
- History of previous hesitancy, poor stream, and nocturia.

Examination findings
- Distressed patient
- Distended lower abdomen
- Palpable bladder, dull to percussion, tender (examining the prostate may reveal enlargement but this does not correlate with prostatic symptoms, or change the management).

Treatment
- Decompression with urethral catheter (Foley):
  - Smaller catheters (12–14F) may be more difficult to pass than larger ones (16–18F)
  - Do not attempt instrumentation of the urethra in the field
- If unsuccessful suprapubic needle decompression is required:
  - Aseptic technique
  - Infiltrate 1% lidocaine two finger breadths above the symphysis
  - Direct the needle towards the anus whilst aspirating
  - Aspirate as much urine as possible
  - May require repeating, but will enable ambulatory evacuation
- Watch for a diuresis (more common with chronic obstruction)
- *Evacuate.*

Renal (ureteric) colic
This is a collection of symptoms produced by ureteric obstruction secondary to a calculus.

Symptoms
- Severe flank pain (unable to get comfortable)
- Radiates around along the course of the ureter into the groin, to the base/tip of the penis or the labia
- Nausea and vomiting are common.

Examination findings
- 'Writhing around' in pain, often holding the flank
- Mild loin tenderness
- Haematuria (on dipstick and occasionally frank).

Treatment
- Pain control:
  - NSAIDs are very effective: diclofenac im or PR (if vomiting)
  - Opiates e.g. tramadol
- Forced diuresis is of no benefit but maintain adequate hydration
- Most calculi pass within a few hours.

Indications for evacuation
- Anuria
- Signs of sepsis
- Unable to control symptoms.

The acute scrotum
Acute scrotal pain and swelling is a true surgical emergency and requires urgent assessment and treatment. A strangulated hernia (□ p. 374) and testicular torsion are the two conditions which must be diagnosed and evacuated.

Testicular torsion
- Any age, commoner near puberty
- Sudden onset of severe scrotal pain
- Associated with vomiting
- Pain on walking.

Examination findings
- Oedematous scrotal skin
- Discoloured with a blue tinge
- No relief when elevated (negative Phren's sign).

Treatment
Scrotal exploration is unrealistic in the wilderness.
   Manual detorsion:
- Lie the patient supine
- Elevate the testis
- Gently untwist, turning the epididymis medially
- If successful relief is swift.

If unable to untwist:
- Strong analgesia
- *Evacuate*.

Epididymitis
- More gradual onset than torsion
- Associated with fever and dysuria
- Relieved by gentle elevation
- Careful palpation reveals a tender, swollen epididymis.

Prostatitis
Prostatitis is an acute infection of the prostate gland by viral or bacterial pathogens. It is an uncommon infection, but can be associated with severe sepsis. Of the bacterial causes, 80% are due to *E. coli*.

Symptoms
- Fever, sweats, rigors
- Perineal pain
- Dysuria, frequency, urgency
- Urinary retention uncommon.

Examination findings
- Pyrexia
- Tachycardia
- Boggy tender prostate on rectal examination.

Treatment
- Treat as bacterial (prolonged courses may be required)
- Ciprofloxacin
- Co-amoxiclav.

Indications for evacuation
- Systemic sepsis
- Poor response to treatment.

Sexually transmitted infections

Definition: any disease transmitted by sexual contact.

Epidemiology: sexually transmitted infections (STIs), although mostly curable, are often asymptomatic, are easily transmissible, can cause serious complications, and can affect anybody.

Incidence: the exact data for infections worldwide is unknown, although the WHO estimated 340 million new cases of STIs globally in 1999, with the largest numbers in South/South-East Asia, sub-Saharan Africa, Latin America, and the Caribbean.

Causes: bacterial STIs include *Chlamydia trachomatis, Neisseria gonorrhea,* and syphilis. Viral STIs include human immunodeficiency virus (HIV), herpes simplex virus (HSV), human papilloma virus (HPV or warts), hepatitis B, and hepatitis C. *Trichomonas vaginalis* is due to a parasitic flagellate protozoan.

Risk factors: any unprotected sexual contact, including skin-to-skin contact (for HSV and HPV), and fluid-to-fluid contact.

Prevention: must be considered prior to travel:
- Hepatitis B vaccination (usually three injections over 6 months).
- Abstinence if possible.
- Avoid sexual contact with higher risk groups (e.g. sex workers).
- Barrier contraception/condoms—take them with you.
- Condoms purchased abroad may not conform to British safety standards and are often smaller and so may break.
- Protected oral sex: some infections (e.g. chlamydia and gonorrhoea) can also be carried in the throat and can be transmitted this way. Use flavoured condoms and dental dams (squares of latex for oral–vaginal/oral–anal contact).

Treatment: for up-to-date STI treatment guidelines see the website of the British Association for Sexual Health and HIV (BASHH): http://www.bashh.org/guidelines.asp.

Urethral discharge

Definition: pus/fluid coming from the tube of the penis.

Causes: most common causes are chlamydia, gonorrhoea, and non-specific urethritis (NSU). HSV can also cause urethral discharge, but would usually be accompanied by painful genital sores/blisters.

Causes and symptoms

Chlamydia
- Caused by bacterium *Chlamydia trachomatis*
- Transmitted via oral/vaginal/anal contact
- 50% of men asymptomatic
- Typically clear/white urethral discharge ± dysuria.

Gonorrhoea
- Caused by bacterium *Neisseria gonorrhoeae*
- Transmitted via oral/vaginal/anal contact
- 10% of men asymptomatic
- Typically yellow/green urethral discharge ± dysuria

Non-specific urethritis (NSU):
(Assuming chlamydia and gonorrhoea are not the cause)
- Up to 30% have no bacterial pathogen.
- Possible causes are *Trichomonas vaginalis* (1–17%), *Mycoplasma genitalium* (20%), urinary tract infection, candida, foreign bodies, chemical irritation (e.g. soaps, washing powders).
- Typically clear/white discharge may only be present on urethral massage ± dysuria.

Investigations: these depend on the equipment available. Ideally, a Gram-stained urethral smear to confirm diagnosis of gonorrhoea and NSU, nucleic acid amplification test (NAAT), or enzyme immunoassay (EIA) test on a first catch urine for chlamydia and gonorrhoea, and culture on urethral swab for gonorrhoea.

Management
- Avoid sexual contact to prevent further transmission
- Ensure partner(s) are informed
- Ideally, test the patient as soon as possible to avoid STI complications
- Consider treating if investigations are not possible and there is uncomplicated infection (no testicular pain, no eye symptoms)
- If patient is treated, suggest full STI screen when returns home.

Treatment
BASHH guidelines suggest:
- Chlamydia: doxycycline 100 mg bd for 1 week *or* azithromycin 1 g stat *or* erythromycin 500 mg four times a day for 7 days (less efficacious than doxycycline and more likely to cause side effects).
- Gonorrhoea: cefixime 400 mg stat *plus* treatment for chlamydia *or* ciprofloxacin 500 mg stat *plus* treatment for chlamydia but high resistance worldwide.
- NSU: treat as for chlamydia. Avoid soaps etc. to genital area.
- If treating blind, consider drug regime that would treat chlamydia and gonorrhoea plus UTI such as ofloxacin 200 mg bd for 1 week.

Complications
- Epididymo-orchitis—inflammation of one or both testes (presentation usually with unilateral testicular pain).
- Sexually acquired reactive arthritis (SARA)—dissemination of bacteria to the joints causing pain ± swelling and stiffness at one or more joints.
- Conjunctivitis.

Vaginal discharge
Definition: fluid coming from the vagina. A 'normal' vaginal discharge is usually clear/milky, does not smell, may change during a woman's cycle, and keeps the vagina healthy.

Changes in vaginal discharge that may indicate a problem are:
- Increase in amount
- Change in colour or smell
- Irritation, itchiness, soreness, or burning.

Causes and symptoms
See Table 12.5.

Investigations

Microscopy of Gram-stained vaginal smears may allow diagnosis of gonorrhoea, *Candida*, and bacterial vaginosis. Direct observation by a wet smear for *Trichomonas*. Ideally more complicated lab tests are administered if they are available.

Management

- Avoid sexual contact to prevent further transmission.
- Ensure partner(s) are informed.
- Ideally, test the patient as soon as possible to avoid STI complications.
- Suggest testing rather than treating blind if possible.
- Consider treating blind if confident of diagnosis (e.g. patient has had same previously) and suitable medication available.
- If patient treated, suggest full STI screen when returns home.

Treatment

BASHH guidelines suggest:

- Chlamydia: doxycycline 100 mg bd for 1 week *or* azithromycin 1 g stat.
- Gonorrhoea: cefixime 400 mg stat *plus* treatment for chlamydia *or* ciprofloxacin 500 mg stat *plus* treatment for chlamydia but high resistance worldwide.
- *Trichomonas*: metronidazole 2 g orally stat.
- Bacterial vaginosis: only treat if symptomatic—metronidazole 400 mg bd for 5 days.
- Avoid soaps/shower gels/scented products to genital area.
- *Candida*: clotrimazole pessary (varying dosages), clotrimazole cream *or* fluconazole 150 mg stat capsule. Avoid soaps/shower gels/scented products to genital area, avoid tight-fitting clothes. Oral treatments and cream are preferable on expedition.

Complications

Untreated chlamydia/gonorrhoea can lead to:

- PID (📖 p. 376)—upper genital tract inflammation, causes low abdominal pain, pyrexia, systemic illness.
- Possible infertility owing to scarring/blocking of fallopian tubes.
- Sexually acquired reactive arthritis (SARA)—dissemination of bacteria to the joints causing pain ± swelling and stiffness at one or more joints.
- Conjunctivitis.

Table 12.5 Vaginal discharge causes and symptoms

Infection	Typical symptoms
Chlamydia	70% asymptomatic
	Purulent vaginal discharge, dysuria, intermenstrual/post-coital bleeding, low abdominal pain
Gonorrhoea	50% asymptomatic
	Increased/change in discharge (especially colour and smell), low abdominal pain
Trichomonas vaginalis	10–50% asymptomatic
	Change in vaginal discharge (varying thickness, sometimes frothy, often yellow/green), vulval irritation, dysuria, offensive odour
Bacterial vaginosis	Thin/watery, white/grey, homogenous, offensive, fishy-smelling discharge. Not STI
Candidiasis (thrush)	Thick, white, curdy 'cottage cheese' discharge, vulval itching, soreness, and erythema. Vulval fissures, external dysuria. Not STI

Genital sores and ulcers (Table 12.6)
Definition: open wound of skin or mucous membrane in genital area.
STI causes:
- Syphilis
- Genital herpes.

Causes and symptoms
Syphilis: caused by bacterium *Treponema pallidum*.
There are three stages:
- Early (primary, secondary, and early latent <2 years).
- Late (late latent >2 years).
- Tertiary (with neurological and cardiovascular involvement).

Syphilis is transmitted via oral/vaginal/anal contact, blood-to-blood contact, or mother-to-baby contact (vertical transmission).
The incubation period is 9–90 days for primary symptoms.

Genital herpes
- Caused by Herpes simplex virus type 1 or 2.
- Transmitted via skin-to-skin contact (oral/vaginal/anal).
- Incubation period is typically 2–10 days but can be years.

Table 12.6 Genital sores and ulcers

Infection	Typical symptoms
Syphilis	Primary: single, painless, indurated ulcer (chancre) with a clean base discharging clear serum. Regional lymphadenopathy
	Secondary: multisystemic involvement, generalized polymorphic rash, often affecting palms and soles
Genital herpes	Painful blisters/sores and ulceration of genital/perianal area. May be accompanied by burning, tingling, itching, dysuria, and urethral/vaginal discharge. Systemic symptoms of fever are common in primary infection. Chronic condition, symptoms can recur

Investigations/diagnosis
In experienced medical practitioners, visual diagnosis is possible. Dark ground microscopy from lesions in early syphilis can confirm infection, otherwise serological test for *Treponema pallidum* is performed. Early false negatives are possible, so repeat if there is high clinical suspicion. HSV viral culture from swab from genital lesions is ideal.

Management
- Avoid sexual contact to prevent further transmission.
- Test patient as soon as possible to avoid complications if STI present.
- Suspected syphilis needs infection confirmation, specialized medical attention, and supervised treatment.
- Consider self-treating herpes if the patient gives a history of HSV, and there appears to be uncomplicated infection (no urinary retention).
- Avoid sharing towels/flannels as there is a very slight risk of transmission.

Treatment
BASHH guidelines suggest:
- *Early syphilis:* 2 × im benzathine penicillin 2.4 MU (day 1 and 8) *or* (if penicillin allergy) doxycycline 100 mg bd for 14 days.
- Treatment differs in pregnancy and HIV.
- *Herpes:* treatment needs to be started within 5 days of the first symptoms.
- Aciclovir 200 mg five times per day for 5 days *or* famciclovir 250 mg three times per day for 5 days *or* valaciclovir 500 mg twice per day for 5 days *and* saline bathing, topical anaesthetic agents, analgesia.

Complications
- Syphilis—reactions to treatment (Jarisch–Herxheimer/anaphylaxis).
- Herpes—urinary retention, secondary bacterial infection.

Differential diagnoses
- Behçet's disease (chronic immune condition. Symptoms of mouth ulcers ± genital ulcers, skin lesions, eye and joint inflammation).
- Chancroid.
- Trauma—possible cause if patient recalls specific incident.

Table 12.7 Genital lumps and other sexually transmitted infections: causes a symptoms

Infection	Typical symptoms
Genital warts	Small, pink/white lumps, sometimes 'cauliflower-shaped', itchy, usually painless. Visually same as warts elsewhere
Molluscum contagiosum	Small, round, 'spots', often have white head or small dimple in centre
Folliculitis	Infected hair follicle causing painful pus-filled swellings in genital area, erythema; may have yellow head

Genital lumps and other sexually transmitted infections
Causes, symptoms, and treatment see Table 12.7

Genital warts
- Caused by human papilloma virus (HPV).
- Transmitted though sexual contact (including skin-to-skin contact).
- Treated with cryotherapy or podophyllotoxin 'paint' (Warticon).
- Psychological distress is the main difficulty; treatment can wait until repatriation as complications are unlikely.

Molluscum contagiosum
- Caused by species of molluscipoxvirus.
- Transmitted though sexual contact (including skin-to-skin contact).
- Avoid sharing towels/flannels/clothing.
- Treatment (if required) with cryotherapy.
- Psychological distress is the main difficulty; treatment can wait until repatriation as complications are unlikely (but can get secondary bacterial infection).

Folliculitis
- Often bacterial cause.
- Common in areas that rub, e.g. buttocks and groin.
- May burst by itself; keep area clean, saline bathing.
- Treat with antibiotics considered if no improvement.

Sexual assault

Definition: any type of sexual act committed without the informed consent of one of the parties

Management: Consider the 4 Ps (Table 12.8).

Table 12.8 The 4 Ps—management of sexual assault

Four Ps	Consider
Police	If patient wishes police involvement this *must* be done first (any examination may compromise forensic examination). Report to local police—forensics within 7 days
Pregnancy	Emergency contraception:
	• Levonelle as soon as possible (up to 72 h)
	• Emergency IUCD fitted up to 5 days (or day 19 of 28-day cycle)
Prophylaxis	Post-exposure prophylaxis following sexual exposure (PEPSE) for HIV (📖 p. 399). Start within 72 h
	Consider prophylactic antibiotics to cover chlamydia, gonorrhea, and *Trichomonas*
	Azithromycin 1 g stat *or* doxycycline 100 mg bd for 1 week
	Cefixime 400 mg stat (*or* ciprofloxacin 500 mg stat but beware resistance)
	Metronidazole 400 mg bd for 5 days *or* metronidazole 2 g stat
	If not vaccinated against hepatitis B, first dose can be given within 3 weeks to cover retrospectively. Rapid course of vaccine preferred (0, 7, 21 days, and 6 months)
Psychological	Strongly consider repatriation owing to likely physical and emotional trauma. Ongoing counselling may be required (📖 p. 506).

Human immunodeficiency virus and prevention

Definition: human immunodeficiency virus (HIV) is a retrovirus that suppresses the body's immune response, and is responsible for acquired immune deficiency syndrome (AIDS), a collection of specific opportunistic infections.

Incidence

HIV is increasing in incidence worldwide. The areas with the highest prevalence of HIV are sub-Saharan Africa, South-East Asia, Russia, the Caribbean, and South America.

Transmission

HIV is present in blood (including menstrual blood), semen, and vaginal fluids. Transmission can occur if infected fluids pass between people. There are three main routes of transmission:

- Unprotected sexual contact (including oral sex).
- Blood-to-blood contact.
- Mother-to-baby.

Risk factors

- Unprotected sexual contact.
- Injecting drug use/sharing injecting equipment.
- Needlestick injuries/contaminated sharps.
- Contaminated blood products.
- Mucous membrane exposure (e.g. splash of blood/semen into the eye).

HIV prevention

- Abstinence from sexual activity.
- Safe sex—condom use for all sexual activity (see STI prevention).
- Avoid sexual contact with higher risk groups (e.g. sex workers, high incidence countries).
- Ensure safe injecting equipment/sharps—take your own with you.

Post-exposure prophylaxis

Consider as a last measure where all other methods of HIV prevention have failed. This comprises a 4-week course of antiretroviral (anti-HIV) medication, started up to 72 h (but ideally ASAP) after possible exposure to attempt to abort HIV infection. It is not guaranteed to work, and medication usually has significant side effects. It was previously used for healthcare workers following needlestick injuries from HIV-positive patients, but is now also considered after sexual exposure (PEPSE; see Table 12.9).

Table 12.9 Situations in which PEPSE would be considered[2]

Sexual activity	Source status		
	HIV-positive	Unknown (area of high prevalence >10%)	Unknown (area of low prevalence <10%)
Receptive anal sex	Recommended	Recommended	Considered
Insertive anal sex	Recommended	Considered	Not recommended
Receptive Vaginal sex	Recommended	Considered	Not recommended
Insertive vaginal sex	Recommended	Considered	Not recommended
Splash of semen into eye	Considered	Considered	Not recommended
Fellatio with ejaculation	Considered	Considered	Not recommended
Fellatio without ejaculation	Not recommended	Not recommended	Not recommended
Cunnilingus	Not recommended	Not recommended	Not recommended

The current recommended drug regime is Combivir bd (zidovudine 300 mg plus lamivudine 150 mg) plus nelfinavir 1250 mg bd (for latest updates refer to http://www.bashh.org.uk). Treatment is very expensive (approximately £1000 for 28 days), so 'starter packs' of 3–5 days could be taken on expedition with immediate repatriation to continue treatment. If expedition does not have PEPSE, some countries may have Combivir available to buy—seek advice in the local area.

Common side effects are diarrhoea, nausea, and vomiting, so antiemetics (domperidone 10–20 mg tds when required) and anti-diarrhoeals (loperamide 4 mg stat followed by 2 mg after each loose motion to maximum of 12 mg in 24 h).

Risk-benefit analysis should be undertaken and decisions made on a case-by-case basis. Consideration must also be given to the possibility of an individual being already infected with HIV and the ability to adhere to (vital) and tolerate the drug regimen, especially in remote areas.

2 Clinical Effectiveness Group (BASHH) (2006). UK Guideline for the use of post-exposure prophylaxis for HIV following sexual exposure. *International Journal of STD and AIDS* 2006; **17**: 81–92.

Gynaecological problems

Gynaecological problems often occur in women who venture into remote regions, even amongst those who have made careful preparations.

Period problems

An 'average' woman loses about 40 ml of blood with each menstrual cycle. Although this amounts to only eight teaspoonsful over 4 or 5 days, coping with this can be surprisingly challenging. There may be no privacy to change sanitary protection and no easy access to water. Some medical advisers encourage young women to start the combined oral contraceptive pill to control menstruation, but this is not the solution[3], particularly in light of the fact that periods often lighten or even stop during the physical demands of an expedition. Introducing the pill can complicate matters if travellers' diarrhoea interferes with its absorption, thus allowing unpredictable and inconvenient breakthrough bleeding; this is particularly likely in those who have newly started taking the pill but it also occurs in those whose periods are usually regulated by it.

Planning

Ideally, each adventurer will have given some thought to her gynaecological needs long before setting out. One option that is often overlooked is to suppress menstruation by arranging 12-weekly Depo Provera injections. This will stop monthly bleeds in most women by the second or third injection. Lack of periods then persist beyond the 3 months between injections, although the woman is, of course, at risk of pregnancy beyond 13 weeks. This contraceptive method has a lot to recommend it amongst travelling women, not least because, being a progesterone-only method, it does not increase the risk of deep vein thrombosis, whereas women taking the combined oral contraceptive pill (or any hormone replacement) have a significantly increased risk; this adds to any risk arising from a long-haul flight, or from ascending to extreme altitude. A progestogen implant (e.g. Implanon) has similar advantages. Both Depo Provera and Implanon need to be organized some time—preferably 6 months—before departure.

Contraceptive types

- *Depo injections* can cause spotting in the first months but thereafter usually suppress menstruation; does not increase DVT risk.
- *Implants* can cause spotting in the first months but thereafter usually suppress menstruation; does not increase DVT risk.
- *Combined pill* increases DVT risk so not good for women ascending to extreme altitude; breakthrough bleeding is often a problem after diarrhoea and in the first 3 months after starting.
- *Progestogen-only pill* can cause spotting, especially in the first month or two; does not increase DVT risk.
- *Intrauterine contraceptive* device tends to increase amount and duration of blood flow; does not increase DVT risk.
- *Intrauterine contraceptive system* can cause spotting in the first months but thereafter usually suppresses menstruation; does not increase DVT risk.
- *Barrier methods* are always worth packing as a back-up and for safer sex.

Pain during the first day or two of a menstrual period is often due to blood clots at the neck of the womb and implies a heavier loss than usual. Sometimes, fluid restriction around the first day of bleeding improves symptoms, and so can iron if a woman is anaemic. Those with recurrent and distressing pain on menstruation will be helped by taking a NSAID preparation regularly for a few days starting a day or two before the onset of bleeding. If a woman complains about her periods, ask whether there is any odour or coloured discharge, which suggests a sexually transmitted infection (see below).

Heavy periods in themselves can be quite debilitating but when combined with a poor diet can lead to anaemia. Anaemia then tends to exacerbate heavy menstrual loss and in turn contributes further to anaemia. Iron tablets are often cheaply purchased overseas, and will act as a good tonic.

Logistics
Plenty of sanitary products need to be packed in waterproof containers (zip-lock bags are ideal) and consideration given to responsible disposal. Burying tampons and sanitary towels in desert environments, for example, can allow retrieval by village dogs or exposure by wind. Some sanitary items compost but some towels contain a lot of plastic and do not; washable products are available (e.g. from http://www.greenbabyco.com). Alternatively, there are devices to collect blood such as the Mooncup (http://www.mooncup.co.uk). This is a small soft cup with a stalk, which fits in the vagina and collects menstrual blood. It removes the need to carry disposables where they might be difficult to obtain, but clean hands are required to take it out and empty it. The user also needs somewhere to dispose of the still-liquid blood and access to water to clean the Mooncup before reinserting it. The solution is perhaps to use both reusable and also some conventional disposable supplies.

Vaginal irritation/discharge
Normal vaginal discharge is colourless and its consistency changes with the menstrual cycle. A woman might complain of a *change* in discharge:

- Yellow or green or foul-smelling discharge implies infection (p. 395).
- Vaginal thrush (see Table 12.5); can be treated with miconazole pessaries or oral fluconazole.
- A fishy odour suggests bacterial vaginosis which is cleared with vaginal clindamycin cream inserted for 7 nights or oral metronidazole.
- Foul-smelling black discharge suggests a forgotten tampon; the discharge settles once the tampon is removed.
- Pregnancy also changes the quality of discharge.
- Finally, mid-cycle bleeding might indicate *Chlamydia* infection and must be investigated or treated with doxycycline 100 mg twice a day for 10 days; make diplomatic enquires about possible contacts.

Urinary tract infections

Ascending infections within the female urinary tract are common in women of all ages (📖 p. 388); they are particularly frequent in those who are sexually active. Mild dehydration of the kind experienced in warm climates seems to predispose to UTIs. Sufferers need to continue to drink in quantity, and take 3 days of oral broad spectrum antibiotic (e.g. cephalexin). If antibiotics are not available, substances which alter urinary pH will help; a teaspoonful of baking soda in a large glass of water is ideal; alternatives are ascorbic acid (vitamin C) or cranberry juice.

Abdominal pain

A woman who complains of significant abdominal pain should be examined especially if the pain is on one side; lateralized lower abdomen pain is often gynaecological in origin but left-sided pain may be caused by gastro-intestinal unease, whilst right-sided pain may be due to appendicitis. A soft abdomen will be reassuring, but vaginal examination is required to exclude problems within the pelvis. An ovarian cyst or fibroid may be palpable during bimanual examination. During vaginal examination, position a finger either side of the cervix so that it can be moved from side to side; if movement of the cervix is painless there is unlikely to be any problem within the pelvis. Equally, pain-free love-making suggests a benign cause for low abdominal pain.

Abdominal pain centred in the right or left lower quadrants

Causes of lateralized abdominal pain that usually require evacuation:

- Right-sided pain may be appendicitis (📖 p. 372), ectopic pregnancy or torsion (📖 p. 375): all are serious.
- Ectopic pregnancy—pain on left or right then often erratic menstrual bleeding sometimes described as 'prune juice' appearance; most often 7 weeks (or more) from last period. There may be a tense abdomen (guarding); shock will soon follow and death is a significant risk.
- Twisted ovarian cyst—management depends upon the severity of the pain and size of the cyst; it needs to be assessed in hospital if the cyst is >5 cm in diameter.
- Hernias (📖 p. 374).

Causes of left- or right-sided abdominal pain that don't usually require evacuation:

- Cystitis—causes malaise and pain on passing urine and sometimes low abdominal pain; blood may be seen in the urine (📖 p. 388).
- Ovulation pain—mid-cycle pain located on one side; tender but no guarding; settles in 36–48 h; treat with pain relief. In the longer term the contraceptive pill will stop the pain.
- Gastroenteritis—often left lower abdominal pain associated with passage of stool or flatus; a bland diet reduces symptoms (📖 p. 380).
- Constipation.
- Irritable bowel disease.
- Kidney stones.

- Endometriosis (anti-inflammatory tablets are helpful).
- Salpingitis—pain may be on both sides, but one side is often worse than the other; it may be accompanied by nausea, vomiting, and often fever. Treat with metronidazole 400 mg twice daily and doxycycline 100 mg twice daily for 14 days. Patients should be investigated on reaching home.

References

Sinclair J, Cohen J, Hinton E (1996). Use of the oral contraceptive pill on treks and expeditions. *British Journal of Family Planning* **22**: 123–6.

Wilson-Howarth J (2006). *Bugs Bites & Bowels*. London, Cadogan.

Wilson-Howarth J (2006). *How to Shit Around the World*. Palo Alto, US, Travelers Tales.

Limbs and back

Section editor
Jon Dallimore

Contributors
Jules Blackham, James Calder, Jon Dallimore,
Carey McClellan, and James Watson

Limb injuries

Limb injuries may be life-threatening and an initial ABC evaluation should be performed, with circulation and respiratory status regularly re-evaluated (see Emergencies, Chapter 6). Consider the possibility of associated pelvic, abdominal, thoracic, or cranial injuries, particularly if the patient is unconscious.

Initial assessment and treatment

- Approach the casualty if safe.
- Ensure that the airway is open, assess the breathing rate, and look for signs of shock (☐ p. 214). Remember the possibility of cervical spine injury with any significant injury above the collarbone, with multiple injuries, and with head injuries resulting in unconsciousness.
- Control any external bleeding with direct pressure.
- Anticipate and treat shock, particularly with thigh fractures. Use a suitable traction splint.
- Remember that painful limb injuries may distract attention from less painful but more significant trunk injuries.
- Expose the affected part and cut off clothing only if *absolutely* necessary given that in some circumstances clothing, waterproofs, etc. will be needed to protect the patient from the environment.
- Look for signs of an interrupted blood supply—pale, pulseless, painful, perishingly cold.
- With fractures/dislocations, attempt manipulation early in an attempt to restore distal circulation. Check pulses and sensation before and after any manipulation.
- Look for nerve damage affecting movement and/or sensation.
- Give painkillers.
- Splint fractures using Sam splint, plaster of Paris, or improvised materials.
- Transfer to suitable shelter.

Improvised splinting materials on an expedition

- Karrimat®
- Paddles
- Skis or ski poles
- Slings and karabiners
- Tree branches
- Sleeping bags
- Ropes.

When applying splints, remember that they must be well padded and must immobilize the joints above and below the injury (Fig. 13.1).

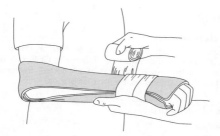

Fig. 13.1 Diagram of a field splint.

Detailed assessment of limb injuries

History

- How did the injury occur? The mechanism is significant; for instance, twisting injuries tend to produce spiral fractures, while a fall onto the heels may produce fractures of the spine or base of skull.
- Did the accident occur in a clean or contaminated environment? Consider intravenous antibiotics.
- When did the injury happen?
- Was the limb trapped or crushed? (Swelling and compartment syndrome are possible; see also crush injuries 📖 p. 257.)
- When was the last tetanus booster? Very important for open fractures.
- Is the patient allergic to anything?
- Does the patient take any medication?

Examination

- Look for contamination and foreign bodies
- Check for pulses and capillary refill time
- Examine carefully for signs of nerve damage—change in sensation, weakness, or paralysis.
- In a wilderness situation, a fracture should be assumed until X-ray studies or clinical examination confirm otherwise.

Capillary refill time

To check for capillary refill press firmly over a finger nail or a bony prominence such as the sternum, forehead, or a malleolus for 5 s to produce blanching. When the pressure is released the colour should begin to return quickly (in less than 2 s). Slow filling indicates that the patient is extremely cold, shocked, or that the blood supply to the limb is interrupted.

Fractures

Fracture classification

Fractures are either *open* if the skin is broken or *closed*. They are *comminuted* if there are more than two fragments. Children's bones may bend, leading to *greenstick* fractures. *Complicated* fractures involve damage to blood vessels, nerves, tendons, or organs.

Features of a fracture

Pain/tenderness
Loss of function
Swelling/bruising
Deformity
Crepitus

Management of fractures in the field

- Stop bleeding
- Treat shock
- Monitor pulse, blood pressure, and urine output
- Give adequate analgesia
- Clean with antiseptic solution and cover exposed bone ends, for example, with Betadine-soaked gauze, and consider the use of antibiotics
- Consider reducing and then immobilize in an appropriate sling or splint
- Evacuate for X-ray and definitive fracture management.

Dislocations

A dislocation is an injury in which the normal relationships of a joint are disrupted. In some dislocations the bone end may be forced out of a socket (shoulder, hip, and elbow dislocations); in others the joint surfaces may simply be displaced (finger dislocations). Fractures, nerve, and blood vessel injuries may also be present with a dislocation.

Management of dislocations in the field

Correction of dislocations can be technically difficult. Attempts to correct the deformity are justified in certain circumstances, particularly in remote areas. If the blood supply to the distal part of the limb is obstructed by a dislocation, reduction must be attempted. Steady, firm traction along the limb's long axis may correct the deformity or at least relieve the obstruction temporarily. Reduction should be attempted as soon as possible because of increasing muscle spasm. After reduction, splint the limb as for a fracture.

Upper limb supports and slings

Collar and cuff (Fig. 13.2)

In the wilderness this may be improvised by passing a long sock around the patient's neck and wrist of the affected side. This can then be secured using a cable tie or piece of cord. This uses the weight of the arm to apply slight traction to the upper arm and should be used for fractures of the humerus.

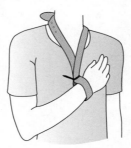

Fig. 13.2 Collar and cuff sling.

High arm sling (Fig. 13.3)

This is mainly used to reduce hand swelling with hand injuries. Avoid excessive flexion of the elbow as this reduces venous drainage of the forearm.

Broad arm sling (Fig. 13.4)

This is commonly used to support the weight of the arm and reduce movement in shoulder and clavicle injuries, dislocations/fractures of the elbow, forearm, and wrist. If used during evacuation of a walking casualty, a swathe around the chest placed on top of the broad arm sling further reduces movement. A broad arm sling may be improvised by pulling the lower edge of a jacket over the arm and then securing with a safety pin.

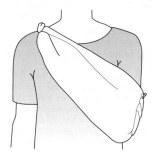

Fig. 13.3 High arm sling.

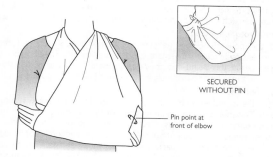

SECURED
WITHOUT PIN

Pin point at
front of elbow

Fig. 13.4 Broad arm sling.

Shoulder and upper arm injuries

Fractured clavicle

This is a common injury following a fall onto the outstretched arm. The clavicle is palpable along its length and there is often obvious deformity and localized tenderness. If the skin over the fracture is tented, then gentle traction with the arm out to the side will reduce the risk of developing an open fracture. Treat with analgesia and a broad arm sling.

Acromioclavicular joint injury

Injury to the acromioclavicular joint commonly follows a fall onto the shoulder. There is usually a characteristic step together with tenderness and swelling at the joint. Treat with analgesia and a broad arm sling. X-rays will show the grade of injury, and the most severe may require surgical treatment.

Anterior shoulder dislocation

The shoulder joint may be dislocated after violent injury (particularly forced abduction/external rotation) or after minimal injury in those with previous shoulder dislocations.

Most dislocations are anterior and are straightforward to diagnose as there is 'squaring' of the shoulder on the affected side and reduced movement, particularly abduction and forward flexion. The humeral head may be palpated antero-inferiorly to the glenoid fossa.

After any shoulder injury examine the area carefully for complications such as damage to the axillary nerve (loss of sensation over the insertion of deltoid—the 'regimental badge area'). Axillary nerve damage merits expert assessment.

Reduction of shoulder dislocations

On an expedition it is reasonable to attempt reduction in the field, preferably with strong analgesia (± sedation such as midazolam). Reduce using the external rotation method or Spaso method (EMJ 1998)[1]. A clunk is often seen, felt or heard, and the shoulder's normal contour is restored.

External rotation method

Hold the patient's elbow next to the trunk and, with the forearm midprone, slowly externally rotate the shoulder to 90°. The shoulder usually reduces at this point; if it does not, forward flex the shoulder slowly. An assistant may help to manipulate the humeral head into position.

Spaso method

Spaso Miljesic and Anne-Maree Kelly first reported the Spaso technique in 1998. This method is simple, needs minimal force, can be performed by a single operator, and is highly effective even in inexperienced hands. The Spaso technique is relatively atraumatic and countertraction is not required.

Lay the patient on the back and give sedation/analgesia as available. Grasp the affected arm around the wrist and lift vertically to 90° shoulder flexion, applying gentle vertical traction. Externally rotate the shoulder slightly. If difficulty is experienced, it may be helpful to use one hand to palpate the head of the humerus and gently push it to assist reduction, while maintaining traction with the other hand.

1 Miljesic S, Kelly AM. Reduction of anterior dislocation of the shoulder. Spaso Technique. *Emer Med* 1998; **10**: 173–5.

Stimson's method

Refers to laying the patient prone with the arm hanging down with a 5-kg weight attached to the wrist/hand. This method may take half an hour or more to achieve reduction.

After reduction of any shoulder dislocation

Re-examine for axillary and radial nerve movement/sensation. Check pulses. Rest in a broad arm sling or collar and cuff. Evacuate for X-rays and orthopaedic follow up/physiotherapy.

Posterior dislocation of the shoulder

This injury is rare and may follow electric shock or convulsions. It is easy to miss. It results from force applied to the anterior shoulder. The shoulder is internally rotated and there is marked loss of movement. Attempt reduction by applying traction and external rotation with the arm at 90° to the body. Manipulation under anaesthesia may be required.

Inferior dislocation of the shoulder (luxatio erecta)

The patient presents with the arm held above the head. Examine carefully for neurovascular status. Attempt reduction by applying traction along the abducted arm, then adduction. If it is not possible to reduce in the field, give strong analgesia, support the arm using padding with sleeping bags or similar, and evacuate for reduction under anaesthesia.

Supraspinatus tendinitis, subacromial bursitis, and rotator cuff injuries

All conditions are caused by acute injury or soft tissue degenerative changes and may be provoked by unaccustomed activity as may occur on wilderness trips. The main symptom is of pain, often following lifting, and onset may be sudden or gradual. Abduction and forward flexion in particular are restricted. There may be a painful arc of movement. Treatment with rest, NSAIDs, and a broad arm sling will usually reduce symptoms. Further assessment will be required if pain and restricted movements persist.

Fracture-dislocation of the shoulder

If crepitus is felt during manipulation of a shoulder dislocation, suspect an associated fracture and desist from further attempts at reduction in the field until the fracture has been identified or excluded by an X-ray. Rest in a broad arm sling, give analgesia, and evacuate.

Fractures of the humerus

These are caused by a fall onto the outstretched arm or onto the elbow. Midshaft fractures can involve the radial nerve as it runs through the spiral groove and result in a wrist-drop. Treatment is with a collar and cuff sling. Any involvement of neurovascular structures, particularly the radial nerve or brachial artery, should prompt urgent evacuation for definitive care.

Ruptured long head of biceps

This can be torn during lifting and may not require large forces. It is seen more commonly in elderly males. There is a characteristic bulge of biceps muscle above the elbow but often little pain; bruising may, however, be extensive. Surgical repair may be considered if the arm is not fully functional.

Elbow and forearm injuries

The elbow may be injured by a direct blow or transmitted forces such as a fall onto the outstretched hand. Full extension without pain makes the presence of fracture or serious injury very unlikely.

Elbow dislocation

This requires considerable force and may be associated with fractures. The radius and ulna are usually dislocated posteriorly. Damage to the brachial artery or radial/ulnar/median nerves may occur. Attempted reduction is justified in a wilderness environment, particularly if evacuation to definitive care will take more than a few hours.

Treatment

After suitable analgesia, apply steady traction to the limb by pulling at the wrist. The elbow is usually flexed at around 30°. Countertraction above the elbow by an assistant is useful, especially if the assistant pushes the olecranon forwards. Rest in a broad arm sling and evacuate for X-ray and further assessment/rehabilitation. If reduction proves impossible, place in a broad arm sling and give analgesia. Monitor radial pulse and assess for nerve damage.

Epicondylitis—golfer's and tennis elbow

Golfer's elbow refers to inflammation around the common flexor origin at the elbow; tennis elbow involves the same process at the common extensor origin. Both conditions are caused by repetitive hand and wrist movements, particularly rowing and paddling on expeditions. On examination there is tenderness at the medial (golfer's) or lateral (tennis) epicondyles of the humerus and pain on gripping.

Treatment

Rest, anti-inflammatory drugs and, where possible, avoidance of the provoking activity.

Olecranon bursitis

The olecranon bursa may become inflamed and painful, sometimes after minor trauma. The lump over the elbow is fluctuant and may be very tender if infected.

Treatment

This condition may take weeks to resolve but usually only requires rest in a broad arm sling and anti-inflammatory drugs. If there is evidence of spreading infection or fever then give antibiotics. Avoid aspiration in the field because of the danger of introducing infection.

Fractures around the elbow

Displaced fractures around the elbow may be associated with neurovascular injury, particularly the brachial artery. Check distal pulses and seek evidence of neurological deficit. Such fractures usually require orthopaedic assessment and often need internal fixation. With the forearm midprone, splint either in the position found, or with the elbow at 90°. Evacuate for X-rays and further management.

Fractured radial head

This injury can only be diagnosed with the help of radiographs but clinically is suggested by a history of a fall onto the outstretched hand and then pain and tenderness on palpating the radial head. Pronation/supination is often very painful. Support the forearm in a broad arm sling and evacuate for assessment.

Fractures of the forearm

These tend to be unstable fractures and may affect the radius and ulna at the same level, at different levels with spiral fractures, or involve a fracture of one bone with associated dislocation at one of the radio-ulnar joints. Check carefully for neurovascular compromise. Treat with analgesia, splinting, and evacuate for definitive care. If there is evidence of an open fracture, clean and dress the wound and give antibiotics.

Wrist injuries

Fractures of the distal radius

These fractures are commonly caused by a fall onto the outstretched hand. There is often obvious deformity together with pain and swelling. Dorsal displacement of the distal fragment is most common—Colle's fracture. All potential wrist fractures on an expedition should be supported in a suitably padded splint and rested in a broad arm sling. Imaging and definitive treatment will be required after evacuation from the field.

Scaphoid fracture

A fall onto the outstretched hand may lead to pain and swelling, together with difficulty gripping. If there is tenderness in the anatomical snuffbox or pain when 'telescoping' the thumb (pushing the straight thumb towards the wrist) a scaphoid injury must be considered. Avascular necrosis, non-union, and osteoarthritis may complicate scaphoid fractures. On an expedition, immobilize in a below elbow splint, and evacuate for X-rays and follow up as long-term disability may result from undiagnosed scaphoid injury.

Wrist sprains

If the mechanism of injury makes a fracture unlikely and if findings on examination are non-specific, it is reasonable on an expedition to treat a tender wrist as for a sprain using a compression bandage, anti-inflammatories, and early mobilization. If there is any uncertainty or if symptoms are not settling, it is safer to assume that there is a fracture and arrangements should be made to image the wrist in a suitable facility.

Tenosynovitis

Inflammation of tendon sheaths may follow repetitive strain injuries. Characteristically there is pain on moving the wrist or thumb and a 'creaking' or 'buzzing' sensation may be felt over the affected tendons, usually on the dorsum of the wrist. Treatment consists of rest in a suitable splint and anti-inflammatories.

Hand injuries

Initial management of hand injuries

- Stop major bleeding using direct pressure and elevation. Consider temporarily inflating a blood pressure cuff (maximum 20 min) around the upper arm.
- Establish the exact mechanism of injury.
- Remove rings early before swelling develops.
- Hand injuries are very painful and adequate analgesia should be given promptly. After neurological assessment consider early use of local anaesthetic, particularly ring blocks for finger injuries (see Fig. 13.6).
- Clean hand wounds carefully (the patient may be able to clean the surrounding area first).
- Open fractures should be treated with careful cleaning and antibiotics.
- Punching injuries with a break in the skin (usually at the knuckles) should be considered to be a bite wound (□ p. 256).
- To avoid later disability, all hand injuries must be carefully assessed and managed.

Examination of the hand

- Record whether the injury affects the patient's dominant hand.
- Compare both hands.
- Look for swelling, deformity, redness, and wounds.
- In the relaxed hand there is increasing flexion from the index to the little finger. A finger which is out of line should raise the possibility of a tendon or nerve injury. Rotation of the digit points to a fracture.
- Ask the patient to make a fist and then fully extend fingers. Look for any obvious motor deficit and crossing of fingers.
- Assess flexor digitorum profundus by holding the proximal interphalangeal joint (PIPJ) extended and asking the patient to flex the finger.
- Assess flexor digitorum superficialis by holding the fingers not being assessed in extension. Ask the patient to flex the finger at the metacarpophalangeal joint.
- Finger extensors can be tested by placing the patient's PIPJs level with a table edge then asking the patient to straighten the finger.
- Test movements at the interphalangeal, metacarpophalangeal, and carpometacarpal joints of the thumb.
- Assess median nerve power by asking the patient to oppose the little finger and the thumb.
- The ulnar nerve may be assessed by abducting or adducting the fingers.
- Check sensation on each side of the digit (digital nerves), in the first web space dorsally (radial nerve), middle finger (median), and little finger (ulnar).

Hand fractures and dislocations

Fractures may be suggested by the mechanism of injury, swelling, bruising, deformity, and loss of normal function. In all cases check for neurovascular deficit. If suspected, immobilize the hand in a boxing glove dressing (diagram 13.5) and broad arm sling. Evacuate for imaging and further treatment.

Finger dislocations

Dislocations can occur at the metacarpophalangeal or interphalangeal joints. After assessing for obvious fractures (small avulsion fractures cannot be diagnosed without imaging), check for any neurovascular damage. It is worth attempting reduction with in-line traction under local anaesthesia. If successful, apply buddy strapping or use a boxing glove dressing (see below).

Thumb dislocations

Attempt reduction, then immobilize in a suitable splint or 'boxing glove' (Fig. 13.5). Evacuate for definitive care as internal fixation may be required if there is an associated fracture.

Ligament injuries

These can occur at the metacarpophalangeal or interphalangeal joints. If the joint is grossly unstable when gently stressing the collateral ligaments, surgical treatment may be required. For most ligament injuries, rest with neighbour strapping will allow healing to occur. Warn patients that swelling may take weeks to settle.

Tendon injuries

Small cuts or lacerations may damage tendons and these injuries may easily be missed unless hand injuries are carefully assessed. (Beware of any injuries caused by glass—evacuation for X-ray is recommended.)

Loss of function is the only reliable sign that a tendon has been damaged, but pain out of proportion to the injury should suggest damage to underlying structures.

Extensor tendon injury

This injury is usually obvious. Partial tendon ruptures are easily overlooked— explore wounds under local anaesthesia or evacuate for full assessment in a bloodless field.

Flexor tendon injuries

Flexor digitorum superficialis flexes the PIPJ. Flexor digitorum profundus flexes the distal interphalangeal joint (DIPJ).

To test these tendons see hand assessment above.

Tendon injuries should be repaired in a suitably equipped hospital, not in the field, because of the danger of infection.

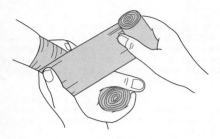

Fig. 13.5 'Boxing glove' dressing.

Finger injuries

Finger injuries

On an expedition fingers can be injured in many ways; they may be crushed in vehicle doors or under heavy weights or during the use of tools/machinery. After release, the digits should be carefully examined (under local anaesthesia if possible), cleaned, and elevated. Possible open fractures should be given an antibiotic such as co-amoxiclav and evacuated for X-ray and further management.

Mallet finger

Rupture of the central slip of the extensor tendon to the distal phalanx results in loss of extension at the DIPJ. This may be associated with an avulsion fracture of the base of the distal phalanx. On an expedition, splint the DIPJ in extension for 6 weeks and arrange for orthopaedic review on return. Do not remove the splint as this will disrupt the healing tendon.

Finger tip amputation

Provided the bone is not exposed and the area of skin loss is <1 cm^2 it may be possible to treat these injuries in the field. After assessment, clean and dress (using Vaseline gauze or similar). Re-examine every 2 days. If the wound is not healing, evacuate for imaging and possible terminalization of bone or skin grafting.

Nail injuries

Finger entrapment or crushing injuries may result in partial or complete avulsion of a nail. The finger should be anaesthetized (Fig. 13.6) and cleaned. The patient may be able to help to clean the finger by immersing in warm, clean water. If the nail is displaced it should be realigned, and the finger dressed and splinted.

Subungual haematoma

Crush injuries to the nail may result in bleeding under the finger nail. The pressure results in throbbing pain which may be relieved by heating a paper clip to red heat and burning a hole in the centre of the nail, using minimal pressure. On an expedition a Leatherman® multi-tool can be used to hold the heated wire paper clip. It may be necessary to reheat the wire on several occasions. Alternatively, a 21G hypodermic needle can be used to drill a hole in the nail. Once the blood has drained the pain is significantly reduced.

Foreign body under the nail

Splinters of metal or wood under the finger nail are common. A ring block may allow removal with splinter forceps or trimming of part of the nail to allow removal.

Paronychia

See hand and nail section in Skin 📖 p. 278.

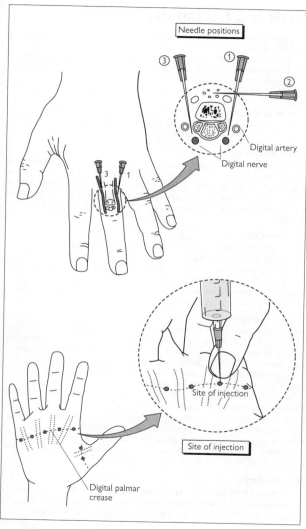

Fig. 13.6 Local anaesthesia of hand.

Pelvic and hip injuries

Many fractures to the lower limbs are high energy injuries and are associated with other injuries:

- Falls from heights may lead to heel, femoral, and pelvic fracture, but 10% have concomitant spinal injury—this may be masked by pain at the obviously fractured leg.
- Fall from heights >2 m and lower limb fracture = spinal injury until excluded.
- Dashboard injury—knee injury in seated passenger during road traffic collision (RTC) associated with femoral fracture and hip dislocation/acetabular fracture.

Pelvic fractures

These follow high energy trauma such as falls and RTC. Considerable force is required to disrupt the pelvis, therefore these fractures are frequently associated with other major thoracic/spinal/abdominal or skeletal injury. Major vessels and pelvic organs lie adjacent to pelvic bones, and these may also be damaged. Mortality rates are approximately 10–20%.

Mechanism of injury

- Lateral compression—deforming force from side-to-side.
- Anterior–posterior compression— this may give rise to the 'open book' fracture where the pelvis opens up; e.g. as a result of a rider hitting the petrol tank of a motorcycle.
- Vertical sheer—usually the result of a fall from a height onto one leg, displacing the hemi-pelvis vertically.

Diagnosis and treatment

Suspect from mechanism of injury, i.e. high energy trauma. On examination there may be pain and hypovolaemic shock (◻ p. 218). The pelvic ring may be unstable, pressing on the front of the pelvis (anterior–superior iliac spines (ASIS)) or compressing sides of the pelvis which causes increased pain and movement of the iliac wings. NB. Repeated examination is not recommended as further disruption may increase bleeding.

Treatment is aimed at stabilizing the pelvis and reducing further haemorrhage/visceral damage during moving of the patient.

- Control lower limbs—splint legs together at knees and ankles. Flex the knees about 20° and pad any bony prominences.
- Splint pelvis—wrap a folded sheet firmly around the pelvis and tie at the front or use a broad belt. Consider use of the Sam sling if available.
- Evacuate urgently and move as little as possible.

Hip fractures

The elderly and those with osteoporotic bones may fracture the neck of the femur with relatively minor trauma; however, the same fracture in younger patients indicates high energy trauma such as a climbing fall.

Diagnosis and treatment

Often there is a history of a fall onto the lateral aspect of the hip. Pain may radiate to the knee and the affected leg may be shortened and externally rotated. Give analgesia; look for and treat shock. A traction splint may improve comfort during evacuation (see Femoral fracture below). If experienced, consider a femoral nerve block (📖 p. 430).

Hip dislocation

These usually follow a fall from a height or dashboard injury in RTCs. The hip joint usually dislocates posteriorly with or without fracture of the acetabulum.

Diagnosis and treatment

There is pain and deformity of the leg, which is shortened and rotated (internally if posterior dislocation). Assess neurological status and distal pulses—hip dislocations may be associated with injury to the femoral or sciatic nerve. If immediate evacuation is possible then splint legs in position and give strong analgesia. If >6 h before evacuation to hospital, then blood supply to the femoral head may become compromised and an attempt at reduction is justified but will require adequate analgesia ± sedation.

Reduction of hip dislocations

In *posterior dislocation,* the assistant places hands as countertraction on the pelvis (anterior superior iliac spine). Flex the hip to 90° with the knee bent and then apply vertical traction with internal rotation. As the hip relocates externally rotate, extend the hip, and continue longitudinal traction to the lower leg. Wrapping a bandage around the lower leg and foot may allow application of 2.5–5 kg skin traction to be maintained. Check neurovascular status post-reduction—relocation may be prevented by entrapment of the sciatic nerve around the femoral neck. The hip may re-dislocate owing to an unstable acetabular fracture. Repeated attempts at reduction are not justified—evacuation is required ASAP for operative intervention.

Femoral fracture

A great deal of force is required to fracture the femur—usually following a fall from a height or RTC. It can be associated with other head, spinal, chest, or abdominal/pelvic trauma.

Diagnosis and treatment

There is pain and deformity of the thigh, together with swelling and fracture crepitus. Assess neurological status and distal pulses. Anticipate hypovolaemia (the patient may lose 1.5 l of blood rapidly even in closed injury). Splint legs in position (splint to un-injured leg); apply traction through a splint if available to maintain alignment and to reduce bleeding into the thigh compartment. Cover any open wounds with sterile dressings, e.g. Betadine-soaked gauze.

Strongly consider a femoral nerve block if suitably experienced.

Blood loss for closed lower limb fractures (average blood volume 5 l) is as follows:
- Pelvis   1.0–4.0 litres
- Femur   1.0–2.5 litres
- Tibia   0.5–1.5 litres

Blood loss for open fracture may be 2–3 times greater.

Femoral nerve block (Fig. 13.7)
- This regional anaesthetic technique provides good analgesia for a fractured femur and is best undertaken before placing the leg in a traction splint.
- The femoral nerve lies lateral to the femoral artery as it passes under the inguinal ligament.

Technique
- Use 10 ml 1% lidocaine or 20 ml of bupivacaine 0.25%.
- Clean the skin.
- Palpate the femoral artery.
- Insert a green needle (21G) approximately 1–2 cm lateral to the artery in a slight caudal direction. Aspirate to check for blood.
- If tingling occurs, withdraw the needle slightly.
- Inject the lidocaine in a fan shape laterally; aspirate before injecting.
- Analgesia takes 10 min or more to develop.

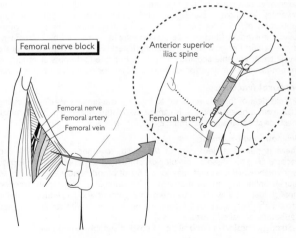

Femoral nerve block

Anterior superior iliac spine

Femoral nerve
Femoral artery
Femoral vein

Femoral artery

Fig. 13.7 Anatomy of femoral triangle.

Knee injuries

Knee injuries on expeditions are relatively common. In all cases take a careful history which may give clues to the diagnosis. Ask about previous knee problems such as swelling, clicking, locking, or 'giving way'.

Examination of the injured knee:

- Look for bruising, swelling, redness, deformity, and compare with the uninjured side.
- Feel for an effusion, warmth, or crepitus. Identify any tender areas—joint line or origin or insertion of collateral ligaments.
- Observe straight leg raising (which assesses the extensor mechanism, below).
- Assess movement—extension (0°), flexion (135°).
- Palpate along the medial and lateral joint lines, and over the fibular head for tenderness.
- Test the joint stability—in 30° flexion support the lower leg and apply valgus and varus stress at the knee (tests collaterals). With the knee flexed at 90°, place the thumbs on the tibial tubercle and rest index fingers behind the knee. With the hamstrings relaxed, gently draw the lower leg forward, looking for any abnormal shift (anterior draw test).
- McMurray's test for meniscal injury—place thumb and index finger on medial and lateral joint lines, flex the knee, and externally rotate the foot followed by abduction and extension of the knee. Pain and a click suggest a medial meniscal injury.

Haemarthrosis

This is relatively common and refers to bleeding into a joint. Rapid tense swelling develops in 1–2 h. They may be *spontaneous* (coagulation disorders and rare vascular tumours) or *traumatic* (80% after anterior cruciate ligament injury, 10% patella dislocation, 10% meniscal injuries/capsular injuries).

Sterile aspiration of the knee (with a needle and syringe under the patella medially or laterally) may alleviate pain and allow thorough clinical examination. Fat globules in the aspirate may indicate an underlying fracture.

Treatment

RICE and analgesia and evacuate for further assessment.

Bursitis

Inflammation of the fluid-filled bursa in front of or below the patella may result from unaccustomed, frequent minor trauma such as kneeling. Rest and NSAIDs usually relieve symptoms. If there are features of spreading cellulitis and a fever, antibiotics should be given (e.g. co-amoxiclav).

Patellar fracture

Sudden knee flexion or a direct blow may result in a fracture of the patella. There is usually pain, swelling (sometimes from a haemarthrosis), and inability to straight leg raise. If suspected, splint the leg almost straight (with 5° of flexion at the knee) and evacuate for imaging and definitive treatment.

Other fractures around the knee

Suspected fractures around the knee should be treated with adequate analgesia and splint, as for patellar fracture. Avoid traction splints if there is a possible fracture in the supracondylar region of the distal femur. Traction may displace the distal part of the fracture posteriorly and damage the popliteal artery.

Patellar dislocation

This is not uncommon and may be a recurrent problem. The patella dislocates laterally and, typically, the patient's knee is held flexed with obvious displacement of the patella. Give analgesia and reduce the patella by pressing with the thumbs on the lateral aspect of the patella as the knee is straightened. Once reduced it may be possible to rehabilitate this injury in the field without evacuation.

Dislocation of the knee

This is a rare injury and huge forces are required to produce disruption of the knee ligaments. There is a high likelihood of nerve and blood vessel damage—check distal pulses and sensation carefully. Treat with strong analgesia and immobilize as for patellar fracture. Keep monitoring foot pulses, as popliteal artery injury may not be apparent initially. If there are signs of vascular compromise, evacuate urgently for vascular surgery.

Ligament injuries to knee

Medial collateral ligament

The medial collateral ligament runs from the medial epicondyle of the femur to 4 cm distal to the knee joint on the medial aspect of the tibia. An isolated rupture usually results from a direct blow to the lateral aspect of the knee in slight flexion. The patient may describe a 'popping' sensation. If there is a rotational component, there may also be injury to the cruciate ligament.

Diagnosis and treatment

- On examination there is tenderness over the medial collateral ligament ± knee swelling. Test valgus stability with knee flexed 20–30° (in full extension the cruciate ligaments stabilize the knee).
- Mild–moderate (<10 mm opening of joint)—rest, ice, compression, and then early increase range of motion/strengthening with physiotherapy.
- Severe (>10 mm opening of joint)—may require hinged brace for 3–6 weeks after initial management and so may benefit from evacuation for definitive care.

Lateral collateral ligament

The lateral collateral ligament runs from the lateral epicondyle of the femur to the head of the fibula. Isolated injuries are rare but are more usually associated with injury to all the lateral capsular ligamentous structures. This may result in marked instability.

Diagnosis and treatment

- Tenderness ± knee swelling. Test varus stability. An isolated lateral collateral ligament injury may be treated as for medial collateral ligament, but more common complex injury may require evacuation for surgery.

Cruciate ligaments

Anterior cruciate ligament injuries account for 50% of documented knee ligament injuries. Posterior cruciate ligament injury is rare (<10% knee ligament injuries). Usually, injuries are caused by non-contact twisting injury, occasionally following hyperextension. There is pain and difficulty weightbearing. Swelling develops rapidly in the first 1–2 h.

Diagnosis and treatment

- There is an acute haemarthrosis following typical history. Examination is often difficult during the acute phase due to pain and swelling.
- Lachman's test will usually be positive—grip the tibia at 30° flexion and pull it anteriorly over the distal femur. There will be no firm end point. There may also be anterior draw and pivot shift. If suspected, evacuate for X-rays and further imaging (MR) or arthroscopy. Younger active individuals may have continuing joint instability and may require reconstruction of the cruciates.

Meniscal injuries

The menisci act as stabilizers for the knee and distribute forces across the articular surfaces. There is usually a history of an axial load with a twisting injury to the knee. 'Degenerative' tears may occur in patients >35 years with very little history of injury.

Diagnosis and treatment

- Patients may complain of the knee 'locking' or 'giving way'. Pain and intermittent swelling may occur. Squatting particularly may aggravate posterior horn tears.
- Physical examination often varies (McMurray's test, above).
- Acute tears may cause marked swelling of knee over 4–6 h and occasionally haemarthrosis. Degenerative tears may settle with physiotherapy.
- Knee arthroscopy is often required if the knee is symptomatic. If the knee is acutely locked, from a loose body, do not attempt to unlock the knee (painful and usually futile). Splint in a comfortable position and evacuate for definitive care.

Knee extensor mechanism injuries

Disruption to any one of these may prevent straight leg raising or active extension of the knee. (NB. Tense knee effusion and pain may also prevent straight leg raise without disruption of extensor mechanism.)

Quadriceps tendon rupture

• 80% occur in individuals >40 years. Normally a gap is palpable close to the superior pole of the patella.

Patellar tendon rupture

• Usually occurs in those <40 years. Tender inferior pole patella.

Patellar and tibial tuberosity fractures

• Usually occur as result of direct trauma.
• Manage with rest, support, and splinting in extension. Tendons usually require operative repair if the extensor mechanism is disrupted. Fractures often require reduction and fixation if displaced.

Lower leg injuries

Tibial fracture

This can occur as a result of a fall, RTC, or twisting injury (particularly when skiing). There is often an associated fibula fracture. Because there is little soft tissue cover, tibial fractures are commonly open.

There is a significant risk of compartment syndrome whether an open or closed injury (see below).

Splint legs in position (splint to the other uninjured leg); apply traction through a splint, if available, to maintain alignment. Cover open wounds with a sterile dressing and give antibiotics during evacuation, e.g. ceftriaxone.

Compartment syndrome

This refers to increased soft tissue pressure within an enclosed soft tissue compartment which can lead to devastating muscle necrosis and nerve damage.

The soft tissues swell but the surrounding envelope does not allow expansion, causing pressure to rise above the capillary pressure. It usually follows fractures or crush injuries (particularly to the lower leg, thigh, forearm, and foot/hand), and is most common following closed fractures to the tibial shaft. Occasionally it occurs as a chronic exercise-induced condition ('shin splints').

Diagnosis and treatment

The soft tissue compartment looks swollen and tense. The most reliable sign is pain on passive stretching of a muscle group within the compartment, e.g. great toe or fingers. Remember the 5Ps—Pain, Pallor, Paraesthesia, Paralysis, and Pulseless, reflecting tissue ischaemia. Pain and local tenderness are the earliest features and are difficult to control with even opiate analgesics. Loss of pulse is a very late sign.

Acute compartment syndrome is an emergency requiring urgent evacuation and surgical decompression. Splint the limb to reduce further trauma and maintain the limb at the level of the heart (i.e. not overelevated or dependent).

Achilles tendon disorders

Achilles tendinopathy

This refers to micro-tears in the Achilles tendon. It usually affects those aged 35–55 years and follows unaccustomed activity such as running, trekking, or jumping.

This occurs in two areas:

- *Non-insertional*—4–8 cm proximal to Achilles insertion into calcaneum. It is probably a result of reduced blood supply and a point of high tension in the tendon. A tender fusiform swelling develops.
- *Insertional*—occurs at insertion of the Achilles into the calcaneum. A hardened bony lump develops, causing painful rubbing and difficulty with shoes/boots. A bony prominence on the posterior–superior aspect of the calcaneus (Haglund's deformity) may be present along with an inflamed bursa (retrocalcaneal bursitis).
- **Treatment**: conservative measures improve symptoms in 90%. In the acute stage, RICE and regular NSAIDs are required.

Consider Achilles stretching exercises and removal of heel tabs in training shoes. A heel-raise to reduce stretching of the tendons can also be considered. There is a small risk of complete rupture.

Acute Achilles tendon rupture

There is a relatively poor vascular supply and high tension approximately 4–8 cm proximal to the insertion into the calcaneum. It affects males> females. Age is usually 35–55 years. The injury occurs during sudden contraction during 'push-off' or traumatic forced dorsiflexion of the ankle.

The patient complains of sudden pain and weakness of plantar flexion at the ankle. A 'gun shot' may be heard as the tendon ruptures. On examination there is tenderness and a palpable boggy gap in the tendon.

Simmonds test-positive—lay the patient prone with foot over end of bed. Gently squeezing the calf causes plantar flexion at ankle in the unaffected side but no or minimal plantar flexion with rupture of Achilles tendon.

Treatment

Initial management is RICE and splint ankle in equinus position, non-weightbearing. Evacuate for expert assessment and management. There is great debate regarding non-operative treatment in equinus cast for 9 weeks (slow recovery and possibly higher re-rupture rate) versus operative repair (wound problems and sural nerve injuries).

Other causes of calf pain

- Shin splints—pain over the anterior tibia following running may be treated with rest and NSAIDs.
- Stress fracture of the tibia—see below.
- Deep vein thrombosis.
- Cellulitis see 🕮 p. 258.

Ankle injuries

Ankle ligament injuries

These commonly occur during a forced inversion injury of the hindfoot. Generally the lateral ligaments are injured—anterior talofibular ligament and calcaneofibular ligament. Bruising and swelling may be severe, occurring within hours. Tenderness is usually maximal laterally.

A fracture may be difficult to exclude clinically; however, the Ottawa rules suggest that X-rays should be arranged if the patient is unable to weightbear (four steps) or if there is tenderness behind the medial or lateral malleolus, over the navicular (proximal to base of first metatarsal), or at the base of the fifth metatarsal. Palpate the fibular head as ankle injuries can cause fracture of the fibular head.

Treatment

RICE and analgesics. Strapping may be beneficial and supporting the ankle initially whilst allowing weightbearing as tolerated. Active exercises should begin immediately to regain full movement.

Ankle fractures

Normally the talus sits in the mortise of the tibia and fibula; twisting may rupture the ligaments or fracture the malleoli. This occurs when the foot is anchored on the ground and the momentum of the body continues forwards. There is swelling, pain, and bruising, with deformity and tenderness along the bony landmarks of the medial and lateral malleoli.

Treatment

If the ankle is obviously dislocated, this may cause pressure necrosis on the soft tissues and neurovascular compromise. Reduction by traction and relocation is indicated urgently (with suitable analgesia). After reduction, check pulses and sensation then immobilize in a suitable splint. Treat with RICE. X-rays are needed to confirm the nature of the fracture. Evacuate for definitive treatment; many displaced ankle fractures will require operative fixation.

Foot fractures and dislocations

Foot injuries can be devastating on trekking expeditions as the victim may require stretcher evacuation. The feet are particularly vulnerable when inadequately protected by lightweight footwear in the tropics or jungle.

Talus and calcaneal fractures

Falls from a height onto the feet can result in fractures around the heel. These may be bilateral and are associated with other significant injuries such as to the spine, pelvis, hips, or knees.

Treatment
• Give strong analgesia, elevate, and immobilize in a splint. Early definitive treatment is necessary to prevent long-term disability.

Metatarsal fractures

Heavy weights such as vehicle wheels or large machinery may break multiple metatarsal bones. Ankle inversion may lead to a small avulsion fracture at the base of the fifth metatarsal.

Treatment
• Check for pulses and evacuate for injury assessment and definitive care.

Lower limb stress fractures

These most commonly affect the metatarsals, but can occasionally occur in the tibia, the calcaneum, or talus. They follow repeated trauma such as occurs in over-training. There is an underlying biomechanical problem that may be resolved with a change in shoes/boots.

Diagnosis and treatment
• Metatarsals—there is gradual onset of pain ± swelling of forefoot without specific trauma. Tenderness is specifically along the bone (usually second metatarsal neck). Early X-rays are often normal but may show callus formation at 3–6 weeks.
• Tibia—shin-splint pain on exercise. Pain may settle after period of rest. May have tenderness along tibia.
• Calcaneum—exertional non-specific heel pain. Squeezing heel causes pain. (NB. Plantar fasciitis may cause pain under the heel when walking, which is normally worse for the first few steps after rest, but there is tenderness specifically at the insertion of the plantar fascia under the heel.) X-rays are normal.

In all cases give analgesia and remove the cause, often necessitating a reduction in training/exercise. Reduce weightbearing with crutches until comfortable and then weightbear as tolerated.

Toe fractures and dislocations

These rarely require any more than 'buddy strapping' to relieve pain for 2–3 weeks. If there is obvious deformity, this may be reduced under ring block (inject 1 ml plain lidocaine 1% on each side of the base of the digit.

Spinal injury

Spinal cord injuries are relatively rare (approximately 17 cases per week in the UK). However, it is vital that the possibility of spinal injuries is considered in all trauma patients:

• High speed injuries.
• Patients with multiple injuries.
• Falls or those who have been hit by a falling object such as a rock.
• Head-injured and unresponsive patients.

The implications of missing one of these can be life-changing or life-threatening for the patient. Manipulation or inadequate management/immobilization of the spinal-injured patient can cause additional neurological damage and worsen outcome.

Injuries most frequently occur at junctions of mobile and fixed sections of the spine (C6,7/T1, T12/L1). In patients with multiple injuries who have a spinal injury, over half will have a cervical spinal injury. About 10–15% of patients with one spinal fracture will be found to have another.

Management

• The aim of spinal management is to prevent any secondary injury to the spinal cord.
• Ensure that the airway is open. Use the jaw-thrust manoeuvre rather than head tilt and chin lift which may create further cervical spine injury.
• If necessary, move the head into a neutral alignment (Fig. 13.8). Stabilize the head and neck manually. If available, use a semi-rigid neck collar such as Stifnek select™ together with sandbags and tape—in the wilderness socks full of sand or soil can be used.
• Assess breathing and look for and treat any life-threatening chest injury (📖 p. 182). Give oxygen if available. Adequate oxygenation and tissue perfusion must be maintained as the spinal cord is very sensitive to hypoxia/hypotension.
• Identify any signs of shock and treat cautiously with intravenous fluids. Ensure an adequate blood pressure (systolic >90mmHg) and pulse rate. If the pulse rate falls below 45 bpm consider atropine 600 mcg iv as minimal stimulation may cause asystole owing to unopposed vagal response.
• Rapidly assess the conscious level with AVPU scale or GCS, look at the pupils, and ask the patient if they can move and feel their fingers and toes.
• Finally, log-roll the patient with great care to allow examination of the back for bruising, laceration, tenderness, and, if in an appropriate environment, perform a rectal examination to assess perianal sensation and anal tone (📖 see p. 138).

Signs of a spinal injury

The patient may complain of:
- Neck or back pain. This may be masked by another more painful injury
- Loss of movement and/or sensation in the limbs
- Sensation of burning/electric shock in the trunk or limbs.

On examination the patient may have:
- Swelling, midline tenderness or a 'step' over the spinous processes.

In the unconscious patient a serious spinal injury may be indicated by:
- Hypotension with bradycardia (neurogenic shock)
- The skin may be warm below the level of the lesion
- Diaphragmatic ventilation
- Differential pain responses
- Flaccid tone
- Priapism (involuntary erection of the penis)
- Loss of sphincter control.

Clearing the suspected spinal injury

Not all patients who are involved in trauma need to have full spinal precautions maintained. The box below indicates when a spinal injury can safely be excluded clinically.

If the patient has any of these signs then imaging of the neck is required before cervical spinal immobilization can be removed.

If it is necessary to move the patient, they should be moved carefully, keeping the spine in alignment throughout and should be kept horizontal if at all possible. This is because blood vessels below the level of a spinal cord injury may have lost their spinal reflexes and so cannot contract in response to hypotension. This can cause a precipitous drop in blood pressure and hence further damage to the spinal cord.

Excluding Spinal Injury ('Clearing the spine')

- No midline cervical tenderness
- No altered level of alertness
- No evidence of intoxication
- No neurological abnormality
- No distracting injury

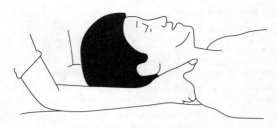

Fig. 13.8 Manual immobilization of the neck.

Incomplete spinal cord injury patterns
- Anterior cord syndrome: loss of power and pain sensation below the injury, with preservation of touch and proprioception.
- Posterior cord syndrome: loss of sensation, but power preserved.
- Brown–Séquard syndrome: hemisecton of the cord producing ipsilateral paralysis and sensory loss below the injury, with contralateral loss of pain and temperature. Occurs more frequently after penetrating injury.

Low back pain

Back pain is a common complaint and on expeditions may be provoked by unaccustomed activity or injuries such as lifting awkwardly, falls, or twisting injury.

Low back pain is very common. Sort into:
- Mechanical back pain.
- Nerve root pain—only concerning if progressive or persistent.
- Serious spinal pathology—will need definitive care.
- Suspected cord compression—needs immediate evacuation.

Consider other systemic disease, such as back pain associated with weight loss, fever/rigors, cough/haemoptysis.

History
- Recent back trauma—note the mechanism of any injury.
- Characterize the pain, noting particularly leg symptoms and aggravating/relieving factors.
- Ask if there is any disturbance of bladder/bowel function.
- Ask about previous back injuries or surgery.
- Presence of red flag signs.

Red flag signs
- Thoracic pain
- Uncontrolled pain, worse at night
- Fever and unexplained weight loss
- Bladder or bowel dysfunction
- History of carcinoma—particularly thyroid, breast, lung, prostate, kidney
- Ill heath or presence of other medical illness
- Progressive neurological deficit
- Disturbed gait, saddle anaesthesia
- Age of onset <20 or >55 years

Examination
'Unwell' patient—immediately assess ABCs and check for presence of pulsatile expansile abdominal mass and presence/absence of femoral pulses (abdominal aortic aneurysm often presents with back pain).

'Well' patient—look for signs of weight loss, scoliosis, and muscle spasm. Watch the patient walk, looking for limping or abnormal posture. Assess spinal movements and note any significant loss. With the patient supine, palpate for tenderness over lumbar spine and sacrum, ribs, and renal angles. Look for muscle wasting in the legs. Perform on both legs:
- Straight leg raise—note angle at which patient detects pain (lumbar nerve root irritation). Normal >70° but compare with other side.
- Check for perineal and perianal sensation. Consider rectal examination to check anal tone.

Neurological examination

	Sensation	Motor	Reflex
L3/4	Medial lower leg	Quadriceps	Knee jerk
L5	Lateral lower leg	Extensor hallucis longus	Hamstring jerk
S1	Lateral foot and little toe	Foot plantar flexors	Ankle jerk

Management
- If red flag sign is found, evacuate for specialist investigation of the cause of the back pain.
- In the absence of red flag signs, even with the presence of nerve root pain, conservative treatment should be effective.
- Manage symptoms with simple analgesics and NSAIDS, and a short course of a low dose of benzodiazepines (2–5 mg diazepam tds for 2 days).
- Advise that symptoms may take 4–6 weeks to resolve.
- Avoid bed rest; encourage gentle, normal movements.
- Consider physiotherapy or manipulation if available.

Physiotherapy

- Most soft tissue injuries will benefit from a short period of rest/protection (splinting) followed by early mobilization to prevent stiffness and to regain full movements.
- Traditionally RICE forms the basis for simple soft tissue injury rehabilitation.
- Rest (for 24–48 h) and ice, if available, applied to the injured part help to reduce swelling and pain. Ice should not be applied directly to the skin but should be wrapped in a damp cloth and applied intermittently for 15 min at a time. If ice is not available, cold packs would be a suitable alternative.
- A crepe or Tubigrip bandage may help to support the injury and will remind the patient about the injury. If the patient must continue to weightbear, compression and ice are beneficial. If complete rest is possible, omit compression and instead elevate and use ice.
- Hand and foot injuries benefit from early *elevation* to reduce discomfort and swelling. However, poorly applied elbow or knee *compression* may be harmful if venous return is affected (risk of DVT).

Mobilization

Gentle range of motion exercises should start as soon as possible. Aim for graded exercises which move joints slightly more each day. Avoid excessive stretching and try to normalize movement as early as possible within the limits of pain. Always provide adequate analgesia.

Advice for the patient

- 1–3 days—rest, ice, elevate.
- 3–14 days—perform regular exercises building up activity, avoiding excessive discomfort or strain.
- 14 days onwards—injury requires less protection. Concentrate on getting the injured part back to full fitness with exercises.
- By 8 weeks all usual activities should have been resumed.

Guide to taping and strapping

Taping or strapping is simply the application of adhesive tape to provide extrinsic stability and/or to offload weakened structures. Its proprioceptive qualities play a significant part in protection and rehabilitation. The principal aim of applying tape is to prevent disability and thus improve otherwise impaired physical function. Techniques can be used for a multitude of musculoskeletal conditions, either following tissue injury or as a preventative measure when a history or risk of injury is present.

Materials

The most commonly used types of taping material are the adhesive elastic type (such as Elastoplast®) and zinc oxide tape (a non-stretch, highly adhesive tape). The indications for each type depend on the aim of the technique being used, but often both types will be used concurrently; for example, elastic adhesive tape is ideal for providing anchor strips as these are often circumferential strips of tape and must stretch to allow contraction of muscle from these anchor strips. Zinc oxide tape can be used to act as a non-stretchy stabilizer to prevent particular joint movements.

In a number of techniques a pre-taping underwrap can be used to prevent direct contact of the tape with the skin. However, it is the traction of the skin–tape interface that is thought to give the techniques their effectiveness and therefore the use of underwrap can be questioned.

Preparation and precautions

Prior to undertaking any taping technique, patients should have undergone a comprehensive assessment of the injury with particular reference to mechanism of injury, precise direction of any resultant instability/weakness, and the phase of healing that is likely to be ongoing. These factors will lead to a clinical decision being made regarding the selection of taping material as well as the technique that is to be applied. Patients should also be questioned as to whether any known allergy to the taping materials is known.

Adequate preparation of the contact area is vital to ensure ease of technique and a good skin–tape interface. The following can be used as a guide:

- The area to be taped should be clean and dry.
- Hirsute areas should be free from hair.
- Areas of broken skin should be covered with a suitable dressing such as Mepore®.
- The patient should be positioned to allow therapist access to the taped area without having to reposition throughout the technique.
- Once the tape is applied, simple checks to observe circulation to the area should be performed.

Acute injuries

Acutely injured joints are at greater risk of further injury owing to the loss of proprioceptive input caused by painful stimuli. The use of taping as an adjunct to improving joint stability extrinsically is commonly used in the sports setting and is aimed at restoring function at an early stage whilst protecting structures from further injury. Adhesive tape has been found to provide compression to acute ankle sprains for up to 10 days post injury (Capasso et al, 1989)[2]. It should be noted, though, that applying tape for such prolonged periods can be counterproductive as it will limit venous flow from the injured area and thus prevent resolution of swelling.

In the presence of swelling around an acutely injured joint, it is often wise to ensure that the circumference of the joint and the surrounding muscular tissues are not completely covered. This allows for further swelling to take place without causing any vascular compromise.

In acute muscle strain, longitudinal taping crossing both the origin and insertion of the muscle can prevent further injury and reduce disability by limiting the muscle's potential to lengthen. This technique, known as *physiological taping*, can also be used during rehabilitation to offload the muscle at the point of stretch and, through the elastic quality of the tape, it can assist muscle contraction.

2 Capasso G., Maffuli N., Testa V. (1989). Ankle taping: support given by different materials. *British Journal of Sports Medicine*; **23**: 239–40.

Preventative taping

The most common use of musculoskeletal taping is as a preventative measure when returning athletes to sporting activity. Taping itself has been compared to functional sports bracing as a means of providing effective joint stability. No difference was found between the overall effectiveness and practicality of taping versus a laced ankle support across a number of sporting activities, but taping has the advantage of being adaptable to the individual athlete or traveller.

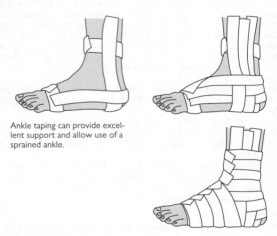

Ankle taping can provide excellent support and allow use of a sprained ankle.

Fig. 13.9 Ankle strapping.

Further reading

MacDonald R (2004). *Taping Techniques, Principles and Practice*, 2nd edn. London, Butterworth–Heinemann.

Infectious diseases

David Warrell

Introduction

The risk of catching a dangerous exotic infection while travelling overseas is small but worrying. Prevention is by far the best strategy.

Find out which important diseases occur in your expedition area by: learning about what is known of the pattern of disease in the area in advance, using literature, websites and local knowledge via your in-country agent, discovering any special vulnerabilities to infections in your team members (📖 p. 58), and preparing accordingly.

Reduce risk by:
• Sensible behaviour.
• Anti-bite measures (clothing, repellents, nets, etc.).
• Vaccination (see Immunizations 📖 p. 32).
• Chemoprophylaxis.

It is wise for expeditions to carry appropriate antimicrobial drugs to treat infections known to be prevalent in the region, so that treatment can be initiated if needed.

Diagnosis in the field

During the expedition diagnosis will depend largely upon history and clinical examination, backed up by a minimum of investigations such as blood or urine dipstick examination or simple microscopy.

Some potential pathogens can be excluded:
• Geographically (see Figs 2.1–2.7 and 14.1–14.7)—for instance, yellow fever does not occur outside Latin America and Equatorial Africa.
• Local medical experience that the disease doesn't occur there.
• Because of assumed immunity from pre-expedition vaccinations.
• Because of the incubation period. A fever starting less than 7 days after entering a malarious area cannot be due to malaria; fever starting more than 21 days after leaving West Africa cannot be Lassa fever.
• On clinical grounds: for instance a fever with lymphadenopathy and rash is not compatible with malaria.
• By carrying out a therapeutic trial (e.g. of antimalarial or anti-rickettsial treatment).
• Suspicion of a serious infectious disease such as bacterial meningitis should prompt initiation of blind antimicrobial treatment and urgent evacuation to the nearest base hospital (see Preparations 📖 p. 136).
• Confirmation of diagnosis, using a wider range of laboratory and other investigations, may be possible after evacuation to a local hospital identified in the planning stage. Depending on the experience and attitude of local doctors and nurses, the expedition medical officer may still have a role and responsibility at this stage, hence the relevance of some of the information about diagnosis and more advanced treatment given below.

Infections are among the commonest medical problems encountered on expeditions. Most involve skin, respiratory tract, conjunctivae, ears, gut (travellers' diarrhoea), and the genitourinary tract, and are readily diagnosed and treated even in a remote location.

- If a particular system is involved, refer to the appropriate section of this handbook (e.g. skin, eye, abdomen).
- If the patient is severely ill, see Sepsis in Chapter 7 (📖 p. 218).
- This section describes some infectious diseases that are common, potentially serious, or inspire great anxiety.
- Infection of particular systems such as gastrointestinal infections, giardiasis, and sexually transmitted diseases, are covered in the relevant chapters

A useful rule of thumb is:

Fever with no signs—treat for malaria (if exposure was possible).
After 48 h still fever but no signs—treat for rickettsia.
After 96 h still fever—evacuate.

Viral infections

Viral hepatitis

At least eight 'hepatitis viruses' (A to G and TT virus or 'TTV', *not* transfusion transmitted virus but named after the initials of the index case!) are currently recognized (see Figs 2.2, 2.3). Many other viruses—yellow fever and other haemorrhagic fever viruses, dengue, Herpes and viruses such as EBV and CMV—can also cause hepatitis. Unvaccinated trekkers and backpackers have a 1 in 50/month risk of catching HAV.

Transmission

- **HAV** is transmitted faecal–orally and rarely by blood transfusion, needle stick, and sexually. Incubation is 4–6 weeks.
- **HBV,** sometimes associated with HDV ('delta agent') is transmitted by transfusion, needle stick, from mother to baby at birth, or sexually. Incubation is 4–24 weeks.
- **HCV** is transmitted by needle stick, transfusion, rarely from mother to baby at birth, and sexually. Incubation is 2–26 weeks.
- **HEV** is transmitted faecal–orally and directly via pork and other animal products. Incubation is about 6 weeks. Many epidemics attributed to HAV are thought to be due to HEV. This condition is potentially fatal in pregnant women.
- **'Non-A, non-E hepatitis'** is transmitted by blood transfusion and needle stick.
- **HGV and TTV** are transmitted by blood transfusion. They are of uncertain pathogenicity.

Clinical

Jaundice appears after a few days of anorexia, nausea, vomiting, fever with chills, weakness, fatigue, headache, aches and pains, and upper abdominal discomfort. Dark urine, pale stools, and pruritis are common. Signs include tender hepatomegaly without splenomegaly, spider naevi, and vasculitic or urticarial rashes. The acute illness lasts days or weeks and in severe cases is complicated by persistent nausea, vomiting, ascites, oedema or liver failure presenting with hepatic encephalopathy. Chronic viral carriage, chronic hepatitis, cirrhosis, and hepatoma are complications of HBV (HDV) and HCV infection.

Diagnosis

Urine dipstick testing reveals bilirubin (early) or urobilinogen. Confirmation is by serology or antigen detection.

Treatment

Evacuation for early hospital treatment with interferon may enhance viral clearance in acute HBV and HCV infections, but there is no specific treatment for acute viral hepatitis. Hepatotoxic drugs and alcohol must be avoided. Rest and low fat diet improve comfort. Corticosteroids and low protein diet have no proven benefit.

Prevention (📖 p. 39)

Effective vaccines are available against HAV and HBV and are strongly recommended to all travellers to developing countries. HBV vaccine is mandatory for medical personnel. Avoidance of HAV and HEV involves food and water hygiene, especially in hyperendemic third world countries.

For the parenterally/sexually transmitted viruses such as HBV and HBC, extreme caution is necessary with blood and blood products unless they have been properly screened. Surgical and dental procedures, ear piercing, tattooing, acupuncture and injections in or out of hospital, unprotected sex, and intimate contact that risks inoculation of blood or tissue fluids, even sharing a tooth brush, are potentially hazardous.

Websites

http://www.cdc.gov/ncidod/diseases/hepatitis/
http://www.hpa.org.uk/infections/topics_az/hepatitis_a/menu.htm
http://www.hpa.org.uk/infections/topics_az/hepatitis_b/menu.htm
http://www.hpa.org.uk/infections/topics_az/hepatitis_c/menu.htm
http://www.hpa.org.uk/infections/topics_az/hepatitis_e/default.htm

Poliomyelitis

Poliomyelitis, caused by the polioviruses (enteroviruses), has been eliminated from the western hemisphere but, in 2006, 2002 cases were reported in African and Asian countries (Fig. 14.1): Nigeria (1129 cases, 56% of the global total), Niger, Somalia, Kenya, Egypt, Yemen, Afghanistan, Pakistan, India (~600 cases), Nepal, Bangladesh, and Myanmar.

Transmission: is faecal–oral.

Clinical: most infections cause only mild upper respiratory tract symptoms, but in about 1% of cases there is aseptic meningitis or flaccid paralysis of one limb or more extensive quadriplegia or bulbar and respiratory paralysis. Other viruses such as enterovirus 71, adenoviruses, and Japanese encephalitis virus can also cause polio-like flaccid paralysis.

Prevention: everyone must be vaccinated and boosted if visiting an endemic area more than 10 years after their previous vaccination. Inactivated vaccine is used increasingly (📖 p. 33–9). Oral vaccine (live, attenuated virus) can cause vaccine-related poliomyelitis (0.5–3.4 cases/1 million vaccines).

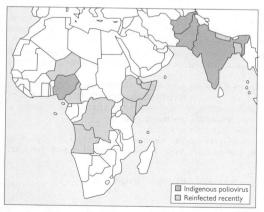

Fig. 14.1 Poliomyelitis distribution.

Viral encephalitides

Japanese (B) encephalitis

This is a common, dangerous, vaccine-preventable, mosquito-borne flavivirus encephalitis of Asia and parts of Oceania (see 📖 p. 41, Fig. 2.4).

Tick-borne encephalitis (TBE)

In Novosibirsk, south-west Siberia, >20 000 tick bites are reported annually. Tick-borne encephalitis occurs throughout a vast area from Germany and the whole of Scandinavia in the west, through eastern Europe, Baltic countries and central Asia to the far west of the Russian Federation (Russian spring—summer encephalitis; see Fig. 2.6). Switzerland reports >100 cases each year, while 3000 clinical cases are reported in Europe and >10 000 in Russia each year. The incidence is increasing in all countries except Austria where an aggressive vaccination policy has proved effective (for distribution see Immunizations 📖 p. 43).

Transmission: hard ticks (*Ixodes ricinus, I. persulcatus*) transmit three subtypes of TBE flaviviruses. Infection can also be acquired by drinking unpasteurized dairy products, especially goats' milk.

Clinical: a feverish illness (myalgia, headache and fatigue) may appear 4–28 days after the tick bite; 1–33 days later about one-third will develop meningitis, meningoencephalomyelitis, myelitis, or meningoradiculitis.

Diagnosis (at the base hospital): can be confirmed by detecting viraemia (early) or serologically.

Treatment is symptomatic.

Prevention: (see Immunizations 📖 p. 43) vaccination (two doses 4–6 weeks apart followed by a booster at 1 year) is effective for those walking and camping in tick-infested coniferous forests of endemic areas, especially during the tick season (May–October and 'Russian spring–summer encephalitis'). In Austria, everyone is vaccinated. Avoid tick infestation (📖 p. 268) and unpasteurized (goats') milk products.

West Nile fever

West Nile fever, caused by a flavivirus, occurs in Africa, Europe, Asia and, most recently, in the US (New York City 1999) where there were around 1000 cases reported in 2006. Kunjin virus is the Australian subtype.

Transmission is by *Culex* mosquitoes, primarily among migratory birds but sometimes to humans, horses, and other mammals and also by blood transfusion.

Clinical: after an incubation period of 3–15 days, about 20% of infected people develop a dengue-like feverish illness. Fewer than 1% have meningitis or encephalitis, although these may prove fatal in elderly patients. Rashes and lymphadenopathy are uncommon.

Diagnosis: confirmation is serological.

Prevention: there is no vaccine. Avoid mosquito bites (📖 p. 265, 478), especially from dusk to dawn. Wear gloves when handling bird carcasses.

Website

http://www.cdc.gov/ncidod/dvbid/westnile/index.htm

Rabies

Rabies ('hydrophobia') is a zoonosis caused by several rhabdoviruses of mammals that can be transmitted to humans by bites. Domestic dogs are the most important source of human rabies worldwide. Other vectors include cats, wolves, foxes, jackals, skunks, mongooses, raccoons, vampire bats (Caribbean and Latin America only), flying foxes (fruit bats), and insectivorous bats. Most of the world is endemic for rabies (see Fig. 2.5).

Rabies-free countries include Antarctica, Scandinavian countries (except Greenland and Svalbard/Spitsbergen), Malaysia, New Guinea, New Zealand, Japan, and some smaller islands. It is especially common in parts of Africa, the Indian subcontinent, South-East Asia, China, and Latin America, causing ~60 000 human deaths each year and untold fear and suffering.

Transmission: virus-laden saliva is inoculated through the skin by a bite or graze. Transmission between humans has been proved only via infected corneal and solid organ grafts from unsuspected rabid donors.

Clinical: the virus spreads from the wound along nerves to reach the CNS, causing fatal encephalomyelitis. The incubation period is usually a few months but can vary from 4 days to many years. Often, the first symptom is itching at the site of the healed bite. Within a few days, headache, fever, confusion, hallucinations, and hydrophobia develop. Attempts to drink water induce spasm of inspiratory muscles and an indescribable terror. Ascending flaccid paralysis is another type of presentation. Rabies encephalomyelitis is inevitably fatal, usually after a few days, but is readily preventable.

Prevention of rabies after possible exposure: avoid all unnecessary and close contact with domestic, wild or pet mammals, especially carnivores, monkeys and insectivorous, fruit-eating, and vampire bats. Irrespective of the risk of rabies, mammal (including human) bites, scratches, and licks on mucous membranes or broken skin should be thoroughly cleaned immediately.

Pre-exposure rabies vaccination is strongly recommended for all travellers to rabies-endemic regions.

- Scrub with soap and water, ideally under a running tap
- Rinse and apply 40–70% alcohol (gin and whisky contain more than 40% alcohol) *or* povidone–iodine.
- Give tetanus toxoid.
- Consider other mammal bite pathogens (e.g. *Pasteurella multocida*), but prophylactic antibiotics (tetracycline, amoxicillin, or co-amoxiclav) are not recommended unless the hands are severely wounded.
- In a rabies-endemic country, if the skin has been broken by the bite or scratch, or if a mucosal membrane or open wound, including a scratch, has been contaminated with the animal's saliva, start post-exposure prophylaxis (see Box, 📖 p. 460). The decision should be made as soon as possible by a doctor working in the area where the bite has occurred. On no account should it be delayed until the traveller's return to their own country. If in doubt, start prophylaxis!

Websites

http://www.dh.gov.uk/assetRoot/04/08/06/57/04080657.pdf
http://www.hpa.org.uk/infections/topics_az/rabies/menu.htm
http://www.cdc.gov/ncidod/dvrd/rabies/
http://www.who-rabies-bulletin.org/
http://www.who.int/rabies/en/

Post-exposure prophylaxis of Rabies

Modern tissue culture vaccines, such as human diploid cell vaccine (Sanofi-Pasteur and Novartis-Chiron), vero cell vaccine (Sanofi-Pasteur) and purified chick embryo cell vaccine (Novartis-Chiron "Rabipur™", "RabAvert™"), are potent and safe. Consider including at least one dose of rabies vaccine in your medical kit.

For those who HAVE received pre-exposure immunization:
- Two booster injections of vaccine should be given on days 0 and 7 but no rabies immune globulin (RIG) is necessary.

For those who HAVE NOT previously received rabies vaccine:
- *Rabies immune globulin (RIG)*—most is infiltrated around the bite wound and the rest given intramuscularly (lateral thigh). Human RIG 20 units/kg body weight Equine RIG 40 units/kg.
  - AND
- Rabies tissue culture vaccine (detailed above):
- **EITHER** intramuscular (deltoid) injections of one vial (0.5ml or 1ml of reconstituted vaccine) on days 0, 3, 7, 14 and 30. **OR** intradermal injections (so that a small papule is produced—see coloured Plate 3 just like with BCG vaccination); divide one ampoule of vaccine between four sites (both deltoids, both thighs, both sides of the umbilicus and above both shoulder blades), ~0.25 ml (in the case of 1ml vials) or ~0.1 ml (in the case of 0.5 ml vials) at each site on day 0, two sites on day 7 (both deltoids) and single site on days 30 and 90.

Early, vigorous cleaning of the bite wound (see above) combined with vaccination and use of RIG has proved very effective in preventing rabies. If no suitable vaccine is available where and when the exposure occurs, the traveller should immediately be repatriated to start post-exposure prophylaxis as a matter of urgency.

No case of rabies has been reported in anyone who was exposed to rabies after receiving pre-exposure prophylaxis, provided that booster shots were given.

Viral haemorrhagic fevers
Yellow fever

Yellow fever is the classic flavivirus haemorrhagic fever. It occurs only in Africa and South America (see Fig. 2.7). Ninety per cent of cases are reported from Africa. In 2005 there were 565 cases with 25% case fatality in South Kordofan, Sudan. In 2006, cases were reported from Brazil, Burkina Faso, Côte d'Ivoire, Togo, and Sudan. There have been as many as 200 000 cases of yellow fever each year, with 30 000 deaths. Deaths of six unvaccinated travellers have been reported in the past 10 years.

Transmission: is by *Aedes* mosquitoes. Jungle (sylvatic) yellow fever is transmitted between monkeys and occasionally humans by tree hole breeding mosquitoes in South America and Africa, while urban epidemics are transmitted between humans by peri-domestic *Aedes aegypti*.

Clinical: after an incubation period of 3–6 days, around 5% of those infected become feverish with chills, headache, photophobia, myalgia, back ache, pain in limbs and knees, nausea, vomiting, epigastric pain, and prostration. Heart rate may be slow relative to the temperature. After a temporary remission, jaundice, generalized bleeding (black vomit, melaena), renal failure, shock, and coma may supervene.

Diagnosis (at the base hospital): leucopenia and thrombocytopenia are typical. Confirmation is by detecting virus in blood or liver tissue (post mortem) or serological.

Treatment: supportive.

Prevention: (see Immunizations 📖 p. 43) vaccination is recommended for all visitors to the endemic area and is a statutory requirement in many countries. For example, you will not be allowed to fly from Ecuador to Brazil without a valid vaccination certificate. The live, attenuated 17D vaccine is contraindicated before the age of 9 months, in pregnant women, and in the immunosuppressed. There have been problems with vaccine supply and safety most recently in the Canary Islands. Yellow fever vaccine-associated viscerotropic disease was first reported in 2001. It affects 0.1–2.5/million vaccinees. Incidences of 0.4 cases of encephalitis and 1.9 cases of Guillain–Barré syndrome (1.9) have been reported per million doses of vaccine.[1]

Websites

http://www.cdc.gov/ncidod/dvbid/yellowfever/index.htm
http://www.nathnac.org/pro/factsheets/yellow.htm

Dengue fever ('break bone' fever)

Dengue viruses are, like West Nile and yellow fever, flaviviruses. There are 50–100 million cases of dengue each year, occurring in almost every part of the tropics, notably in South-East Asia, South America, and the Caribbean, and increasingly in urban areas (Fig. 14.2).

Transmission: mosquitoes such as *Aedes aegypti* and *A. albopictus* transmit the four types of dengue virus from human to human.

Clinical: in most foreign travellers, dengue causes an acute fever associated with headache, backache, pains in the muscles and joints ('break bone' fever), and a rash. A reddish blotchy rash that may blanch on pressure often appears after a temporary lull in the fever. Petechial haemorrhages may be found in the skin and conjunctivae.

Severe dengue: 200 000–500 000 cases of severe, life-threatening dengue (dengue haemorrhagic fever and dengue shock syndrome) occur each year, with 5% case fatality, usually in children born and being brought up in endemic areas who are suffering their second infection with a dengue virus type different from that causing their first attack. However, severe and even fatal, apparently primary, dengue infections have been seen in adults, including travellers. After 2–7 days of fever, spontaneous bleeding (nose, gums, gastrointestinal) leads to shock, haemoconcentration, and thrombocytopenia.

Diagnosis (at the base hospital): is supported if the blood count shows leucopenia with relative lymphocytosis and thrombocytopenia often with raised liver enzymes and may be confirmed serologically.

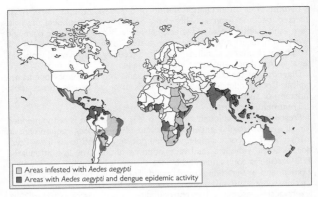

Fig. 14.2 Global distribution of dengue.

Treatment: for primary dengue only symptomatic treatment is needed (bed rest, control of fever and pain with paracetamol). Suspected severe dengue warrants immediate evacuation and correction of hypovolaemia, hypoglycaemia, and electrolyte and acid–base homeostasis but avoidance of corticosteroids, heparin, NSAIDs, and aspirin. Supportive treatment reduces case fatality to <1%.

Prevention: wear sensible clothing (see malaria below) during the daytime biting period and apply DEET-containing repellents to exposed skin surfaces. A vaccine is expected soon (http://www.cdc.gov/ncidod/diseases/submenus/sub_dengue.htm).

Apart from yellow fever and dengue haemorrhagic fever, there are a number of other notorious viral haemorrhagic fevers, none of which is preventable by vaccination.

Lassa fever (West Africa) and Bolivian, Argentine, and Venezuelan haemorrhagic fevers

These fevers are caused by Arenaviruses and are acquired through contact with urine of peri-domestic or feral rodents.

Transmission: between humans is by contamination with infected blood, needle sticks, and sexual contact.

Symptoms: after an incubation period of 6–21 days, Lassa fever presents with insidious fever, malaise, headache, and painful sore throat with visible exudative pharyngitis, conjunctivitis, backache, chest pain, cough, nausea, vomiting and diarrhea, but no jaundice (despite hepatitis), bleeding or rash. Hypovolaemic shock (associated with facial oedema) may supervene after about 1 week. Early antiviral treatment with ribavirin (tribavirin) reduces case fatality 5- to 10-fold.

Prevention: is by avoiding all contact with rodents (including not eating them) and rodent-contaminated accommodation and food in endemic areas. No vaccine is available. In West Africa there are thought to be 300 000–500 000 cases of Lassa fever, with 5000 deaths each year. In parts of Liberia and Sierra Leone, the prevalence of Lassa fever among hospital admissions is 10–16%. The overall case fatality rate is 1%, up to 15% among hospitalized patients. Pregnant women and their fetuses are at very high risk. Worldwide about 20 cases of imported Lassa fever have been described, the most recent from Sierra Leone to Germany and Nigeria to South Africa.

Websites

http://www.who.int/mediacentre/factsheets/fs179/en/index.htm
http://www.cdc.gov/ncidod/dvrd/spb/mnpages/dispages/vhf.htm
http://www.who.int/mediacentre/factsheets/fs_marburg/en/index.htm

Marburg and Ebola viruses (Filoviruses)

These filoviruses have caused epidemics of highly fatal haemorrhagic fever (1850 cases with over 1200 deaths) in Equatorial Africa, most recently in Angola in 2005 where 378 cases with 329 deaths (case fatality 88%) were reported mainly in Uige Province, Kamwenge in Western Uganda in July 2007 (Marburg) and Kasai Occidental, Democratic Republic of the Congo in September 2007 (Ebola). The natural reservoir is unknown, but virus has been isolated from monkeys and recently from a fruit bat.

Transmission: between humans during the devastating epidemics has resulted from contamination with infected blood, needle sticks in hospitals, and sexual contact.

Symptoms: after an incubation period of 3–20 days there is sudden fever, headache, myalgia, arthralgia, conjunctivitis, prostration, abdominal pain, vomiting, diarrhea, and a generalized papular, desquamating, erythematous rash but no jaundice (despite hepatitis). Severe bleeding and hypovolaemic shock begin on about the fifth day. Case fatality ranges from 50 to 90%.

Prevention: is by avoiding epidemic areas, contact with patient's blood, and risk of parenteral infection by needles and sharps.

Bunyavirus zoonoses

Crimean–Congo haemorrhagic fever (CCHF) occurs in Eastern Europe, the Middle East, Africa, and Asia (recently in Kazakhstan and north-eastern Turkey). CCHF is transmitted by tick bites from farm and other animals and by needle sticks in hospitals. In 2006, hundreds of suspected cases were reported in Stavropol (Central Caucasus), Russia. After 3–7 days' incubation period, there is sudden fever, headache, photophobia, nausea, vomiting, generalized body pains, thrombocytopenia, leucopenia, and severe bleeding with a case fatality of 15–80%. Treatment with ribavirin may be helpful. No vaccine is available. Avoid tick bites (📖 p. 270) and parenteral exposure.

Hantavirus haemorrhagic fever with renal syndrome (HHFRS or Korean haemorrhagic fever) occurs in Europe, especially Scandinavia, Germany (Puumala virus) and the Balkans, and Asia.

Hantavirus pulmonary syndrome (HPS) occurs in the Americas.

HHFRS is spread by aerosol from rodent urine or bites. After a long incubation period (12–16 days, up to 2 months), fever, facial flushing, and subconjunctival haemorrhages develop, followed by shock and renal failure. The case fatality is up to 15% (50% in HPS). These infections are not transmitted between humans. Treatment is early ribavirin and supportive treatment (dialysis). Avoid rodent contact and human-to-human spread in HPS. No vaccines are generally available.

Rift valley fever (RVF) occurs in Africa and the Middle East. RVF is spread from camels and domestic ruminants by mosquitoes and contamination by infected blood in abbatoirs. In 1997–8 and 2006–7, there were epizootics in Kenya, Tanzania, Burundi, and Somalia. In the recent epidemic, 684 cases with 155 deaths were reported in Kenya (case fatality 23%), 264 with 109 deaths in Tanzania (41%) and 114 with 51 deaths in Somalia (45%). After 3–6 days' incubation, there is acute fever, mucocutaneous haemorrhages, conjunctivitis, photophobia, eye pains, blinding retinitis, and lymphadenopathy, with occasional progression to disseminated intravascular coagulation (DIC), severe bleeding, encephalopathy, hepatorenal failure, and death. Veterinary vaccines are marketed. Avoid mosquito bites and contact with infected animal blood.

Websites

http://www.who.int/topies/haemorrhagic_fevers_viral/en/
http://www.cdc.gov/ncidod/diseases/hanta/hps/index.htm
http://www.cdc.gov/MMWR/preview/mmwrhtml/rr5109a1.htm

Chikungunya fever

'Chikungunya' means 'that which bends up' in Makonde, an East African language, referring to the crippling arthralgia that characterizes the disease. A massive epidemic of this dengue-like *Aedes* mosquito-transmitted alphavirus infection has raged in India (>1.3 million cases), adjacent countries, Kenya and Indian Ocean islands [Comoros, Mauritius, Seychelles, Madagascar, Mayotte, and Réunion (34% of the population infected)] since 2006, and in 2007 it reached Gabon in Central Africa. This epidemic was caused by a new variant virus. More than 800 cases were imported into France and 100 into the UK from Réunion and the other islands popular with tourists. In August 2007, local transmission of chikungunya by *Aedes albopictus* mosquitoes was confirmed around Ravenna in Italy, resulting in ~200 cases and one death.

Clinical: after 2–4 days' incubation there is sudden fever, headache, malaise, conjunctivitis, arthralgia, arthritis (ankles and small joints), myalgia, and low back pain with rash in half the cases. Rashes are very variable: erythematous (blanching), vesicular, bullous, dyshydrotic, keratolytic, purpuric, and hyperpigmented, associated with facial oedema, erythema nodosum, and aphthous ulcers. Joints may be severely and persistently involved with effusions and bursitis. A useful sign is pain on squeezing the wrists (tenosynovitis). Severe and occasionally fatal features are meningoencephalitis, Guillain–Barré polyradiculopathy, myocarditis, hepatic dysfunction, and renal failure.

Prevention: an effective vaccine has been developed in the US but is not generally available. Anti-mosquito measures are the only protection.

Zika virus infection

This flavivirus causes a mild dengue-like illness. A total of 120 confirmed and probable cases occurred in Yap, Micronesia, in March–May, 2007.

Reference

1 McMahon AW, Eidex RB, Marfin AA, *et al.* Neurologic disease associated with 17D–204 yellow fever vaccination: a report of 15 cases. *Vaccine* 2007 Feb 26; **25**(10): 1727–34.

Bacterial infections

Brucellosis

This globally prevalent zoonosis of goats, sheep and camels (*Brucella melitensis*), cattle (*B. abortus*), and dogs (*B. canis*) has been eliminated from <20 countries. More than 500 000 new cases of *B. melitensis* infection are reported each year.

Transmission: the main risk of infection, except for farmers, is ingestion of milk products, especially soft white goats' cheeses, and raw meat.

Clinical: after an incubation period of 1 week to several months, every system can be involved and so the range of symptoms is enormous. Commonly there is acute or insidious persistent fever with chills, arthralgias, septic arthritis, back ache, spinal tenderness signifying osteomyelitis, granulomatous hepatitis, meningoencephalitis, endocarditis, and epididymo-orchitis and other genitourinary infections.

Diagnosis: at the base hospital or after return home in the case of long incubation periods, blood, marrow, and other cultures (prolonged, using special media) and serology (IgG agglutinins difficult to interpret) may prove diagnostic.

Treatment: doxycycline (oral 100 mg twice/day) and rifampicin (oral 600–900 mg/day) for 45 days or doxycycline for 45 days and streptomycin (0.5–1.0 g/day im) for 2 weeks are the most effective regimens.

Prevention: avoid all unpasteurized milk and milk products, especially cheeses and undercooked meat products in parts of the world where brucellosis is prevalent, such as Africa, the Middle East, and Latin America (e.g. the Canta valley outside Lima, Peru).

Diphtheria

Diphtheria (*Corynebacterium diphtheriae*) usually infects the upper respiratory tract or skin (📖 p. 272) and its toxin can affect the heart, nerves, and kidneys. Although largely eliminated by childhood vaccination, diphtheria still occurs in developing countries and has increased in the former Soviet Union.

Transmission is from human-to-human by aerosol or contact with respiratory tract secretions.

Clinical: after an incubation period of 2–5 days there is inflammation of mucosae, usually of the fauces, nasal cavity, trachea, larynx or bronchi, development of the classic greyish-yellow pseudomembrane, local lymphadenopathy, and swelling of the neck ('bull neck'). Diphtheria can cause skin ulcers apparently indistinguishable from simple bacterial ulcers, but they have an area of anaesthesia round them which can be detected by testing pinprick sensation (see Skin 📖 p. 272).

Treatment: high dose benzyl penicillin (12 g each day in six divided doses) or erythromycin will eliminate the infection but antitoxin is needed for severe toxic effects, and emergency tracheostomy or needle cricothyroidotomy (📖 p. 181) may be needed to relieve airway obstruction. Suspected diphtheria warrants immediate evacuation.

Prevention: (📖 p. 35) childhood immunization in combination with tetanus and pertussis is routine in most countries. For boosting immunity in adult travelers, adsorbed diphtheria (low dose) and tetanus vaccine (formol toxoids) is recommended for adults and adolescents.

Leptospirosis

Leptospirosis is a zoonotic infection by *Leptospira icterohaemorrhagiae* and related spirochaetes affecting rats, dogs, pigs, sheep, cattle, other mammals and humans in most parts of the world. Increasing numbers of cases are being detected in South Asia. Leptospirosis is an occupational disease of farmers and sewer workers. Those involved in fresh water sports (canoeing, sailing, water skiing) and exposure to watery, flooded environments are also at risk. During the 10-day Eco-Challenge-Sabah 2000 multisport endurance race, 26% of 304 athletes caught leptospirosis.

Transmission: infection is acquired when broken skin or intact mucosae are in contact with fresh water contaminated by infected mammals' urine.

Clinical: the incubation period is 2–26 (mean 10) days. Most infections are subclinical or mild but in about 10% severe features, including jaundice, hepatorenal failure, pulmonary haemorrhage, and shock may develop. Symptoms include fever, rigors, headache, myalgia, backache, painful tender calves, meningism, and gastrointestinal and pulmonary haemorrhages. Jaundice and subconjunctival haemorrhages are common signs.

Treatment: early treatment with oral doxycycline (100 mg twice daily for 1 week) for suspected mild disease and high dose parenteral benzyl penicillin may be effective.

Prevention: doxycyline in the dose taken for malaria prophylaxis (100 mg each day) or 200 mg once each week is protective.

Lyme disease

Lyme disease is named after Lyme, Connecticut, USA. In North America, there are about 20 000 new cases reported each year, making it the most common vector-borne disease. It occurs particulary in north-eastern, mid-Atlantic, and north-central states in people aged 5–14 years and 45–54 years. Elsewhere, it occurs in Europe, especially Estonia, Latvia, Lithuania, Russia, and northern Asia. A total of 482 cases were reported in Estonia in 2006, 154 of them on Saaremaa island. *Borrelia burgdorferi* causes the disease in North America while in Europe, *B. garinii* causes classic Lyme neuroborreliosis (Bannwarth syndrome) and *B. afzelii* causes a less distinctive clinical picture.

Transmission: from mice, deer, and other mammals to humans is by bites of hard (*Ixodes*) ticks.

Clinical: after an incubation of 7–10 days, a red macule/papule and later an expanding red ring (erythema migrans) usually appears around the tick bite site (Coloured Plate 4) and is associated with local lymphadenopathy, fever, chills, headache, myalgia, arthralgia, and meningism. The classic erythema migrans does not always appear. Unilateral facial nerve palsy, radiculopathy, carditis with heart block, arthritis, and other rashes may occur.

Diagnosis is confirmed by serology at the base hospital.

Treatment: early treatment with oral doxycycline 100 mg twice daily for 14–21 days is curative. About 15% of patients show a mild exacerbation of symptoms (Jarisch–Herxheimer reaction) within 24 h of starting treatment.

Prevention: anti-tick measures (see Skin 🕮 p. 268) are important. Chemoprophylaxis before tick attachment is not justified and afterwards only within strict criteria.[1] An effective (OspA) vaccine was developed in the US but is no longer used.

Meningitis

Bacterial (pyogenic) meningitis is an acute infection involving the meninges and CSF. Common causes in younger people are the meningococcus (*Neisseria meningitidis*), pneumococcus (*Streptococcus pneumoniae*), and *Haemophilus influenzae* b (Hib). Meningococcal meningitis is common across the sub-Sahelian zone of Africa, extending from Senegal to the Sudan ('meningitis belt'; see Fig. 2.1), where there are annual cold season epidemics of group A or C disease. Epidemics occur elsewhere, for example in 1970 in north-western Uganda contiguous with north-eastern Democratic Republic of Congo, southern Sudan and Niger (serogroup X) (check http://www.promedmail.org for up-to-date information). In China and South-East Asia, *Streptococcus suis* is an important cause in those working with pigs or pork.

Other causes of acute meningitis include viruses (e.g. *Herpes simplex*, enteroviruses, mumps, etc.); causes of more insidious meningitis are tuberculosis, fungi (e.g. *Cryptococcus*) and even worms (e.g. *Angiostrongylus*).

Transmission: by aerosol from infected carriers or cases.

Symptoms:
- Sudden fever
- Severe headache
- Photophobia
- Nausea
- Vomiting
- Diarrhoea
- Myalgia.

Meningococcal meningitis

A petechial/purpuric rash is characteristic. It is initially macular, often starts on the forearms or shins, and may be visible on the conjunctivae (Coloured Plate 5). It spreads over the trunk and face, and may become vasculitic with geometrical areas of skin necrosis (Coloured Plate 6). Stiff neck (meningism) is the diagnostic sign of meningitis. Ability to flex the neck so that the chin touches the chest or shake the head from side to side virtually excludes meningism. Impairment of consciousness and seizures (children) are ominous developments. Very rapid evolution to classic meningococcal septicaemia (profuse rash, shock, bleeding, peripheral gangrene, multiple system failure) occurs in a minority of cases.

Pneumococcal meningitis

There may be an obvious source of infection (e.g. pneumonia, otitis media).

Diagnosis: Unless the diagnosis can be rapidly confirmed by lumbar puncture and CSF examination (unlikely in most expeditions), suspicion of bacterial meningitis warrants immediate, parenteral, preferably intravenous, antibiotic treatment, and urgent evacuation to the base hospital.

Treatment: ceftriaxone or cefotaxime (2 g iv or im 12-hourly) are the antibiotics of choice, covering all causes of bacterial meningitis except *Listeria monocytogenes* (special risk in pregnant women and some immunosuppressed patients; add ampicillin). Benzyl penicillin 2.4 g iv or im 4-hourly is effective for meningococcal infection. If parenteral treatment is impossible, amoxicillin 2 g 4-hourly, or chloramphenicol 100 mg/kg each day in four divided doses can be given by mouth. If *H. simplex* (viral) meningitis is suspected, aciclovir should be given.

Prevention: (🕮 p. 33) Hib vaccine (since 1992) and meningococcal group C vaccine (since 1999) have been routinely offered to children in Britain. Travel to the African meningitis belt (see Fig. 2.1) or other areas of current epidemic meningocical meningitis, justifies group A,C,W135,Y vaccine ('ACWY Vax')(see Immunizations 🕮 p. 37). Contacts are treated with ciprofloxacin (500 mg single dose) or rifampicin (600 mg twice daily for 2 days).

Plague

About 2500 cases and 190 deaths from plague are reported each year (case fatality 7.7%), mainly from Madagascar and other African countries, and south Asia, but a few are from the western USA (Fig. 14.3). Plague is flea-borne from rodents to humans. Warning of an impending epidemic is a die-off of rats, mice, marmots, etc.

Prevention: if your expedition is going to a notorious plague area (see website below) and an epidemic is in progress, consider going elsewhere or taking preventive measures such as avoiding rodents and their parasites, and taking chemoprophylaxis (doxycycline, ciprofloxacin, or co-trimoxazole). No vaccines are currently available.

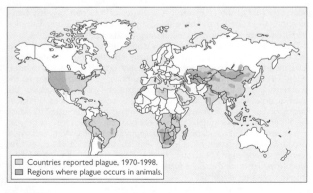

☐ Countries reported plague, 1970-1998.
■ Regions where plague occurs in animals.

Fig. 14.3 World distribution of plague, 1998.

Website

http://www.cdc.gov/ncidod/dvbid/plague/
http://www.britishinfectionsociety.org/documents/meningitisAlgorothm03.pdf

Tuberculosis

Mycobacterium tuberculosis is the world's most prevalent bacterial infection, affecting 2 billion people. The incidence is 8 million new cases and 1.6 million deaths each year, 23% of which are in India and 17% in China. Throughout most of Africa, Eastern Europe, Asia, and Latin America the incidence exceeds 50/100 000 of the population/year. All these figures are increasing as a result of the HIV pandemic.

Transmission: this is by aerosol created by coughing and, to a lesser extent, by ingestion of *M. bovis*-infected (unpasteurized) milk.

Clinical: typically, if the immune response is inadequate, infection involves the lungs (apical cavitating pneumonia), mediastinal nodes or pleura during the period up to 2 years after exposure or much later from reactivation of latent infection. Pericardium, lymph nodes (e.g. scrofula of the cervical nodes), kidneys, genital tract, bones, joints, gut or peritoneum, spleen, brain or meninges (tuberculous meningitis) or any other organ may be affected. Fulminant miliary or disseminated TB is most common in children and immunocompromised patients. More commonly, TB develops insidiously. No symptom is diagnostic, but a chronic productive cough lasting for weeks and associated with malaise, weakness, wasting, and the classical fever and night sweats are typical presentations of pulmonary TB, the commonest form of the infection.

Diagnosis (at the base hospital): confirmed by staining or culturing *Mycobacteria* in sputum or elsewhere or detecting characteristic histopathology in biopsies. A strongly positive Mantoux test suggests active infection but a negative result is uninterpretable.

Mantoux test: inject 0.1 ml of solution, containing 2 Tuberculin Units of Statens Serum Institut (SSI) tuberculin RT23, intradermally into the volar surface of the forearm. After 48–72 h, measure the diameter of palpable induration (*not* of the red weal!). A diameter of >15 mm suggests active infection; 6–15 mm may be caused by previous BCG immunization (http://www.immunisation.nhs.uk/files/mantouxtest.pdf).

Treatment: quadruple therapy with isoniazid, rifampicin, pyrazinamide, and ethambutol or streptomycin is usually effective, but emerging drug resistance is worrying. Recently, extensively drug-resistant tuberculosis (XDR-TB) has been reported from 37 countries. This is resistant to the two most important first-line drugs isoniazid and rifampicin, any of the fluoroquinolones, and at least one of the aminoglycosides amikacin, kanamycin, or capreomycin. Treatment with other antibiotics to which the XDR may be susceptible, such as ethionamide, cycloserine, viomycin, or para-aminosalicylic acid, produces disappointing results. WHO estimates 25 000–30 000 new cases of XDR-TB/year. In South Africa 314 cases have been detected, with 214 deaths. In the initial outbreak among 53 HIV-infected patients in ZwaZulu Natal, 52 died, with a median survival of only 16 days after diagnosis.

Prevention (see Immunizations 🔲 p. 43): intradermal BCG vaccination (Coloured Plate 3) provides very variable but potentially valuable protection against TB (especially miliary TB and tuberculous meningitis in children) and leprosy. Those born in hyperendemic countries should have been given BCG at birth (look for the scar). Routine Mantoux (tuberculin skin) testing (see above) and BCG vaccination of Mantoux-negative expedition members is recommended if the destination is in a hyperendemic area and if the programme involves mixing with local people in crowded high risk environments such as hostels, prisons, refugee camps, hospitals or clinics. HIV-immunocompromised people should consider taking prophylactic isoniazid (300 mg each day with pyridoxine 50 mg/kg each day) or rifampicin (which interacts with some HAART drugs!) and pyrazinamide.

http://www.nice.org.uk/guidance/index.jsp?action=byID&r=true&o=10980

Typhoid and paratyphoid (enteric fevers)

Infections by *Salmonella typhi* and *S. paratyphi* A, B, and C are still common in the Indian subcontinent, Viet Nam, and Indonesia (100–1000 cases/ 100 000 population/year). Worldwide, there are an estimated 15–30 million cases and 500 000 deaths each year.

Transmission: is by faecal–oral spread from water and food infected by human carriers (up to 1% of the population in some communities).

Clinical: after an incubation period of 3–60 (usually 7–14) days, the illness starts insidiously with fever, headache, malaise, abdominal discomfort, some bowel disturbance (often constipation but sometimes diarrhoea), cough, sore throat, and epistaxis. Signs include a slow pulse rate in relation to the fever, hepatosplenomegaly, a blanching macular rash on the abdomen (rose spots (Coloured Plate 7)), rhonchi in the chest, and abdominal tenderness (especially right iliac fossa). Untreated patients may develop severe complications in the second to fourth weeks of illness: perforation, intestinal haemorrhage, shock, and coma.

Diagnosis is by blood, stool, urine or bone marrow culture. Widal test is unreliable but newer Typhidot® IgM test is promising.

Treatment: fluoroquinolones, such as ciprofloxacin 0.5–1.0 g each day in two divided doses for 7–14 days, are usually effective.

Prevention: strict food and water hygiene (📖 Chapter 3, p. 89) are crucial. Effective injectable and oral vaccines are available and strongly recommended for all expeditions to developing countries (see Immunizations 📖 p. 43).

Typhus

Rickettsial bacteria cause a large variety of arthropod-borne acute febrile diseases in most parts of the world, usually with a distinctive rash. Louse-borne epidemic typhus (*Rickettsia prowazeckii*) remains an epidemic threat in poorer countries, mite-borne scrub typhus (*Orientia tsutsugamushi*) is prevalent throughout South-East Asia (Fig. 14.4), tick-borne Rocky Mountain spotted fever (RMSF) (*R. rickettsii*) is one of the most dreaded infections in North America, and tick-borne African tick fever (*R. africae*) is commonly acquired by safari travellers in Southern Africa.

Transmission: is by tick or mite saliva during their blood meal, by louse or flea faeces inoculated through skin or mucosae by scratching.

Clinical: after an incubation period of 4–14 (average 7) days, fever, chills, headache, photophobia, nausea, vomiting, abdominal pain and cough may develop. This is followed 3–5 days later by a generalized maculopapular and eventually petechial rash (Coloured Plate 8). A papule appears at the site of the infected bite in spotted fevers such as African tick fever (Coloured Plate 9), RMSF and Mediterranean boutonneuse fever and in scrub typhus (Coloured Plate 10). This evolves into a black-scabbed eschar with lymphangitis and local lymphadenopathy. Severe multisystem complications may ensue.

Diagnosis: confirmation is serological.

Treatment: early treatment with oral doxycycline 200 mg or chloramphenicol 2 g in four divided doses each day for 2–3 days is appropriate for clinically suspected rickettsial infections. The therapeutic response is often dramatic and diagnostic.

Prevention: vaccines are not generally available. Doxycycline in the dose taken for malaria prophylaxis (100 mg each day) or 200 mg once each week is protective. Scrub typhus is suppressed rather than eradicated and so it may appear after cessation of chemoprophylaxis. Prevention of tick, louse, flea, and mite infestation is crucial (📖 p. 266–268).

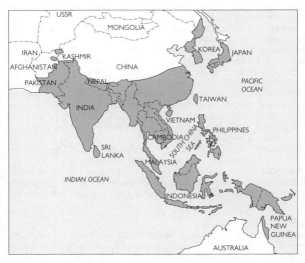

Fig. 14.4 Distribution of scrub typhus.

Website

http://www.cdc.gov/ncidod/dvrd/rmsf/index.htm

Reference

Wormser GP, Dattwyler RJ, Shapiro ED, *et al.* The clinical assessment, treatment, and prevention of lyme disease, human granulocytic anaplasmosis, and babesiosis: clinical practice guidelines by the Infectious Diseases Society of America. *Clin Infect Dis.* 2006 Nov 1: **43(9)**: 1089–134. Epub 2006 Oct 2. Erratum in: *Clin Infect Dis.* 2007. Oct 1; **45(7)**: 941.

Malaria

Malaria occurs throughout the tropics: north to southern Turkey, south to north-eastern South Africa, west to Mexico, and east to Vanuatu in the western Pacific, an area inhabited by more than 40% of the world's population (Fig. 14.5). It was reintroduced into Jamaica in 2006.

Malaria causes more than 500 million cases of fever each year, 75% in Africa, 25% in South-East Asia. It kills 1–2 million people each year, the majority young children and pregnant women in sub-Saharan Africa.

Four species of malaria parasites commonly infect humans: *Plasmodium falciparum,* causing life-threatening malignant falciparum malaria, and *P. vivax, P. ovale,* and *P. malariae,* causing the three benign malarias. Monkey malarias cause some human infections (e.g. *P. knowlesi* in Borneo Malaysia).

Transmission

Female *Anopheles* mosquitoes bite between dusk and dawn, transmitting malaria while they suck human blood. Transmission transplacentally (congenital malaria) and via blood transfusion, marrow and organ transplant, needle stick, and nosocomially through contaminated injections is also reported.

Imported travellers' malaria: 1758 cases of imported malaria were reported in the UK in 2006, 78% of which were caused by *P. falciparum.* Since 1977, an average of nine deaths has been reported each year, mostly in people who have taken no prophylaxis. A total of 1324 cases of imported malaria was reported in the US in 2004, with four deaths. Most deaths could have been prevented by better education of the travellers, use of approved methods of prevention, and prompt medical attention when they fell ill.

Incubation

The minimum interval between an infective mosquito bite and the first symptom (incubation period) is about 7 days, but most travellers with falciparum malaria become ill within a month of returning home; exceptionally, there may be a delay of more than a year. More than 1% of vivax infections present more than a year after leaving the tropics.

Symptoms

- Acute severe fever with rigors
- Severe headache
- Pain in muscles and back
- Nausea
- Diarrhoea
- Loss of appetite
- Postural hypotension
- Prostration
- There is no sore throat, rash or lymphadenopathy. Classic periodicity of fever (every other day—tertian—in falciparum, vivax, and ovale malarias, every third day—quartan—in malariae malaria) is uncommon, but recurrences of fever at the same time every day—quotidian—is typical.

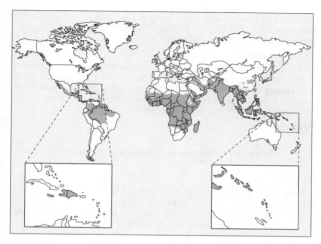

Fig. 14.5 Distribution map for malaria.

Signs
- There may be none.
- Petechiae, tender enlarged liver and spleen, pale conjunctivae, and jaundice are worth looking for.
- Falciparum malaria in non-immunes (those who have not acquired temporary immunity to malaria through repeated infections) can be a rapidly evolving and potentially life-threatening disease (exceptionally, first symptom to death in 24 h). Worrying features are severe prostration, impaired consciousness (cerebral malaria), seizures, profound anaemia, deep jaundice, hypoglycaemia, shock, renal failure, spontaneous systemic bleeding (suggesting DIC), and respiratory distress.

Diagnosis
http://www.malaria-reference.co.uk/
Suspect malaria in anyone who develops acute fever more than 7 days after entering, or within a few months of leaving, a malarious area whether or not they have taken prophylaxis. Consider unusual risks of infection, such as 'runway', 'airport', 'needle stick', and transfusion malarias.

Classic microscopy remains the best way of confirming the diagnosis. Thick and thin blood films, preferably made from finger prick blood at the bedside rather than from blood stored in anticoagulant, are stained with Field's or Giemsa stains and examined (oil immersion, high power). If negative, repeat daily for 72 h before rejecting the diagnosis of malaria. On an expedition, rapid malaria antigen tests may be a convenient alternative to microscopy. They are quick, sensitive, and species-specific (http://www.rapid-diagnostics.org/rti-malaria-com.htm). The NOW® Malaria Test (http://binax.com/NOWmalaria.shtml) is available in the UK.

'Paracheck Pf' (Orchid Biomedical Systems, Goa, India) and 'SD BIOLINE malaria antigen test' (Standard Diagnostics Inc., South Korea) are not available in the UK but are recommended.

Differential diagnosis

At the base hospital, malaria must be distinguished from other tropical fevers (typhoid, typhus, relapsing fevers, leptospirosis, dengue, and other viral haemorrhagic fevers), less exotic infections such as glandular fever (EBV), pyogenic bacterial infections, meningitis, viral hepatitis, viral encephalitis, HIV seroconversion illness, and heatstroke.

Treatment

> **Suspected malaria warrants immediate evacuation.**

Falciparum malaria
- Assume chloroquine-resistant *P. falciparum* infection.
- For adults who can swallow and retain tablets:
    - Artemether-with-lumefantrine (Riamet, Co-artem or Co-artemether): adult and children >12 years and >35 kg in weight dose four tablets at 0, 24, 36, 48, and 60 h *or*
    - Proguanil hydrochloride-with-atovaquone (Malarone): adult dose four tablets [children 11–20 kg 1; 21–30 kg 2; 31–40 kg 3 tablets] daily for 3 days *or*
    - Quinine sulphate: adult dose 600 mg (three tablets) [children 10 mg/kg] 8 hourly for 5–7 days followed by either doxycycline 200 mg for 7 days or clindamycin 450 mg three times daily [children 20–40 mg/kg in three divided doses] for 5 days.

Severe falciparum malaria
For adults unable to swallow and retain tablets or who have severe prostration, impaired consciousness, jaundice, profound anaemia, hypoglycaemia, renal failure, spontaneous systemic bleeding/DIC, black urine or respiratory distress:
- Sodium artesunate is the drug of choice; however, it is not licensed or available in some countries (http://www.cdc.gov/malaria/features/artesunate_now_available.htm): loading dose 2.4 mg/kg by iv injection followed by 1.2 mg/kg by iv injection daily for a minimum of 3 days, followed by oral antimalarial.
- Quinine dihydrochloride; loading dose 20 mg/kg by iv infusion over 4 h (or im), then maintenance dose 10 mg/kg by iv infusion over 4 h (or im) 8-hourly until able to swallow tablets. Complete the course with quinine sulphate followed by either doxycycline 200 mg for 7 days (*not* for children or pregnant women) or clindamycin 450 mg three times daily (children 20–40 mg/kg in three divided doses) for 5 days. *Quinine may cause hypoglycaemia!*
- Artemether: loading dose 3.2 mg/kg by im injection followed by 1.6 mg/kg by im injection for a minimum of 3 days followed by oral antimalarial.

Benign malarias
For adults, chloroquine (BASE!) 600 mg (usually four tablets) (children 10 mg BASE/kg) followed by 300 mg after 6–8 h (children 5 mg BASE/kg) followed by 300 mg daily for 2 days (children 5 mg BASE/kg) (total dose~25 mg BASE/kg body weight). Eradicate liver cycle with primaquine (see below) (beware of G6PD-deficiency!). In New Guinea and adjacent areas of Indonesia (for example, Lombok), *P. vivax* has become resistant to chloroquine. A double dose of chloroquine or the standard dose of mefloquine, followed by a 4-week course of primaquine, can be used to treat such resistant infections.

Prevention of malaria

Assessing the risk

Within malarious countries, the areas of malaria transmission may be patchy, depending on environmental factors such as temperature, altitude, vegetation, and season. Thus there is no malaria transmission in some African capital cities that are at a comparatively high altitude, such as Addis Ababa and Nairobi, and in other areas malaria transmission occurs only during a brief rainy season. Seek reliable local advice about malaria transmission where and when the expedition will take place. Even within a transmission area, the risk of being bitten by an infected mosquito can vary from less than once per year to more than once per night. The chances of catching malaria during a 2-week visit without any protection have been estimated at about 0.2% in Kenya and 1% in West Africa.

People who are especially vulnerable to malaria (see Table 14.1) should seriously reconsider whether they really need to enter the malarious area.

Table 14.1 Principles of personal protection against malaria

Awareness of risk: vulnerable individuals, such as pregnant women, infants, splenectomized or otherwise immunocompromised people, should avoid entering a malarious area.

Anti-mosquito measures: kill, exclude, repel, and avoid mosquitoes.

Sensible clothing: long sleeves and long trousers between dusk and dawn.

Diethyltoluamide (DEET)-containing insect repellent applied to exposed skin.

Insecticide (pyrethroid)-impregnated mosquito bed net or screened (air-conditioned) accommodation sprayed with insecticide each evening.

Vaporizing insecticide in the sleeping quarters (burning mosquito coil, electrical, knock-down insecticide).

Chemoprophylaxis: mefloquine (Lariam) or other drugs, depending on the particular geographical area (see ☐ p. 479).

Standby treatment: co-artemether, quinine or Malarone.

In case of feverish illness within a few months of return: see a doctor and mention malaria specifically!

Avoid all alternative/homeopathic remedies for prevention or treatment of malaria.

http://www.hpa.org.uk/infections/topics_az/malaria/homeopathic_statement_260705.htm

Anti-mosquito measures

Sleeping quarters: malaria-transmitting mosquitoes bite in or near human dwellings during the hours of darkness and so the risk of infection can be reduced by insect-proofing sleeping quarters or by sleeping under a mosquito net. Individual, lightweight, self-supporting mosquito nets are available. Protection against mosquitoes and other biting invertebrates (sandflies, lice, fleas, bed bugs, ticks) is greatly enhanced by soaking the net in a pyrethroid insecticide such as 10% permethrin (75 ml or 200–500 mg per m^2 of material every 6 months). Screens and curtains can also be impregnated with insecticide. In addition, bedrooms should be sprayed in the evening with a knock-down aerosol insecticide (e.g. Etofenprox, Malathion, Deltamethrin) to kill any mosquitoes that may have entered the room during the day. Mosquitoes may also be killed or repelled by vaporizing synthetic pyrethroids (D-Allethrin, S-Bioallethrin, trans-Fluthrin) on an electrical vaporizing mat (such as No Bite and Buzz Off) where electricity is available, or over a methylated spirit burner (Travel Accessories UK Ltd, PO Box 10, Lutterworth, Leicester LE17 4FB, UK). Burning cones or coils of mosquito-repellent 'incense' may also be effective.

Protective clothing: to avoid bites by any flying insect, long-sleeved shirts and long trousers afford better protection than vests and shorts. To avoid malaria-transmitting mosquito bites, this sensible clothing should be worn, particularly after dark. Cotton clothes and ankle bands can be impregnated with DEET and other materials can be impregnated with permethrin insecticide.

Repellents: exposed areas of skin should be rubbed or sprayed with repellents containing NN-diethyl-m-toluamide (DEET) or *p*-methane-diol ('Mosiguard Natural'). Insecticide-containing soaps ('Mosbar', Simmons Pty Ltd, Box 107, Chadstone, Victoria 3148, Australia) and suntan oil are available.

Antimalarial chemoprophylaxis

The emergence of drug-resistant strains of *P. falciparum* has made chemoprophylaxis much more difficult. Chloroquine-resistant strains of *P. falciparum* now predominate in most parts of the tropics except in Mexico and Central America, north-west of the Panama Canal, Haiti, and the Dominican Republic (Hispaniola).

Compliance: the failure of travellers to take their antimalarial tablets regularly, and in particular to continue taking them for long enough after leaving the malarious area (4 weeks for all but Malarone which need only be taken for 7 days), also reduces the effectiveness of chemoprophylaxis. During bouts of vomiting and diarrhoea (travellers' diarrhoea), these drugs may not be adequately absorbed.

Choice of drug: risk of contracting malaria should be balanced against the relative efficacy and risk of side effects of a particular prophylactic drug.

Chemoprophylactic drugs and combinations

Mefloquine (Lariam)

Mefloquine is effective against most multiresistant *P. falciparum* strains but has some unpleasant side effects: nausea, stomach ache, and diarrhoea in 10–15% of people who take it; insomnia and nightmares; giddiness and ataxia (unsteadiness and incoordination) in some; and a rare 'acute brain syndrome' (psychosis and even seizures).

Contraindications include a history of previous adverse reactions to this drug, hypersensitivity to quinine, depression, neuropsychiatric disease, epilepsy, pregnancy, and breastfeeding. Airline pilots, scuba divers, and those whose work demands manual dexterity should choose another drug unless they have already proved tolerant of mefloquine.

Adult dose is 250 mg once a week.

Start weekly mefloquine 4 weeks before leaving for the malarious area in case side effects demand a change in treatment. All antimalarial drugs that kill parasites in the bloodstream must be continued for 4 weeks after return so that late-emerging parasites (hepatic merozoites), protected as long as they remain in the liver, are eliminated when they enter the circulation.

Atovaquone–proguanil (Malarone)

This is a safe, effective, but expensive drug. Malarone acts on liver stage parasites and so need be taken for only 7 days after leaving the malarious region. The dose is one tablet each day for adults.

Doxycycline (Vibramycin)

This tetracycline antibiotic has proved useful for prophylaxis in areas where mefloquine resistance is prevalent, such as the Thai–Cambodian border region. It gives some protection against other travellers' diseases such as typhus, leptospirosis, and some types of travellers' diarrhoea. One 100 mg tablet a day should be taken. Side effects include photosensitive rashes, skin irritation, diarrhoea, and oral/oesophageal or vaginal thrush. It is not suitable for pregnant women and children.

Proguanil (Paludrine) and chloroquine (Avloclor, Nivaquine, Malarivon)

Proguanil—adult dose two tablets (each of 100 mg) every day—and chloroquine—two tablets (each of 150 mg BASE) once a week—is no longer recommended for Africa, the Amazon region, South-East Asia, Assam, and Oceania but remains effective prophylaxis elsewhere. It is safe in pregnancy and (in a lower dose) in children. The only side effects are rare mouth ulcers, mild indigestion, and hair loss. The combination is available in the UK as Paludrine/Avloclor (AstraZeneca).

Chloroquine taken for up to 5–6 years continuously in the dose recommended for prophylaxis against malaria does not cause damage to the eyes, but those who have taken it for more than 6 years continuously (total cumulative dose approaching 100 g) should have their vision checked.

Choice of prophylactic drugs in different geographical areas
See http://www.hpa.org.uk/publications/PublicationDisplay.asp?PublicationID=87&TandC=true&

- Middle East, West Asia, Indian subcontinent (except Assam), parts of South America (except Amazon region of Brazil), and China: use proguanil and chloroquine.
- Mexico, Central America, Haiti, Dominican Republic, and parts of South America (except Amazon region of Brazil): use proguanil and chloroquine.
- Africa, Amazon region of Brazil, South-East Asia (except Thai–Cambodian border region), and Assam: use mefloquine, doxycycline or Malarone.
- West Pacific and New Guinea: use mefloquine, doxycycline or Malarone.
- Thai–Cambodian border region: use doxycycline or Malarone.
- Turkey, Egypt, and Mauritius (rural, seasonal only): use chloroquine or proguanil.

Pregnant women

During pregnancy it is vital for the expectant mother to take antimalarials or, preferably, to avoid entering a malarious area. The hazards of getting malaria, particularly *P. falciparum* malaria, during pregnancy are great. The remote hazard of adverse effects to the baby of the antimalarial drugs is far outweighed by the advantages. Proguanil and chloroquine are safe. Mefloquine may be an acceptable alternative where there is a high risk of infection and this combination is ineffective. Doxycyline and Malarone should be avoided during pregnancy.

> No antimalarial drug offers absolute protection. Much depends on compliance. Travellers who become feverish and ill, especially in the early months after their return should consult a doctor and mention the possibility of malaria. If there is any doubt, referral to an infectious/tropical disease unit for exclusion of malaria is an urgent necessity. Antimalarial prophylactic drugs should be stopped until the diagnosis is confirmed or rejected.

Standby treatment for malaria in high-risk areas

Travellers to remote malarious areas who have no ready access to hospitals and diagnostic laboratories should carry a course of standby treatment to be taken if they develop a malaria-like fever. This must not delay their seeking medical treatment at the base hospital as soon as possible. Appropriate drugs for standby treatment are:

- Artemether-with-lumefantrine (Riamet, Co-artem or Co-artemether): adult dose four tablets at 0, 24, 36, 48, and 60 h *or*
- Quinine sulphate: adult dose 600 mg 8-hourly for 5–7 days followed by either doxycycline 200 mg for 7 days or clindamycin 450 mg three times daily for 5 days *or*
- Proguanil hydrochloride-with-atovaquone (Malarone) four tablets daily for 3 days (Unless this is being taken for prophylaxis).

Prevention of the 'benign' malarias (*P. vivax, ovale* and *malariae*)

Weekly chloroquine or mefloquine prevent *P. vivax, ovale,* and *malariae* malarias. However, *P. vivax* and *P. ovale* can establish themselves in the liver despite chloroquine prophylaxis, and may re-emerge to cause relapsing infections months or years later. Primaquine, adult dose 15 mg a day for 2 weeks, eradicates latent liver infection (hypnozoites) and should be given to travellers who have spent more than a few months in areas where these species are endemic (beware of G6PD-deficiency!). In parts of Indonesia, particularly Irian Jaya, and in Papua New Guinea, Thailand, the Philippines, and the Solomon Islands, Chesson-type strains of chloroquine-resistant *P. vivax* require a 4-week course of primaquine.

Useful websites and other information

http://www.who.int/malaria/docs/TreatmentGuidelines2006.pdf
http://www.hpa.org.uk/infections/topics_az/malaria/Treat_guidelines.htm
http://www.britishinfectionsociety.org/documents/malariatreatmentBIS07.pdf
http://www.britishinfectionsociety.org/documents/malariapreventionBIS07.pdf
http://www.britishinfectionsociety.org/documents/malariaAlgorithm07.pdf
http://www.hpa.org.uk/publications/PublicationDisplay.asp?PublicationID=87&TandC=true
http://www.cdc.gov/malaria/index.htm

Advice about malaria can be obtained from the following tropical medicine units:
Malaria Reference Laboratory (Health Protection Agency) London, UK.
Tel: +44 (0) 20 7636 3924 (advice on prophylaxis only).
Tel: +44 (0) 20 7927 2427 (advice on laboratory diagnosis).
Fax: +44 (0) 20 7637 0248.
Tel: +44 (0) 9065 508908 (24-h 100 p/min).
http://www.nathnac.org.

Hospital for Tropical Diseases, London, UK.
Emergency Admission Tel: +44 (0)20 7387 9300 and ask for the Duty Doctor on Bleep 5845.
Tel: +44 (0)845 155 5000 and ask for Duty Tropical Diseases Doctor.
Fax: +44 (0)20 7388 7645.
http://www.thehtd.org

Liverpool School of Tropical Medicine, Liverpool, UK.
Tel: (0900–1700 h) +44 (0) 151 708 9393.
Tel: (24 h; ask for tropical/ID physician on call) +44 (0) 151 706 2000.
Fax: +44 (0) 151 708 8733 or +44 (0) 151 705 3368.
http://www.liv.ac.uk/lstm/travel_health_services/travel_clinic/index.htm

Oxford Centre for Clinical Vaccinology and Tropical Medicine, John Warin Ward, Churchill Hospital, Oxford, UK.
Tel: (24 h; ask for I D consultant on call) +44 (0)1865 741 841.

Other protozoal infections

Leishmaniasis

Leishmania can cause a spectrum of skin, mucosal membrane, and visceral infections in humans and animals in the Mediterranean, Middle East, Africa, Asia, and in North, Central and South America (Fig. 14.6). An estimated 1.5–2 million cases of cutaneous leishmaniasis and 500 000 cases of visceral leishmaniasis (kala-azar) occur each year.

Transmission: leishmania are transmitted from infected humans or animals by the bite of tiny sandflies (*Phlebotomus, Lutzomyia*).

Clinical: cutaneous leishmaniasis: days to months after the infected sandfly bite, a nodule appears that grows, crusts, and ulcerates over weeks to months. The classic 'oriental sore' is 1–5 cm in diameter, painless with raised edges and granulating apple jelly base, and small satellite lesions on an exposed area (Coloured Plate 11). Lesions may slowly heal or persist, recur, and spread.

Mucocutaneous leishmaniasis: infection with some Latin American *Leishmania* presents with a cutaneous ulcer but (sometimes years) later destructive lesions develop in the nasopharyngeal mucosa.

Visceral leishmaniasis (kala-azar): there is fever, massive splenomegaly, hepatomegaly, wasting, hypersplenism, and secondary bacterial infection. Post-kala-azar dermal leishmaniasis may develop, after apparent recovery. HIV-immunosuppressed patients are especially vulnerable.

Diagnosis: scrapings from the nodular edge of the sore are stained with Giemsa and examined microscopically. Mucosal lesions are biopsied. Kala-azar can be confirmed serologically (direct agglutination test or rK39 dipstick test (http://bmj.com/cgi/doi/10.1136/bmj.38917.503056.7C) and in hospital, Leishman–Donovan bodies are sought in splenic or bone marrow aspirate, liver or lymph node biopsy or buffy coat.

Treatment for cutaneous leishmaniasis: small sores can be excised, larger ones can be injected with sodium stibogluconate ('Pentostam') twice weekly for 2–3 weeks or the lesions can be left to heal. For infections acquired in Latin America; unless *L. brasiliensis, L. panamensis,* and *L. guyanensis,* which carry the risk of mucosal involvement, can be excluded; prolonged courses of intravenous treatment with drugs such as Pentostam, pentamidine, paromomycin (*L. aethiopica*), ketoconazole or fluconazole (*L. major, L. mexicana*) are needed. For kala-azar, oral miltefosine or prolonged courses of intravenous treatment with drugs such as Pentostam or amphotericin B are needed.

Prevention: avoid bites by nocturnally active sandflies tiny enough to penetrate ordinary mosquito nets but deterred by pyrethroid-impregnated bed and face nets, wear sensibly ample clothing and apply DEET-containing repellent to skin, cotton clothing, and ankle bands.

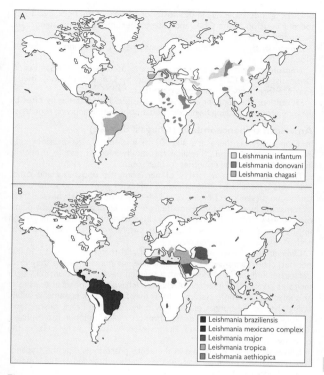

Fig. 14.6 Leishmaniasis distribution.

African trypanosomiasis (sleeping sickness)

An estimated 40 000 new cases of sleeping sickness occur each year in a number of smallish areas scattered throughout West, Central, East, and southern Africa (Fig. 14.7). There is currently a resurgence of the disease in Angola, Central African Republic, Uganda, Nigeria, and adjacent countries following the breakdown of control measures. A few foreign travellers, especially to the game parks of eastern and southern Africa, have been infected.

Transmission: tsetse flies (*Glossina*) transmit the trypanosomes causing Gambian sleeping sickness (*Trypanosoma brucei gambiense*) between humans and those causing Rhodesian sleeping sickness (*T. b. rhodesiense*) between humans and animal reservoir hosts (game, antelopes, etc.).

Clinical: a small ulcer with a scab ('chancre') may appear at the site of the infected tsetse fly bite and, within the next few days, intermittent fever begins, associated with headache, loss of appetite, and enlargement of lymph glands, especially in the posterior triangle of the neck. Eventually, there is invasion of the CNS, and patients become apathetic, sleepy, and eventually comatose.

Diagnosis: by finding motile trypanosomes in lymph node aspirates, blood or CSF.

Treatment: pentamidine or suramin are used before CNS invasion. Drugs used after CNS invasion (detected by CSF examination), melarsoprol, eflornithine, and nifurtimox are toxic.

Prevention: chemoprophylaxis is not feasible. Avoid tsetse fly bites by wearing sensible clothing (light-coloured, not blue) and applying repellents.

American trypanosomiasis (Chagas' disease)

In Latin America, there are 300 000 new cases of *Trypanosoma cruzi* infection each year and 20 million chronically infected people, especially in Brazil, Peru, and the countries further south.

Transmission: from a variety of peri-domestic opossums and other mammals is usually by inoculation of faeces of giant blood-sucking triatomine bugs (see Insect bites 📖 p. 264–5) and not by their bites. Rarely, transmission by drinking juices made from berries of açaí or bacaba palms or cane sugar 'garapa' in which infected bugs have been accidentally ground up, by blood transfusion and other parenteral routes, trans-placentally, and via breast milk has been documented.

Clinical: bugs frequent traditional mud and thatch huts (up to 10 000 per hut). They drop onto the faces of sleeping humans where they feed, defaecate, and infect. Waking with a swollen painful eye (Romaña's sign) indicates conjunctival infection. A chancre (chagoma) appears at the site of skin infection. A febrile systemic illness may follow and, eventually, debilitating chronic megaorgan effects may develop in the heart, oesophagus, bowel, ureters, and elsewhere after invasion, multiplication in macrophages and destruction of autonomic innervation. Cardiac arrhythmia is the commonest mode of death.

Diagnosis: can be confirmed in the acute phase by finding the trypanosomes in blood smears, by isolating them in clean bugs fed on the patient's blood ('xenodiagnosis') or by serology.

Treatment: early benznidazole ('Rochagan' Roche) 5–7 mg/kg each day in two divided doses for 60 days is essential in an attempt to limit invasion of tissues.

Prevention: in endemic areas, avoid sleeping quarters conducive to bug infestation, or apply repellents to exposed surfaces and sleep under a pyrethroid-impregnated net (📖 p. 264–5). Avoid uncooked palm or cane sugar juices that have been left unprotected.

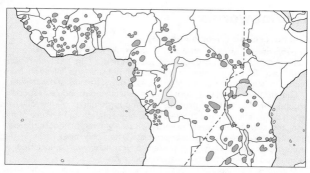

Fig. 14.7 Distribution of African trypanosomiasis.

Filarial worms

Onchocerciasis (river blindness)

In parts of east, west, central and southern Africa, Yemen, Mexico and Central America, and north-eastern South America (Fig. 14.8), pernicious little black flies (e.g. *Simulium damnosum*) transmit this infection from human to human in the vicinity of fast-flowing rivers, streams, and waterfalls.

Clinical: the adult filarial worms live in subcutaneous nodules, especially around the waist. They produce enormous numbers of microfilariae which cause irritation and changes in the pigmentation and texture of the skin and damage the eyes, eventually causing river blindness. Foreign travellers have contracted onchocerciasis after only brief stops in the transmission zone. They may present a year later with a localized or generalized itchy red macular/maculopapular rash.

Diagnosis: eosinophilia is usual. Microscopic examination of skin snips taken from affected areas reveals wriggling microfilariae. ELISA and PCR are sensitive and specific.

Treatment: ivermectin (dose 150 mcg/kg repeated annually) is effective, but may cause a temporary but damaging exacerbation of lesions in the eye and skin, and should therefore be supervised in a hospital. Ivermectin resistance was recently reported from Western Ghana.

Prevention: wear light-coloured clothing (long sleeves and long trousers) and apply DEET-containing repellents to exposed areas of skin. Avoid unnecessary stops and camping near *Simulium*-infested waters.

Elephantiasis (lymphatic filariasis)

Throughout vast areas of tropical America, Africa, Asia, and the western Pacific, mosquitoes (*Culex* and *Anopheles* spp.) transmit filarial infections that cause fever and chronic inflammation with obstruction of the lymphatic system, producing grotesque lymphoedema of the limbs and scrotum and other complications such as chyluria, lymphuria, and pulmonary eosinophilia (Fig. 14.9). Mosquito vectors can be controlled by insecticides, etc. and exluded by using mosquito nets; population-based chemoprophylaxis with diethylcarbamazine has proved effective. If your expedition is going to an endemic area, find out more from the websites given below.

Websites

http://www.filariasis.org/index.htm
http://www.cdc.gov/ncidod/dpd/parasites/lymphaticfilariasis/index.htm
http://www.who.int/mediacentre/factsheets/fs102/en/

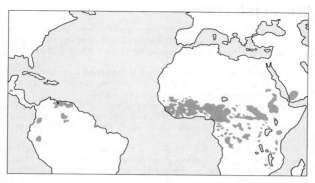

Fig. 14.8 World distribution of onchocerciasis.

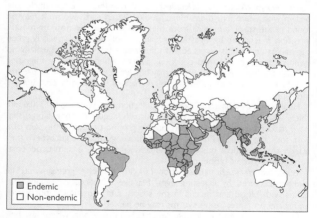

■ Endemic
□ Non-endemic

Fig. 14.9 Distribution of lymphatic filariasis.

Worm infections

Passing a wriggling worm-like object in the stools, or even worse vomiting one up, is a singularly unpleasant experience. Intestinal worm infections are enormously prevalent in developing countries where they cause much debility.

Transmission: is by ingesting eggs or cysts in food (e.g. *Ascaris*, tape worms, liver flukes) or by human contact (e.g. pin worms), or percutaneously by filariform larval worms (hook worms and *Strongyloides*).

Diagnosis: is established by identifying the worm that has been passed. It may be suspected in someone with anorexia, malaise, and weight loss who looks anaemic. Confirmation is by identifying specific helminth eggs in the stool.

Prevention: is by ensuring that all food, especially meat, fish, and green vegetables and salads, is thoroughly cooked, that people wear proper shoes, especially in areas contaminated by human faeces, and that latrines are properly constructed.

Round worms (nematodes)

'Round worm' (Ascaris lumbricoides) (12–35 mm long, 2–6 mm thick, pale brown with white longitudinal lines) looks like an earth worm. It may be found in the stool, emerging from the anus, or even the nose or mouth. Infection is acquired by ingesting eggs in uncooked food, especially green vegetables and salads fertilized with human faeces. There are usually no symptoms except for mild cough or asthma when larvae are migrating through the lungs. Rarely, a worm may block the appendix, bile or pancreatic duct, causing acute inflammation. A mass of worms may obstruct the intestine.

Hook worm (Ancylostoma, Necator): infection (7–13 mm long, 0.3–0.6 mm thick, white, grey, reddish brown) is usually acquired when larvae that have hatched from human stools on the ground penetrate the skin of a bare foot and travel via lymphatics and the lungs into the gut where they attach to the jejunal mucosa. Symptoms (tiredness, anaemia, oedema) result from chronic blood loss.

Whip worm (Trichuris): infection (30–50 mm long, greyish-white or pink) is acquired by ingesting eggs. Massive infections cause anaemia, colitis with blood and mucus in the stools, and sometimes appendicitis and rectal prolapse. Visible worms may be passed.

Pin worms (Enterobius vermicularis) (2.5–13 mm long, white) lay their eggs around the anal verge, causing intense nocturnal pruritus ani, scratching and excoriation of perianal skin, and insomnia. Eggs contaminate the microenvironment and are spread among the family by ingestion or inhalation. The host is reinfected by licking contaminated fingers. Diagnosis is confirmed by microscopic detection of eggs stuck to strips of sellotape applied to the anal margin on waking.

Treatment: all these round worm infections can be treated with albendazole 400 mg single dose or mebendazole 100 mg twice each day for 3 days. However, those with hookworm infection may need haematinics for iron deficiency, and treatment of pin worm infection should include the whole household and must be repeated after 1 week.

Flukes

Schistosomiasis (bilharzia)

This fluke infection occurs in Africa, the Middle East, eastern South America, China, and South-East Asia (Fig. 14.10). Infection is acquired through contact with fresh water from lakes and sluggish rivers, usually by bathing or washing with water taken from these sources. Infected humans contaminate the lake by defecating or urinating into it and infect, in turn, the intermediate snail hosts. Snails release tiny cercariae into the water which burrow through the skin of bathers.

Clinical: the earliest symptom of possible infection is 'swimmer's itch', experienced soon, sometimes minutes, after contact with infected water. Some people develop an acute feverish illness associated with an urticarial rash and blood eosinophilia a few weeks after infection ("Katayama fever"). Later symptoms include passing cloudy or frankly blood-stained urine or dysentery and, rarely, ascending paralysis and loss of sensation in the lower limbs. Travellers usually get worried about bilharzia when they get back from their trip and remember bathing in forbidden lakes or hear that another member of the party has been diagnosed as having schistosomiasis.

Diagnosis: search for characteristic ova in stool, urine (midday, centrifuged, end-stream sample is optimal) or rectal biopsy, or by a blood test.

Treatment: is fairly simple with one to two doses of praziquantel (Biltricide).

Prevention: avoid bathing in sluggish fresh water sources in endemic areas. Local advice may be misleading. Lake Malawi, officially declared free of bilharzia, has been the source of many imported cases of bilharzia in the UK over the last few years.

Screening of returned travellers: although routine screening is not indicated, groups of people travelling with and presumed to have shared the same exposure as a confirmed case deserve to be tested, as do those who were at particularly high risk (see Diagnosis above). Ova can be detected as soon as 3–4 weeks after exposure.

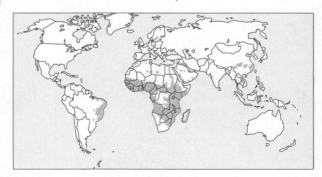

Fig. 14.10 Geographic distribution of schistosomiasis.

Liver flukes

Liver fluke (*Clonorchis, Opisthorchis*) (7–25 × 3–5 mm) infections acquired by eating fresh water fish are very common in South-East Asia and China. Liver fluke *Fasciola hepatica* (20–30 × 8–13 mm) and intestinal fluke *Fasciolopsis buski* (20–75 × 8–20 mm) infections result from ingestion of metacercariae attached to water cress, water chestnuts and other fresh water plants. Anorexia, right upper quadrant abdominal pain, tenderness and hepatomegaly, and episodes of cholangitis are typical of liver fluke infection, while nausea, anorexia, abdominal discomfort, lienteric diarrhoea (passing undigested food) are typical of heavy *F. buski* infections.

Treatment: praziquantel 25 mg/kg three times daily after meals for 2 days is effective.

Tape worms (cestodes)

Beef (*Taenia saginata*) (4–12 m long, 5–7 mm thick whitish, semi-transparent) or pork (*T. solium*) (3–8 m long, 5–7 mm thick, yellowish) tape worms are acquired by eating inadequately cooked meat containing viable cysticerci (e.g. 'measly' pork). Passing a long tape worm through the anus or seeing the elongating and contracting whitish reproductive segments (proglottids) (18–30 × 5–7 mm) in the stool or vomitus are the commonest symptoms, but nausea, abdominal pain relieved by eating, pruritus ani, and weight loss are common. (Cerebral) cycticercosis, a complication of *T. solium* infection, presents with seizures.

Treatment: niclosamide 2 g as a single morning dose or praziquantel 10–20 mg/kg as a single dose after breakfast is effective.

Emerging infections

Over the past decade, a number of entirely new pathogens have emerged as important causes of (sometimes epidemic) human disease; some known pathogens have mutated into drug-resistant strains and others have re-emerged. Members of expeditions to remote areas might, like 'sentinel animals', be exposed to some of these known emerging and unknown reclusive pathogens enzoonotic in wild animals. They should be aware of current epidemics to assess risk and plan prevention.

A free online journal is devoted to these infections: http://www.cdc.gov/ncidod/EID/

Other useful websites
http://www.promedmail.org/pls/promed/
http://www.cdc.gov/mmwr/
http://www.who.int/wer/en/

Severe acute respiratory syndrome (SARS)
Infections caused by the SARS corona virus emerged in China in November 2002. The last case was reported in China in April 2004, but SARS could re-emerge at any time. The epidemic affected >8000 patients in 25 countries in five continents, with a case fatality of 10%.

Transmission is by droplets and close human-to-human contact, especially in hospitals. A wild mammalian reservoir, possibly in bats, is suspected but has not been confirmed.

Clinical: after an incubation period of 1–14 (average 4) days, fever, myalgia, malaise, chills, non-productive cough, breathlessness, pleurisy, and watery diarrhoea may develop. The diagnosis can only be suspected in a patient who fails to respond to antibiotic treatment and has an epidemic or contact history.

Diagnosis is confirmed by serology after about 10 days of illness. No effective specific treatment or prophylaxis is known.

Prevention is by avoiding epidemic areas and especially hospitals and by wearing face masks. Markets in which wild mammals are sold for food in China pose a hypothetical risk of infection.

Websites
http://www.who.int/csr/sars/guidelines/en/
http://www.cdc.gov/ncidod/sars/
http://www.hpa.org.uk/infections/topics_az/SARS/menu.htm

Avian influenza
Avian flu is caused by H5N1 influenza virus which naturally infects wild birds and has caused large outbreaks in domestic poultry. Since the first human cases were reported from Hong Kong in 1997, 350 cases have been reported to WHO from 14 countries in Asia, Europe, the Near East, and Africa, with 217 deaths (case fatality 62%), the most in Indonesia and Viet Nam. Over 90% of cases have been <40 years old.

Transmission is by close contact (aerosol) with infected birds and eating their uncooked blood or meat. Suspected human-to-human spread is very rare.

Clinical: typical 'flu-like' symptoms such as fever, cough, sore throat, myalgia, conjunctivitis, and pneumonia with acute respiratory distress requiring mechanical ventilation.

Treatment: oseltamivir and zanamivir are effective for treatment and prevention of H5N1 viruses, but resistant strains have already been discovered.

Prevention: watch the epidemic news (see below) and avoid contact with poultry and wild birds as far as possible, especially commercial or backyard poultry farms and live poultry markets. Do not eat uncooked or undercooked poultry or poultry products, including dishes made with uncooked poultry blood. H5N1 vaccines are being developed. If there is an epidemic, prophylactic/therapeutic oseltamivir will be distributed by WHO and perhaps by some embassies in affected countries. Wear a face mask (preferably N-95) in high risk environments.

Websites

http://www.hpa.org.uk/infections/topics_az/influenza/avian/default.htm
http://www.who.int/csr/disease/avian_influenza/en/
http://www.cdc.gov/flu/avian/
http://www.britishinfectionsociety.org/documents/PandemicFlu06.pdf

Other emerging viruses

Australian bat lyssavirus, closely related to classic rabies virus, was discovered in 1996 in flying foxes (fruit bats) and other bats. It has caused two known human deaths in people who handled bats.

New paramyxoviruses are a group of viruses associated with flying foxes and other bats in South Asia and Australia. They include the Nipah virus that caused an epidemic of encephalitis, mainly among pig farmers in Malaysia and Singapore in 1999. In total, 258 cases were reported with a case fatality of 40%.

Human bocavirus is a newly recognized parvovirus associated with lower respiratory tract infection in children in Europe, Thailand, China, Japan, and Australia.

Monkey pox virus, previously known as a rare cause of a febrile small-pox-like disease in children in equatorial Africa, caused a multistate outbreak of >70 human cases in USA in 2003. Pet prairie ('dogs') marmots had apparently been infected by rodents imported from West Africa.

WU virus is a newly discovered polyoma virus causing acute respiratory tract infections in Queensland, Australia.

Mimivirus is the largest known virus and a possible cause of pneumonia.

Emerging bacteria

New antibiotic-resistant strains of bacteria are constantly emerging:
http://www.cdc.gov/drugresistance/

Some examples are: penicillin-resistant pneumococci; methicillin and vancomycin-resistant *Staphylococcus aureus*, which may be community-acquired, and Panton–Valentine Leukocidin (PVL)-positive strains of *S. aureus*; carbapenem-hydrolyzing metallo-beta-lactamase (MBL)-producing

Pseudomonas aeruginosa that are resistant to all beta-lactams except monobactams; extended spectrum beta-lactamase (ESBL)-producing *E. coli* and *Klebsiella pneumoniae*; vancomycin- and teicoplanin-resistant *Enterococcus faecium*; multiresistant gonococci; fluoroquinolone-resistant typhoid bacilli (*Salmonella typhi*) and tetracycline-resistant scrub typhus (*Orientia tsutsugamushi*). *Acinetobacter baumannii* is an intrinsically multi-resistant bacterium associated with some recent blast victims from Afghanistan and Iraq. It has caused some nosocomial outbreaks.

Rhodococcus equi can cause severe lung disease in HIV-immunocompromised people, and *Arcanobacterium haemolyticum* causes bacterial pharyngitis. Both are diphtheria-like bacteria. Emerging rickettsia-like organisms include *Ehrlichia chaffeensis* which causes human monocytic ehrlichiosis, *Anaplasma phagocytophilum* (human granulocytic anaplasmosis), and *Ehrlichia ewingii* (human granulocytic ehrlichiosis). *Stenotrophomonas maltophilia* is one of very many other unfamiliar bacterial species mentioned in the literature.

Other emerging pathogens

Pythiosis: caused by the aquatic fungus *Pythium insidiosum*, is being recognized as a cause of human eye, skin, and systemic infections in tropical countries.

Scedosporium prolificans is a fungal opportunist and *Fusarium* has caused keratitis in contact lens wearers.

Cyclosporiasis: since 1996, the coccidian protozoan, *Cyclospora cayetanesis*, has been increasingly recognized as a cause of giardiasis/cryptosporidiosis-like gastrointestinal symptoms in travellers. There have been some epidemics related to imported berries, herbs, and salads.

Balamuthia mandrillaris is a free-living amoeba of tropical fresh water environments that can cause devastating cutaneous, nasal, and intracerebral disease.

Microsporidiasis: many species of protozoan *Microsporidia* (e.g. *Encephalitozoon* spp.) are now recognized as causes of keratoconjunctivitis and gastrointestinal, biliary, urinary and respiratory tract, and muscle infections in severely immunocompromised people.

Psychological and psychiatric problems

Section editor
Jon Dallimore

Contributors
Karen Forbes, Michael Jones, Debbie Lovell Hawker,
James Moore, and Ian Palmer

Introduction

Expeditions by definition involve travel, usually into remote areas by lone travellers or groups. Very small groups are likely to consist of companions who are previously acquainted in other settings, and an informal process of selection may have occurred. Those in larger groups may have had little contact with other participants prior to the expedition. The longer the expedition the greater the likelihood that relationship problems will surface and start to cause psychological difficulty and this is most likely to occur if members with pre-existing psychological morbidity are selected (see Team selection 📖 p. 14 and Psychiatric illness 📖 p. 67).

Stressors in the wilderness

Cultural adjustment

During an expedition, contact with indigenous peoples may be limited or very intense. The opportunity for developing understanding of different cultural values may be limited by language barriers unless fluently bilingual interpreters are present.

Factors which may reduce cultural transitional stress include:
- Previous exposure to that culture and knowledge of local languages.
- Understanding cultural adaptation and local values and customs.
- A flexible, resourceful temperament, and the ability to tolerate ambiguity with a good sense of humour.

All these factors should be borne in mind when screening potential expedition team members.

The physical demands of the expedition

The physical demands of the expedition are likely to cause a lowered reserve for dealing with other stressors, including making new relationships within the group.

If participants are first timers on an expedition they may be unprepared for the intensity of contact involved in sharing tents or cramped sleeping accommodation. Experienced members may be intolerant of the difficulties experienced by those unused to, for example, close quarter living, jungle style sanitation, the reduced opportunity for keeping clean, and the absence of home comforts. If possible, a team building exercise before the expedition should be considered to see how people may adapt to the physical demands of the expedition.

Psychological considerations before the expedition

Assessing vulnerability

Some form of psychological health screening of potential expedition members is highly desirable and becomes increasingly important for longer expeditions. An acute psychosis, although rare, may cripple the progress of an expedition to a very remote area whilst repatriation is organized. Removal of the ill person may also impair the skill base of the group.

The purpose of health screening should be explained to the candidate. It should be clear who will see the report and candidates should give their informed consent for a report to be released. No screening process will ever distinguish perfectly between those who will thrive on an expedition and those who will develop problems; however the risks of serious adverse events can be reduced with some simple measures.

- Application forms—forms should be prepared carefully and be constructed so that all questions have to be answered (see Pre-existing medical problems 📖 p. 59). General practitioners completing medical forms should be informed that any psychological history is fundamentally important, and that non-disclosure may be detrimental to the safety and the health of the applicant.
- Work references—references may be particularly important because they are provided by people who are in regular contact with the candidate when they are not necessarily on their best behaviour. Any offer in a written reference to comment verbally should always be explored.
- Interview—an interview is often at the core of any selection process and should be integrated into the process rather than occurring when a provisional decision has already been made which is unlikely to be altered. Panel members should be those involved in the expedition, have previous experience in the field in similar situations, and awareness of small group dynamics and their importance to the mental health of teams.
  Subjects to consider during interview
  - *Employment history:* relationships at work and the reasons for job changes should be explored. Candidates who give up easily may not be the best team members for a physically and psychologically demanding expedition.
  - *Personal and family mental health history:* the assessor should ask about any consultations with the GP for any form of emotional ill health and any previous referrals for psychiatric help or counselling, as well as any untreated episodes.
  - *Substance abuse:* any abuse of alcohol or drugs should be noted. Insight into any past difficulties, and healthy strategies for dealing with any future problems would balance concerns about previous substance abuse.

Unsuitability because of psychiatric history

Each expedition will be different, and the ability to help those with complex psychological needs will depend on the location, purpose, duration, staffing levels, and medical competence of the team.

- Serious mental illness, e.g. schizophrenia, bipolar disorder, hypomania, depression: people with schizophrenia are more prone to psychotic breakdown when their environment is altered. Bipolar and manic disorders often require potent medication for control, and failure to take medication may lead to relapse.
- Any current untreated psychological disorder: psychological disorders should have been treated and followed by a symptom-free period where the individual has been able to cope with other stressful situations.
- Anxiety or depression: repeated episodes of anxiety and depression will raise concern.
- Recent loss events: it is wise to delay moving into the high stressor environment posed by expeditions after recent bereavements, divorce, or broken relationships.
- Eating disorders: previous anorexia or bulimia must have been controlled for a year or two such that the applicant has healthy eating routines and is maintaining a satisfactory BMI.
- Deliberate self-harm and previous suicide attempts: a recent psychiatrist's report may be required to ensure that the individual is safe to travel to a remote area, has resolved any outstanding issues, and will not be a risk to themselves.

Psychopathologies

Psychopathology in people working overseas, even after rigorous selection, is common, and those engaged in expeditions and other prolonged visits into wilderness locations are at risk.

Anxiety disorders

Anxiety may be generalized or focused on particular concerns such as snakebite or flying. Features are as for panic disorder (see below).

Anxiety about health is normal when travelling internationally, but can be a problem if it becomes extreme or remains despite reassurance. It may be exacerbated on expeditions which are isolated from competent medical help.

Aviophobia (fear of flying) is experienced by up to 20% of air passengers. Behavioural therapy and, in particular, systematic desensitization, is a very effective treatment, and medication such as beta-blockers can complement physical techniques and cognitive strategies to overcome the fear. Details of UK-based courses and online resources are at: http://www.gatwick-airport-uk.info/fear-of-flying.htm.

Panic disorder is the presence of recurrent panic attacks; a discrete period of intense fear or discomfort, involving at least four of the following symptoms:

- Palpitations
- Sweating, shaking
- Shortness of breath
- Feeling of choking
- Chest pain
- Nausea/abdominal symptoms
- Dizziness
- Feelings of unreality or being detached from oneself
- Fear of losing control or going crazy
- Fear of dying
- Numbness or tingling sensations
- Chills or hot flushes.

Management of anxiety or panic consists of calm reassurance and, in the case of rapid breathing, breathing in and out of a bag. If symptoms persist, an expert opinion should be sought. Anxiolytic drugs or/and psychological therapies may be advised.

Depression

It is important to distinguish clinical depression from the misery which all people experience from time to time. Homesickness, concerns about how one may cope, and fatigue may all produce similar symptoms during an expedition. Depression may follow a clear trigger such as bereavement but it may have no obvious precipitant.

Characteristic features of clinical depression include:

- Low mood (particularly in the morning)
- Lack of motivation and low energy levels
- Poor sleep, particularly early morning wakening
- Weepiness

- Preoccupations with worries
- Guilty feelings
- Possible suicidal thoughts and/or plans.

Management of depressed people is likely to require expert help in the form of psychological therapy and/or medication, particularly if there are suicidal features. Repatriation may be required.

Psychosis and acute confusional states

Psychoses are severe mental illnesses and are rare, but they can develop while travelling and may be provoked by medication such as mefloquine (Lariam) or illicit drugs such as marihuana, amphetamines, and cocaine. However, it is important to remember that physical illness may be the cause for abnormal behaviour:

- Protozoal tropical infections—malaria, African trypanosomiasis (sleeping sickness), and amoebic dysentery.
- Bacterial infections—enteric fever (typhoid) and meningitis.
- Other causes—hypoglycaemia, head injury.

Features of psychosis/acute confusion include:

- Bizarre behaviour
- Paranoia
- Disinhibition
- Hallucinations, delusions
- Thought disorder
- Pressure of speech
- Disorientation in time, place, and person
- Lack of insight.

Management of acute psychotic illness requires rapid evacuation and expert assessment, and usually treatment with psychotropic medication. Consider sedation with chlorpromazine 50 mg/8 h PO or lorazepam 1–2 mg PO.

Psychological reactions to traumatic events

Most expeditions will be completed with only minor untoward events. However, anyone taking a group into the field, particularly those responsible for young people, must be aware of how to care for the group's psychological welfare should illness, accident or, at worst, death occur. These events might occur within the group whilst on expedition, but it is also possible that leaders might be responsible for informing an expeditioner of events that have occurred at home.

Possible traumatic events include:
- Grave illness or injury
- A member of the team going missing
- A hostage situation
- The death of a relative, close friend at home or fellow expeditioner.

In some situations the whole group will have witnessed what has happened. In others the leader may have to inform the members of the group about the traumatic event or its repercussions. The box on 'Breaking Bad News' gives some guidance on how to do this (📖 p. 155).

When a traumatic event occurs, leaders should assume that only 15% of their group will react effectively, many (70%) will be stunned and bewildered, and 15% may react with incapacitating anxiety or hysteria. The leader needs to identify quickly how people are reacting and use them appropriately; those reacting effectively may be needed to help in rescue efforts or to ensure the safety of the bewildered majority.

What should the leader do?

In the event of a disaster, the care of the victim is the first priority; however, other group members, the leader, rescuers, family and friends, and expedition organizers will all react psychologically. The psychological care of the victim and the rest of the group and self-care are the leader's responsibility, but he or she also has a role in the care of the wider group in providing accurate information in a timely fashion.

Care of the victim

Whilst an ill or injured group member is awaiting evacuation, their physical comfort, security, and dignity must be maintained; for instance, ensuring they are covered and have privacy. If the person is conscious they should be kept informed of what is happening. They may be very distressed or bewildered. It is important to be patient, honest, to allow them time to talk, and to accept what may be muddled and rapidly changing thoughts and emotions, and reassure them these are normal.

If the victim is unconscious, their right to privacy and dignity must still be respected. It should also be assumed they can hear; they should have company, be kept informed, and be spared pessimistic conversations happening around them.

Care of the group

Having ensured the initial safety of the group, the leader is responsible for ensuring their needs for food, water, and shelter are met, and then for providing a supportive environment. In a small, functional group this may be relatively simple and possible on a one-to-one basis.

In a larger group, particularly if fault or blame might be apportioned around the cause of the traumatic event, the task will be more difficult and the leader might choose to arrange a debriefing meeting 24–48 h after the event, after the practicalities of medical care, evacuation, and informing relatives have been completed. The primary aim of this meeting would be to facilitate a supportive emotional environment and get a functional team home.

Such a meeting requires:
- Sensitive leadership.
- Ground rules about honesty, confidentiality, and not apportioning blame.
- Encouragement for everyone to speak.
- Encouragement of discussion of feelings and fears.
- Acknowledgement of loss and grief.
- Identification of those not coping.
- Strategies to support those not coping.
- Agreement from the team about the next steps (whether to continue the expedition or to go home, for example).
- Agreement from the team about how to support others in a positive way.

Reactions to traumatic events or bad news

Group members witnessing or being involved in a traumatic event and an expeditioner given bad news from home will react in similar ways.

To be bereaved is to be deprived of someone or something of value. We may grieve for a person, but we may also grieve for other losses, such as friendship, hope, or our perceptions of safety and immortality. People who are grieving have feelings of numbness, sadness, anxiety, anger, guilt, or yearning; they may experience physical sensations of a 'flight or fright' reaction, with dry mouth, hollow stomach, breathlessness, or tachycardia; they may be confused, bewildered, disbelieving, and disorientated. In close relationships they may even have auditory or visual hallucinations of the person who has died. Their behaviour may be altered, with crying, restlessness, loss of appetite, sleep disturbance, and absent-mindedness, which could compromise the individual's safety on an expedition.

The vast majority of people who are bereaved of someone close to them, or who experience a traumatic event, recover with time and the support of family and friends. Bereavement and loss are a normal part of life. In the aftermath of such an event, individuals should be reassured that the jumble of emotions, sensations, thoughts, and behaviours they are experiencing is normal and does not mean there is something wrong with them or they are 'going mad'. Expeditioners who are so distressed by grief they might compromise their own or the group's safety might have to be evacuated, but there may be good arguments for keeping a supportive group together.

It is important to stress that difficulty with grieving or post-traumatic stress disorder (PTSD) may occur even with good leadership, because of the person's pre-existing personality or mental health, or because of the nature of the event. The leader's job is to provide a supportive environment so that recovery is encouraged, where possible, and to get the team home safely.

Post-traumatic stress disorder

Symptoms of PTSD may develop after experiencing 'a stressful event of an exceptionally threatening or catastrophic nature'. Sufferers involuntarily re-experience the event or aspects of it and these 're-experiencing symptoms' may feel very real, frightening, and distressing. Victims often have recurrent flashbacks or nightmares and may avoid triggers reminding them of the event or return continuously to why it happened or how it could have been avoided. They may have emotional numbing or be in a constant state of alertness, being fearful, irritable, easily startled, and having difficulties with concentration and sleeping. Some develop chronic mental health problems.

Who develops post-traumatic stress disorder?

The chances of developing PTSD are higher in women than men and differ according to the traumatic event. The risk of developing PTSD is highest after rape (about 20% in women), other sexual attack, being threatened with a weapon, and kidnapped or taken hostage. About 10% of people seeing accidents, death or injury, and natural disasters will go on to develop PTSD.

The recovery environment

People are most likely to recover after a traumatic event if they experience positive and supportive responses from those around them. Blaming and negative thoughts about the event are unhelpful. Reactions which avoid victims thinking about, appraising, and 'working through' the events, such as not talking about them, denial, suppressing painful thoughts, or ruminating on an aspect of the incident may hinder recovery and predispose to PTSD.

Serious psychological threats

The most extreme psychological threats of an expedition relate to death, serious accident or illness, road traffic accident, mugging/carjacking, or, rarely, kidnapping/hostage-taking.

Kidnapping and hostage-taking are very rare but probably represent the most extreme and sustained form of psychological (and sometimes physical) abuse. Surviving abduction highlights some of the key psychological strategies which can be employed to minimize psychological trauma.

Surviving kidnapping

Unfortunately, kidnapping and hostage-taking remain prevalent in many areas of the world. It is important to be aware of any such risks in the locations to be explored. Clear contingency plans are advisable. A reputable 'survival in hostile region' course may help in learning how to avoid becoming captured (AKE run courses: see http://www.ake.com).

All kidnappings are undertaken for gain, usually after careful surveillance. Captors are criminal and/or political; whilst of perceived value, captives of criminals are relatively safe. The fate of political hostages is less knowable. Kidnappers' previous behaviour is the best predictor of outcome. Kidnapping is not personal; most victims are a pawn in another's game. The aim of those kidnapped is to survive.

Kidnapping may be conceptualized in three phases:
- Capture
- Incarceration
- Release.

Capture

Kidnappers obtain compliance through extreme violence, dominance, and uncertainty. Capture and release are the most dangerous times of kidnapping. Escape is best attempted at capture, preferably in response to a plan. If escape is impossible, heroics should be avoided. Weapons should not be used, unless the captive is skilled in their use. Sensory deprivation may be used to isolate the captive and is disorientating, by design. After the initial shock of abduction, there may be a short-lived euphoria at having survived, followed by a pattern of enforced sensory deprivations, intimacies, threats, abuse, and hardships.

On abduction:
- Be calm, composed, patient, polite, and cooperative
- Obey all orders
- Keep quiet unless spoken to
- Move slowly and deliberately—ask first
- Listen closely to what is going on
- Keep clothes and belongings if possible
- Rest/sleep/eat/drink whenever possible/offered
- Inform captors of any medical requirements.

Incarceration

Immediately establish a routine that focuses on maintaining physical and mental hygiene, health, and fitness. Physical health requires eating the food and drink offered. Physical fitness improves resistance to infection, raises mood, and may allow for a successful escape attempt. Mental fitness requires awareness of uncontrollable (external) and controllable (internal, self-induced) stressors. A positive frame of mind is important. Release is the most likely outcome; someone will be working for release of hostages.

A primitive existence will develop, centred upon bodily functions, sleeping, and eating in an atmosphere of intimidation and ruthlessness. Self-questioning and blame are destructive to self-esteem and self-worth, and lead to inertia, depression, and despair. Emotional lability is common. Any pre-existing psychological or psychiatric predispositions may be triggered. Physical activity is the best counter to this.

Compassion is required for those who are not coping well. Captors' attempts to 'split' the group will severely worsen the situation for all captives. Maintaining clear lines of communication and interest in each others' welfare is protective. The intimacy engendered by enforced proximity and shared adversity may lead to deep personal attachments/antipathies. A group leader should be appointed if taken as a group.

Captors vary in their abilities to mistreat their charges. Dehumanization promotes maltreatment. Trying to understand captors and developing rapport by active listening and drawing attention to your human needs, e.g. hunger, thirst, and bodily functions may be beneficial.

To prevent dehumanization:
- Remain calm and courteous.
- Develop rapport and negotiate (with care) for basic needs.
- Act to maintain self-respect and dignity.
- Avoid whining, begging, or arguing.
- Prepare for a long captivity.
- Seek information on captors, time, place, deadlines.
- Look for humour in all things and help each other.
- Keep the mind active:
  - Chess, writing/reciting poems, plots of/for plays, films, novels.
- Focus on previous good experiences.
- What to do if/when.
- Monitor body language.
- Do not believe all given information.
- Maintain religious or spiritual beliefs—without irritating others.

Release

Maintain belief in rescue, and be patient. Peaceful resolution is the default option, as violent conclusion will involve killings. Deadlines are dangerous for all parties. Any escalation of violence by kidnappers will increase the likelihood of an armed solution. Thus always assume there are plans for a forceful solution. Think ahead; obtain as much information as possible about deadlines. Armed forces are most likely to enter through windows or doors, thus stay away from portals, locate a safe place, and wait.

On hearing gunfire or explosion:
- Go to ground
- Keep your hands visible at all times
- Make *no* attempt to help
- Make *no* sudden movements

- Follow all instructions immediately
- Rescuers will assume you are a kidnapper—expect extremely firm handling
- Never exchange clothing with captors.

There is a natural euphoria on release. This may be tempered if locally employed individuals remain behind or were killed. Relationships formed during captivity may influence the healing process. Problems present before capture will remain unresolved. Depending on the event, consideration should be given to the competing physical, psychological, and social variables, and the variety of interested parties involved, e.g. family, friends, colleagues, employers, pressure groups, politicians, doctors, and media.[1]

1 Palmer I (2004). What to do if you are taken hostage. *BMJ Career Focus* **329**:157–8.

Recreational drugs

Worldwide, levels of drug abuse are rising, with evidence suggesting illegal drug use in up to one-third of some groups of travellers. Experimentation has been associated with travel/expeditions in all age groups. Do not assume that expedition members are immune to inquisitive behaviour such as this, especially if the expedition finds itself located amongst bushes of wild plants such as marihuana.

The consequences of drug misuse on expedition are considerable, ranging from life-threatening illness to life-threatening judicial sentencing. In addition, the consequences might not be confined to the individuals participating, but also to other non-participants on the expedition.

When managing drug abuse on expedition, consider the implications of involving local authorities, especially the police. Advice should be sought carefully and involve the expedition leadership team. However, decisions such as these should not prevent the patient from receiving life-saving hospital treatment.

General approach
Management
- Immediate resuscitation of the patient (BM, BP, temperature).
- Prevent further absorption of drug where possible.
- Medical and nursing care, including:
  - Rule out organic, psychiatric, and medicinal reactions as cause of signs and symptoms of drug misuse (see below).
  - Removal and safe storage or destruction of drugs.
  - Consider further expedition participation and repatriation of individual.

Considerations
- Drugs are not always taken alone—always consider alcohol.
- The patient's condition might change suddenly—don't get caught out!

Drug categories and treatments
Stimulants
- Amphetamines (speed, meths, bennies, dexies, uppers, pep pills, diet pills, co-pilots, hearts).
- Amphetamine derivatives (MDMA—3,4 methylenedioxymethamphetamine, ecstasy, e, xtc, Dennis the menace, Mitsubishi, Porsche).
- Cocaine (blow, Charlie, coke, crack, gold dust, Bolivian marching powder).

Clinical features
- Nausea and muscle pain
- Tachycardia and tachyarrhythmias
- Hypotension/hypertension
- Mydriasis and blurred vision
- Ataxia
- Muscle spasm—particularly in the jaw
- Urinary retention
- Hyperthermia

- Mood change:
  - Confusion
  - Highly stimulated/agitated appearance
  - Euphoria.

Management
Without sedatives or antihypertensives or antipyretics, field management of somebody under the influence of amphetamines or amphetamine derivatives will be purely supportive.
- Management of hyperpyrexia is imperative
- Consider diazepam 0.1–0.3 mg/kg PO for anxiety/agitation
- Consider:
  - Tepid sponging, wet sheet, and fanning
  - iv fluids; beware hypertension.

Opioids
- Diamorphine (heroin, Chinese, rocks)
- Morphine
- Codeine
- Pethidine
- Methadone
- Fentanyl.

Clinical features
- Drowsiness leading to coma
- Respiratory depression
- Hypotension
- 'Pin-point' pupils
- Nystagmus
- Ataxia
- Risk of convulsions with pethidine.

Management
- Maintain airway
- Monitor respiratory rate and effort:
  - Provide respiratory support where necessary
  - Give oxygen
- Monitor HR, BP, BM, temperature and GCS.

Specific treatment
Cardiac arrest in these circumstances is normally secondary to respiratory arrest.

If severe respiratory depression (RR<10), give naloxone at a dose of 0.8–2 mg iv repeated every 2–3 min until RR≥10, and maintain an adequate airway. NB. The half-life of naloxone is short, therefore respiratory depression might recur. Careful monitoring of the patient after naloxone for up to 6 h is imperative. In addition, administration of reversal agents can cause acute withdrawal symptoms, including marked agitation, diarrhoea, and abdominal cramps.

Hallucinogenics
- LSD—lysergic acid diethylamide (acid)
- PMA—paramethoxyamphetamine
- 2C-B—4-bromo-2, 5-dimethoxyphenethylamine
- Mushrooms (*Amanita muscaria*) or other hallucinogenic flora
- Cannabis (dope, ganja, homegrown).

Clinical features
- Mydriasis
- Tachycardia
- Sweating and fever
- Hallucinations
- Acute anxiety and paranoia
- Acute psychosis
- Seizures.

Management
- Mainly supportive—quiet reassurance, calm, and quiet environment
- In severe agitation, consider sedative agents (im lorazepam 1–2 mg and/or im haloperidol 5–10 mg)
- Symptoms should fade within 3–8 h depending on drug and dose ingested.

Hypnotics
- Nitrazepam, temazepam, flunitrazepam.

Clinical features
- Respiratory depression
- Hypotension
- Slurred speech
- Drowsiness/↓GCS
- Nystagmus and double vision
- Ataxia and hypotonia

Severe poisoning
- Coma
- Cardiorespiratory arrest (rare).

Management
- Maintain airway
- Monitor respiratory rate and effort:
  - Provide respiratory support where necessary.
  - Give O2.
- Monitor HR, BP, BM, temperature, and GCS.

After the expedition

For the majority, expeditions are positive experiences which enhance self-esteem and, in young people, contribute to maturity. Expeditions will change all those involved; the individual and those they interact with at work, socially, and at home. It takes time for the 'system' to readjust to the returnee and vice versa. Readjustment requires acceptance, adjustment, and accommodation.

If participants on a recent expedition are not readjusting to their return to their usual environment, the following may be important:

• Full physical and mental state examination and appropriate treatment. Persistent physical symptoms for which there is no demonstrable organic cause occur regularly amongst expatriates, including those who have been on expeditions. It is vital that physical causes are thoroughly excluded with a detailed medical history and physical examination and appropriate investigations. Once this process is complete, other factors which may be generating symptoms can be explored.
• Persistent psychological symptoms commencing during the expedition should prompt referral to a GP or an appropriate mental healthcare professional.
• Re-establishment of relationships, social functioning, productive employment, and communications.
• Mourning where appropriate.
• Acceptance that change is irrevocable and inevitable, but not necessarily negative.

Risks from animals

David Warrell

Animals capable of severe trauma

Animals, especially large ones, wild and domesticated, should always be treated with respect and not approached unnecessarily. Tigers, lions, leopards and other big cats, hyenas, domestic dogs, jackals, wolves, bears, elephants, rhinos, hippopotamuses, buffaloes, bison, domestic cattle, moose, elk, other large deer and antelopes, domestic and wild pigs, rams, tapirs, chimpanzees, baboons, ostriches, cassowaries, and even ferrets have killed people.

Learn about the local hazards by asking the residents. Be vigilant at all times. Beware of wandering alone and unprotected between dusk and dawn when most attacks by large mammals occur. Travel in groups, do not stray from vehicles, and do not take dogs with you; they attract large predators. A look-out armed with a large caliber rifle (preferably >0.35 mm) is essential if you are working in the open in country inhabited by big game animals.

Bears

All bears, even giant pandas, are potentially dangerous carnivores. Mothers with cubs are responsible for 80% of attacks on people. In North America, where backpackers and campers in national parks are victims of daytime/evening attacks, black bears (*Ursus americanus*) were responsible for about 5.8 attacks and 0.3 deaths/year, while brown bears (*U. arctos*), including grizzlies and Kodiak bears, were responsible for about 1.65 attacks and 0.6 deaths/year in the 1990s. Brown bears also kill and injure people in Romania, Scandinavia, and other parts of Europe. Polar bears (*U. maritimus*) are the most predatory, aggressive, and dangerous of all, killing six people in Canada (1965–85), and attacking 50 people in Svalbard (Spitzbergen, Norway) (1973–86) (📖 p. 592–3). Asian sloth bears (*Melursus ursinus*) killed 48 people and injured 687 in Madya Pradesh, India (1989–94).

Prevention

In bear country, hikers should travel in groups, making plenty of noise so that the bears are not taken by surprise. Never approach bears (e.g. to photograph them), especially those with cubs, and keep away from animal carcasses and garbage tips which attract scavenging bears. Signs of irritation include standing up, hissing or growling, yawning, and head swinging. If a bear approaches or charges you, avoid eye contact and do not attempt to hide, run away, or climb a tree. When it is within a distance of 30 feet, it may be repelled by discharging a pepper spray (10% capsicum oleoresin) towards its eyes. If this fails and the attacker is a grizzly bear, roll into a ball, interlocking your hands behind your neck, protecting your face with your elbows, and your back with your backpack. Stay in this position for long enough to ensure that the bear has really left. If the attacker is a black bear, growl, shout, and fight back with any available weapon. Do not store food in camp but hang it in a tree >100 yards/metres away, >14 feet (4 metres) from the ground and >4 feet (1.25 metres) away from the tree trunk. In polar bear country, carry a firearm and flares, and know how to use them.

Website
http://www.canadianrockies.net/backpack.html#bear

Big cats

Attacks by lions, tigers, leopards, American mountain lions (cougar, puma), jaguars, and other large felines are increasing in many areas. Historically, Kenya and Tanzania were notorious for lion attacks. In 1898, two lions killed about 140 workers building the Mombasa–Nairobi railway bridge over the Tsavo river, while between 1932 and 1946, 15 lions killed about 1000 people around Njombe in southern Tanzania. A total of 563 human deaths and 308 injuries was reported in south-east Tanzania in the 15 years from 1990 to 2005. Lions may be attracted to farms by marauding bush-pigs but end up killing farmers sleeping in shelters in their fields in the evening or night. In Gujerat, India, lions killed 28 people (1978–91) but the case fatality of attacks was only 14.5% compared to ~100% for African lions. In North America, there are an average of 5.6 mountain lion attacks and 0.8 deaths each year. From 1900 to 1907, a tigress killed 436 people across the Nepal–Indian border near Champawat. In the Sundabans (India–Bangladesh border), tigers kill up to 100 people every year in daylight attacks. In India and Pakistan, individual man-eating leopards have claimed hundreds of lives through nocturnal attacks. They sometimes enter dwellings.

Prevention
Boma-fence (a fence or stockade made of wooden stakes) long-term camps in lion-infested areas and burn campfires at night. Tigers nearly always attack villagers from behind. Wearing a face-like mask on the back of the head has reduced attacks in the Sundabans. Big cats are best observed from a vehicle, hide, or from the back of an elephant. Firearm protection is necessary in dangerous areas. If all else fails, fight for your life, using any available weapon and making as much noise as possible.

Camels and horses

Domesticated and wild beasts of burden can lethally kick, bite, crush, and bolt! Treat them with great respect and stand well clear unless you are an expert.

Dogs and wolves

Bites by domestic dogs are common worldwide. More than 200 000 patients bitten by dogs attend hospital in England and Wales each year. In the US, dogs are responsible for 80–90% of all animal bites and each year bite 4.7 million people (1.8% of the population), 800 000 of whom (0.3% of the population) require medical attention; 12 are killed. Children are especially vulnerable. Walkers and joggers in both urban and rural areas frequently encounter aggressive dogs guarding their owners' properties.

Unless they are rabid, wolves usually keep away from humans and rarely attack, but there have been fatalities, especially in children, in Europe (Estonia, Poland, Spain, Russia, Belarus), Iran, India, and North America.

Prevention

Avoid dogs' territories as far as possible. Carry a heavy stick or club and fill your pockets with stones. If attacked, avoid eye contact. Do not run away but shout, protect yourself with your backpack, and fight back with sticks and stones.

Website

http://www.cdc.gov/ncipc/duip/biteprevention.htm

Elephants

Elephants, especially bulls in 'musth' (an annual period of increased testosterone production that causes black oily discharge from temporal glands, urinary incontinence, priapism, green algal staining of the penis, and extreme aggression), are some of the most dangerous and unpredictable animals on earth. They kill 100–200 people each year in India and about 30 people each year in Kenya. Humans may be thrown, trampled, or impaled.

Prevention

Always treat elephants with extreme respect and caution even if they are working or performing animals. Stay in the vehicle or downwind, avoid cows with calves, and bulls obviously in musth. Look for early warning signs of irritation before a charge; spread ears, raised swaying head and tail, lowered trunk, trumpeting; and retreat to your vehicle or other refuge while you can.

Hippopotamuses

These massive and irritable herbivores wallow in water by day and come ashore to graze by night. Some show carnivorous and cannibalistic tendencies. In Africa, especially in Kenya, Tanzania, Niger, and Botswana, they are notorious for capsizing canoes and drowning their occupants (usually fishermen), for trampling people under foot and, in water or on land, inflicting terrible bite wounds with their 50 cm-long canines. However, there is no evidence for the claim that they kill more people than do other African mammals or crocodiles. Recently reported deaths included a man swimming to retrieve a duck he had shot and a woman who got between a grazing hippo and her calf.

Prevention

Avoid swimming, diving, and canoeing in hippo-infested waters; never block a grazing hippo's retreat to the water and beware of cows with calves.

Hyenas

Campers resting by day or sleeping in the open at night in Africa have been seized by the head and severely mauled by hyenas. Attacks and deaths are reported from Malawi, Mozambique, and Kenya.

Pigs and peccaries

Wild, domesticated, and feral pigs are armed with sharp tusks and can attack swiftly and unexpectedly, especially in Melanesia. Penetrating abdominal injuries with prolapse and strangulation of the intestine, pneumothorax, open fractures, laceration of tendons, and artery and nerve injuries have been described.

Prevention

For protection against these lethal animals in Papua New Guinea, an expert's considered advice was: 'carry two spears'.

Crocodiles and alligators

Since 1948, 391 attacks and 19 fatalities from alligator (*Alligator mississippiensis*) attacks have been reported in the US. Florida is worst affected. Nile crocodiles (*Crocodilus niloticus*) kill about 1000 people each year in Africa, while in northern Australia 27 deaths from 60 attacks by the salt water crocodile (*C. porosus*) have been reported since 1876. In March 2006, Dick Root, the doyen of American infectious diseases specialists, was seized by a crocodile from a canoe on the Limpopo River, Botswana and was never seen again. It is extremely foolhardy for travellers to bathe in rivers regarded as dangerous by the local inhabitants. A Peace Corps worker in Ethiopia did this in 1967, and was promptly killed and eaten by the resident crocodile. Massacres have occurred historically (reputedly, the army of Perdiccas, one of Alexander's generals, when crossing the Nile during the war against Ptolemy in 321BC and the Japanese army off Ramree Island, Burma in the second world war) and recently after flooding in Ethiopia. Many victims are killed outright and their bodies are never recovered. Those reaching hospital usually survive but most will require debridement, amputations, and skin grafting. Forty per cent are left with permanent deformities. Fatalities are increasing in Ethiopia, Tanzania, Malawi, and PNG. *Pseudomonas, Enterococcus, Aeromonas, Clostridium, Serratia, Citrobacter, Bacteroides, Burkholderia*, and *Vibrio*, including *V. vulnificus*, have been implicated in crocodile/alligator bite infections (see Skin marine wounds 📖 p. 276).

Prevention

Walkers should keep well away from the water's edge. Avoid footpaths by lakes, rivers, and waterfalls. If camping near water, do not attract crocs by throwing in waste food. Do not bathe between dusk and dawn. Canoeing is hazardous in croc-infested waters. If attacked on land, run. If attacked in the water, fight back, hitting the animal on the nose and eyes with any available weapon.

Sharks

Since 2000, there have been only about 60–80 confirmed unprovoked attacks by sharks and an average of 4.3 fatalities each year (case fatality ~8%). Most attacks are in North American, Australian, and South African waters. In the US, there were 592 attacks, with nine fatalities, between 1948 and 2005, affecting mainly surfers and swimmers. The highest risk is off Florida. Great white (*Carcharodon carcharias*) (length ~16 m, weight 2250 kg), tiger (*Galeocerdo cuvier*) (5.5 m, 900 kg), and bull (*Carcharhinus leucas*)

(3.5 m, 360 kg) sharks are the most dangerous, but more than 70 species which grow longer than about 2 m are potentially lethal. Sharks can inflict truly appalling wounds, resulting in devastating blood loss from severed arteries, causing shock, and the risk of drowning. Common targets are buttocks, thighs, or shoulders.

Prevention

Avoid bathing in shark-infested waters, between sand bars and the deep ocean, where dead fish have been thrown into the water, where many sea birds are feeding, and where there is sewage effluent. Reduce risk by bathing in groups, close to the shore, only in daylight, and not if you are injured or menstruating. Do not wear jewellery or brightly coloured or patterned clothing. Avoid looking like a seal, a major prey species of dangerous sharks, when you are lying on a surf board. Neither splash excessively nor swim with pet dogs. If attacked by a shark, fight back, hitting it on the nose and clawing at its eyes and gills. Surface swimmers and surfers are usually targeted rather than divers. Scuba divers who encounter sharks can avoid attacks by descending to the ocean floor, hiding beneath rocks or reefs, and staying in groups. Various chemical and electrical-field repellents and chain mail protective suits have been developed.

Websites

http://www.flmnh.ufl.edu/fish/sharks/statistics/2006attacksummary.htm
http://www.sharkattacks.com/

Other fish

Most fish can inflict a painful and damaging bite if handled carelessly on a line or in a net, with a high risk of infection (see Skin 📖 p. 276). In the great river systems of South America, piranhas are capable, at the very least, of biting a chunk out of a foot or hand trailed over the side of the boat. Tiny catfish (Portuguese 'candirú', Spanish 'canero'), their tropism for the gills of the large fish that they parasitize confused by the smell of urine, may, like aquatic leeches, penetrate the urethra, vagina, or anus of bathers, especially women who are menstruating. At Hospital Santa Rosa, Puerto Maldonado, Peru, some half a dozen cases are seen at the local hospital every year. Indo-Pacific marine gar fish or needle fish (*Tylosurus*) can leap out the water at night, attracted by a light, and fatally impale the fisherman.

Prevention

Prevention of all these unusual hazards is to take local advice and to take sensible precautions (e.g. don't bathe in the nude!).

Treatment of trauma caused by animals

First aid of severe injuries

- Secure the victim out of danger and out of the water.
- Control bleeding.
- Close perforating injuries with pressure dressings.
- Start iv fluid volume repletion.
- Evacuate to the base hospital.
- Assume that all injuries are infected. Clean wounds urgently and thoroughly with soap and water, and apply iodine and alcohol solutions. For multiple/severe dog- and cat-bite wounds and bites of face and hands, start prophylactic co-amoxiclav, doxycycline, or erythromycin. For other bites, use penicillin, an aminoglycoside (e.g. gentamicin for 48 h) and metronidazole; for marine wounds see Skin 📖 p. 276.
- Cover risk of tetanus and rabies.

Emergency treatment at the base hospital

- Replace blood loss.
- Attend to local mechanical complications such as fractures, tension pneumothorax, damage to large blood vessels, perforation of the bowel, and lacerations of other abdominal viscera.
- Débride or amputate dead tissue, removing animals' teeth, etc.
- Irrigate and drain.
- Delay primary suturing for 48–72 h, except for head and neck wounds which should be sutured immediately.

Further reading

Woodroffe R, Thirgood S and Rabinowitz A. (eds) (2005). *People and Wildlife. Conflict or coexistence?* Cambridge, Cambridge University Press.

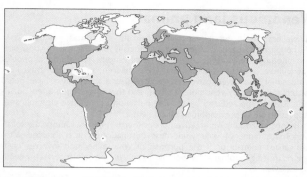

Fig. 16.1 Map of venomous land snake distribution.

Venomous land animals

Travellers' fears about venomous animals are usually exaggerated. Although most parts of the world, especially the tropical regions, are inhabited by animals with potentially lethal venoms, it is the local people (agricultural workers, hunters, and their children) rather than travellers who suffer. However, travellers, explorers, and researchers have been bitten and stung by venomous animals, and there have been a few fatalities. Risk can be reduced by sensible behaviour, protective clothing, and education about prevention and treatment.

Before embarking on an adventurous journey, find out about the local venomous fauna of your wilderness destination. If it is infested with dangerous animals or if the purpose of your expedition involves high exposure (e.g. zoological or botanical surveys in a rain forest), proceed as follows:

- Decide whether to take your own supply of antivenom (antivenin, antivenene or anti-snake-bite serum); this is justified only if the expedition is at high risk of venomous bites and stings, the area is more than a few hours' evacuation time from medical care, and your party includes someone capable of injecting the antivenom and dealing with an anaphylactic reaction.
- Check the availability of antivenom at the nearest (base) hospital.
- Identify a national centre for antivenom production, supply, and treatment (see end of chapter for addresses and websites of foreign manufacturers). Antivenoms for bites by foreign snakes cannot be ordered in UK except from Sanofi Pasteur MSD Ltd. (Tel: 0800 16 96 796; Fax: 0800 085 5511). Expect 4–6 months delay in fulfilling orders.
- Acquire the necessary knowledge about preventing and treating envenoming. Educate the expedition members at an early stage about prevention and first aid, and rehearse treatment and evacuation of bite/sting victims.

Snake bite

Snake bite is an important cause of death in agricultural communities in some parts of West Africa, Burma, the Indian subcontinent, New Guinea, and among indigenous Amerindians of the Amazonian region. Most parts of the world are inhabited by venomous snakes (Fig. 16.1). The medically important groups are elapids, vipers, pit vipers, and burrowing asps (Figs. 16.2, 16.3 and 16.4).

Europe
- Vipers only, e.g. adder *Vipera berus*.

Africa and the Middle East
- Elapids, e.g. cobras and spitting cobras (*Naja*), mambas (*Dendroaspis*).
- Vipers (Fig. 16.3), e.g. saw-scaled vipers (*Echis*), puff adders (*Bitis*), desert horned-vipers (*Cerastes*).
- Burrowing asps (*Atractaspis*).

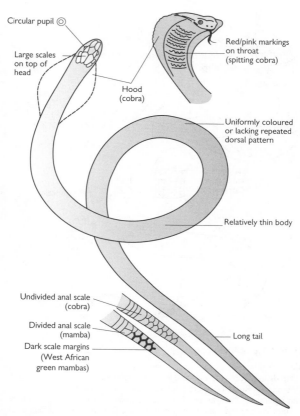

Circular pupil ⊙

Large scales
on top of
head

Hood
(cobra)

Red/pink markings
on throat
(spitting cobra)

Uniformly coloured
or lacking repeated
dorsal pattern

Relatively thin body

Undivided anal scale
(cobra)

Divided anal scale
(mamba)

Dark scale margins
(West African
green mambas)

Long tail

Fig. 16.2 Typical African elapid snake.

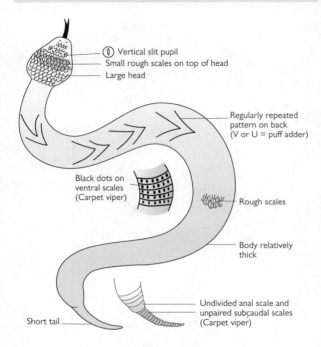

Fig. 16.3 Typical African viper.

Asia
- Elapids, e.g. cobras (*Naja*) and kraits (*Bungarus*).
- Vipers, e.g. Russell's vipers (*Daboia*), saw-scaled vipers (*Echis*).
- Pit vipers, e.g. Malayan pit viper (*Calloselasma rhodostoma*), green tree vipers, habus, and mamushis (*Cryptelytrops, Trimeresurus, Gloydius,* etc.).

Australasia
- Elapids only, e.g. taipans (*Oxyuranus*), black snakes (*Pseudechis*), brown snakes (*Pseudonaja*), tiger snakes (*Notechis*), death adders (*Acanthophis*).

The Americas
- Elapids, e.g. coral snakes (*Micrurus*).
- Pit vipers, e.g. lance-heads (*Bothrops*), moccasins (*Agkistrodon*), bushmasters (*Lachesis*), rattlesnakes (*Crotalus*).

The Indian and Pacific Oceans
- Elapids, e.g. sea snakes.

Clinical features

The following are the main groups of clinical features [and the snakes that cause them]:

- Local pain, swelling, bruising, blistering, regional lymph node enlargement, and tissue damage (necrosis) [vipers, pit vipers, burrowing asps, some cobras].
- Incoagulable blood (20 minute whole blood clotting test—see below) and spontaneous systemic bleeding (from gums, nose, skin, gut, GU tract) [vipers, pit vipers, Australasian elapids].
- Shock (hypotension) [vipers, pit vipers, burrowing asps].
- Descending paralysis progressing from ptosis and external ophthalmoplegia to bulbar and respiratory muscle paralysis [elapids, a few vipers and pit vipers].
- Generalized skeletal muscle breakdown (rhabdomyolysis) (generalized myalgia, muscle tenderness, and myoglobinuria-black/'Coca-Cola-coloured' urine positive for blood on stix testing) [sea snakes and a few other elapids, vipers, pit vipers].
- Acute renal failure (oliguria/anuria, ECG changes of hyperkalaemia) [sea snakes, a few vipers and pit vipers].

Treatment of snake bite

First aid treatment of snake bite must be applied immediately by the victim or other people who are on the spot.

First aid treatment of snake bite

- Reassure the bitten person
- Do not interfere with the bite site in any way
- Immobilize the bitten person as far as possible, especially the bitten limb using pressure-immobilization (see below)
- Arrange transport to medical care
- Treat pain with paracetamol or codeine tablets (not aspirin or NSAIDs!)
- *Do not* attempt to catch or kill the snake
- Avoid all traditional and 'quack' remedies

- **Reassure** the patient, who may be terrified by the thought of sudden death. Only a small minority of snake species are dangerous and even the most notorious species often bite without injecting enough venom to be harmful. The risk and rapidity of death from snake bite has been greatly exaggerated. Lethal doses of venom usually take hours (cobras, mambas, sea snakes) or days (vipers, rattlesnakes, and other pit vipers) to kill a human, not seconds or minutes as is commonly believed. **Correct treatment is very effective**.
- **Remove** tight rings, bracelets, and clothing from the bitten extremity before it becomes swollen.
- **Immobilize** the whole patient, especially the bitten limb, with a splint or sling. Pressure-immobilization (see below) is an effective way of achieving this, but correct application requires training.

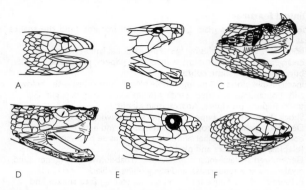

Fig. 16.4 Snake fangs: A Sea snake, B Cobra, C Viper, D Pit viper, E back-fanged snake (boomslang), F Burrowing asp.

- **Transport** the victim to medical care (e.g. to the expedition doctor, clinic or base hospital), as quickly, safely, passively, and comfortably as possible. Vehicle, boat, bicycle, stretcher or even fireman's lift is suitable. The patient must keep as still as possible to avoid exercising any part of the body, especially the bitten limb. Don't waste time before starting the journey; get going!
- **Do not** attempt to catch or kill the snake, but if it has been killed already take it with you; it is useful clinical evidence. **However, it must not be handled with bare hands even if it appears to be dead.**
- **Do not** use traditional methods (incisions, suction, tourniquets, electric shock, cryotherapy, instillation of potassium permanganate crystals, black/snake stone, etc.). They are useless and potentially harmful.
- **Do not** give aspirin or non-steroidal anti-inflammatory agents. They can cause bleeding.

Pressure-immobilization

Pressure-immobilization is indicated for bites by rapidly paralysing elapid bites, but in most case in the field, snake identification is uncertain. **Immediate application of pressure-immobilization is therefore recommended for all cases of snake bite**. Pressure-immobilization can be removed later if the snake is reliably identified as a viper or non-venomous snake. The aim is to empty and compress the lymphatic vessels draining the bite site. This can be achieved with an external pressure of 50–70 mmHg (roughly equivalent to the tight binding of a sprained ankle), thus preventing the lymphatic flow from transporting large molecular weight neurotoxins into the systemic circulation where they may cause rapidly evolving respiratory paralysis.

Firmly bind the whole of the bitten limb, starting around the fingers or toes and finishing at the axilla or groin. Use a series of stretchy crepe bandages (10 cm wide, 4.5 m long) and incorporate a splint (e.g. SAM® splint) (Fig. 16.5). Don't bind it too loosely! If it is too tight and acts like an arterial tourniquet, the limb will become ischaemic, cyanosed, and painful, and peripheral pulses at the wrist or ankle will be impalpable.

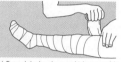

a) Apply a broad pressure bandage from below upwards and over the bite site as soon as possible. Do not remove trousers, as the movement of doing so will assist venom to enter the bloodsteam, keep the bitten leg still

b) The bandages should be as tight as you would apply to a sprained ankle. The patient should avoid any unnecessary movements

c) Extend the bandages as high as possible (ideally up to the groin)

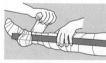

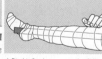

d) Apply a splint to the leg, immobilizing joints either side of the bite

e) Bind it firmly to as much of the leg as possible. Walking should be restricted

f) Bites on the hand and forearm: bind to the axilla, use a splint to the elbow, and use a sling

Fig. 16.5 Pressure-immobilization method.

Indications for antivenom treatment

Any of the following:
- Spontaneous systemic bleeding (see above).
- Incoagulable blood: failure of the patient's blood to clot solid when placed in a new, clean, dry, glass vessel and left undisturbed for 20 min *or* persistent bleeding (more than 30 min) from the fang punctures or other wounds, including venepuncture sites.

- Shock: low or falling blood pressure or cardiac arrhythmia.
- Paralysis (see above).
- Black/dark red-brown/'Coca Cola-coloured' urine (indicating rhabdomyolysis or massive haemolysis; see above).
- Local swelling: involving more than half the bitten limb *or* swelling after bites on the fingers and toes *or* swelling after bites by snakes whose bites have a high risk of causing necrosis.
- Mild local swelling alone is not an indication for antivenom. Never give antivenom unless you have adrenaline (epinephrine) available to treat early anaphylactic reactions to the antivenom (see below).

Choice of appropriate antivenom

Before giving antivenom make sure that its range of specificity includes the snake likely to have bitten your patient.

Most antivenoms are polyvalent and are able to neutralize venoms of all the medically important venomous species of the region for which it is intended. For example, in India, all antivenoms cover the 'big four' venomous species: cobra, common krait, Russell's viper, and saw-scaled viper; in Latin America many antivenoms cover the local lanceheads, rattlesnakes, and bushmaster (*Lachesis*). Monovalent antivenoms can be used if only one dangerous species occurs in the area (e.g. adder *V. berus* in UK, Netherlands, Belgium, and Scandinavia), if the snake has been reliably identified, or if a diagnostic clinical syndrome of envenoming appears. For example, in the northern third of Africa, incoagulable blood is diagnostic of saw-scaled viper (*Echis*) bite.

Administration of antivenom

- For optimal effect, administer by slow iv injection (2 ml/min) or iv infusion diluted in 250–500 ml isotonic fluid over 30–60 min.
- Initial dose depends on the type of antivenom, species of snake, and severity of symptoms: typically four to five 10 ml ampoules.
- Repeat initial dose after a few hours if life-threatening bleeding, shock, or paralysis is undiminished or if the blood remains incoagulable when retested after 6 h.
- Watch the patient closely for 2 h after starting antivenom for signs of anaphylaxis: fever, itching, urticarial rash, angioedema, vomiting, breathlessness and wheezing, increase in pulse rate, and fall in blood pressure.
- Treat anaphylaxis immediately with adrenaline/epinephrine, adult dose 0.5 ml of 1 in 1000 solution im (thigh muscle); this can be repeated after 10 min if it is not effective. Asthmatic reactions require additional inhaled bronchodilator.

Only in an extreme emergency should untrained people administer antivenom; for example, when the victim is many hours away from medical care, develops severe envenoming (see above), and is deteriorating (Fig. 16.6). Deep intramuscular injections at multiple sites into the front and side of the thighs (not the buttocks) can then be used. Injection sites should be massaged to increase absorption, but firm pressure must then be applied to injection sites to prevent haematoma formation.

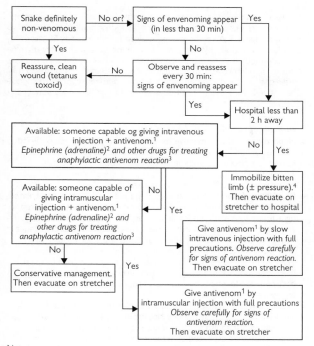

Notes:

1 *Antivenom* means appropriate specific antivenom for the species of snake involved.

2 *Epinephrine (adrenaline)* means 0.1% (1:1000) adrenaline for intramuscular injection (adult dose 0.3–0.5 ml).

3 *Other drugs for treating anaphylactic antivenom reaction* means anthistamine and hydrocortisone for intravenous injection.

4 *Immobilise bitten limb (± pressure)* means immobilization of the bitten limb with a splint or sling, *Pressure* means use of the pressure immobilisation method (Figure 16.5) using a long crepe bandage, This should be used unless a bite by a neurotoxic elapid snakes can be excluded.

Fig. 16.6 Algorithm to guide use of antivenom in remote wilderness situations.

Paralysis caused by Asian cobras and Australasian death adders sometimes responds to anticholinesterases such as edrophonium, neostigmine, or physostigmine. Atropine 0.6 mg is given iv followed by 10 mg edrophonium (Tensilon) by slow iv injection or 0.02 mg/kg neostigmine bromide/methylsulphate (Prostigmin) by im injection (all adult doses). If there is an improvement in muscle power within the next 20–30 min, treatment can be continued with subcutaneous neostigmine methylsulphate, 0.5–2.5 mg every 1–3 hours up to 10 mg/24 h maximum (adult dose).

Treatment of complications
- *Hypovolaemic shock:* massive external bleeding or leakage of blood and tissue fluid into a swollen limb may leave the patient with an inadequate circulating volume so that the blood pressure falls. Transfusion with plasma expanders such as Gelofusine™ or Haemaccel™ or 0.9% saline may be needed.
- *Respiratory failure:* from respiratory muscle paralysis must be treated with assisted ventilation; mouth-to-mouth or Ambu bag connected to a tight-fitting face mask, endotracheal tube or laryngeal mask airway, whatever is available and can be used effectively in the circumstances.
- *Acute renal failure:* some patients become anuric or oliguric soon after bites by Russell's vipers, some pit vipers, and sea snakes. They must be managed conservatively until they reach the base hospital. Correct hypovolaemia by giving intravenous fluid until the JVP becomes visible when the patient is propped up at 45° but avoid excessive fluid replacement.
- *Wound infection* may be introduced by the snake's fangs or by ill-advised tampering at the bite site producing local inflammation (difficult to distinguish from envenoming) or an obvious abscess which should be aspirated. A tetanus toxoid booster is appropriate immediately after the bite. Obviously infected or necrotic wounds should be treated with antibiotics such as co-amoxiclav or chloramphenicol.
- *Surgical complications:* at the base hospital, necrotic tissue should be debrided and the skin defect covered with split skin grafts. Fasciotomy to relieve suspected compartment syndrome (e.g. anterior tibial compartment) is very rarely indicated and should be considered only after normal haemostasis has been restored with adequate antivenom treatment and raised intracompartmental pressure confirmed by direct measurement (e.g. using a Stryker pressure monitor).

Spitting cobra-induced eye injuries
In Africa and parts of south-east Asia, there are spitting cobras that, as a defensive strategy, spray their venom forward from the tips of their fangs for a metre or more towards the glinting eyes of an aggressor. Venom falling on the conjunctivae causes an agonizing chemical conjunctivitis with profuse watering, leucorrhoea, and blepharospasm. Corneal ulceration, infection, and permanent blindness may result.

Emergency treatment

Irrigate the eye(s) immediately with generous volumes of any available bland fluid, ideally water under the tap (but milk or even urine is better than nothing: 'Please urinate into my eye'!). 1% adrenaline eye drops relieve the pain dramatically. Paracetamol can be given by mouth. Ideally, the eye should be examined by instilling fluorescein (or by slit lamp at the base hospital) to exclude corneal abrasion. If in doubt, prophylactic chloramphenicol or tetracycline eye ointment should be applied for several days. Topical antivenom, local anaesthetic, and corticosteroid should not be used.

Prevention of snake bites

Snakes never attack humans without provocation and so the risk of snake bite can be reduced as follows:

Do:

- Avoid all snakes and snake charmers.
- Open and shake out sleeping bags and clothing before use.
- Tap boots before wearing to dislodge any unwanted inhabitants.
- Check ground before sitting at the base of trees.
- Wear boots, socks, and long trousers when walking in undergrowth or deep sand.
- Wear boots and use a torch when walking off or on the track at night, especially after heavy rain and also when visiting the latrine at night (many snakes are most active at night).
- Be cautious and wear gloves when collecting fire wood.
- Remember that banks and streams are common snake haunts.
- Travel with a local guide who is much more likely to see camouflaged snakes.
- Sleep off the ground (camp bed or hammock) and under a tucked-in mosquito net if possible. Otherwise use a sewn-in ground sheet and mosquito-proof tent or tuck the net under your sleeping bag. This will protect against nocturnally prowling kraits (Asia) or spitting cobras (Africa) which often bite people while they are asleep on the ground.

Do not:

- Put hands blindly down inside rucksacks—empty out contents.
- Put hands or poke sticks into burrows or holes.
- Put hands up onto branches or ledges that can't be seen.
- Swim in rivers matted with vegetation in which snakes may be hiding or in muddy estuaries where there are likely to be sea snakes.
- Straddle logs—better to step up onto them then over.
- Disturb, corner, provoke, or attack snakes. Never handle them, even if they are said to be harmless or appear to be dead (a severed head can bite!).
- Move if you do corner a snake by mistake. Keep absolutely still until it has slithered away. This demands enormous *sang froid*, but snakes strike only at moving objects.

Lizard bite

Until recently, the Gila monster (*Heloderma suspectum*) (up to 60 cm long) of south-western USA and adjacent Mexico, and the Mexican beaded lizard or escorpión (*H. horridum*) (up to 80 cm) of western Mexico south to Guatemala were regarded as the only venomous lizards. However, some iguanas (*Iguanidae*), monitors (*Varanidae*) [notably the Komodo dragon (*Varanus komodoensis*)] and glass/alligator lizards (*Anguidae*) have now been shown to secrete venomous saliva. Helodermids' venom glands and grooved fangs are in their lower jaws. Bites are rare. The lizard hangs on like a bulldog and is difficulty to disengage (try intense heat under its chin or instilling strong alcohol into its mouth). There is immediate severe local pain followed by tender swelling and regional lymphadenopathy, weakness, dizziness, tachycardia, hypotension, syncope, angioedema, sweating, rigors, tinnitus, nausea, and vomiting. No fatal cases have been confirmed. Byetta™ (exenatide), a new glucagon-like-peptide-1 homologue from Gila monster venom used in type-2 diabetes mellitus, can also cause angioedema.

Treatment
Antivenom is not available. A powerful analgesic may be required. Hypotension should be treated with plasma expanders and perhaps adrenaline or a pressor agent such as dobutamine.

Arthropods

Bee, wasp, hornet, yellow jacket, and ant sting (Hymenoptera)
Stings by hymenoptera are a very common nuisance in many countries. Bees (*Apidae*) and wasp-like insects including yellow jackets and hornets (*Vespidae*), occur world-wide. Fire ants (*Solenopsis*) inhabit the Americas and jumper ants (*Myrmecia*) are found in Australia (especially Tasmania). Stings by all these hymenoptera can cause rapidly developing, potentially-lethal, systemic anaphylaxis in approximately 2–4% of the population who have become sensitized to their venoms. Other people may develop delayed, massive and persistent local swelling and inflammation which is unpleasant but not life-threatening.

Clinical
Symptoms of anaphylaxis can evolve in seconds. They include urticaria, angioedema, shock, unconsciousness, bronchoconstriction, gastrointestinal symptoms (nausea, vomiting, diarrhoea), double incontinence, and, in women, uterine contractions. Venom-specific IgE is detected by radio-allergosorbent test (RAST) or prick skin/patch testing, confirming hypersensitivity (see Treatment of anaphylaxis 📖 p. 220).

Prevention
People who have had anaphylaxis must carry a self-injectable adrenaline apparatus (EpiPen™, Anapen™) with them all the time. Most people who carry these pens have little idea how to use them in an emergency (Fig. 16.7). The technique should be practised with an EpiPen™ Trainer. Allergic subjects should wear an identifying tag (e.g. MedicAlert™ or MediTag™) to indicate their problem (e.g. 'allergic to wasp stings—give adrenaline') in case they are found incoherent or unconscious.

Those with a history of systemic anaphylaxis to a sting who are RAST or skin test-positive for the appropriate venom can be effectively desensitized before the expedition. Control of the hypersensitivity takes about 8 weeks, while cure takes 3–5 years.

1. Pull off the grey safety cap, as shown in diagram (a).

2. Hold the Auto-Injection as shown in diagram (b) and place the black tip on your thigh, at right angles to your leg. Always apply to the thigh.

3. Press hard into your thigh until the Auto-Injection mechanism works and hold the device in place for 10 seconds. The EpiPen® unit can then be removed. Massage the injection site for 10 seconds

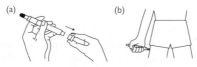

(a) (b)

Fig. 16.7 Epipen™ technique.

Mass attacks

In tropical countries, rock climbers and other travellers have been attacked by large swarms of angry bees. Fatal falls have resulted (e.g. on Wase Rock, Jos, Nigeria in the 1970s). In Zimbabwe, a man survived 2000 bee stings despite terrible symptoms of massive histamine release. Some of these accidents could have been prevented if local advice had been sought. Thundery weather is known to upset bees.

In the face of an attack, run away very fast, ideally into undergrowth, or immerse yourself under water. For climbers, a fall is the greatest danger. Secure yourself first, then use anorak, rucksack, or tent for protection. In South America there have been many deaths from mass attacks by furious swarms of Africanized honey bees ('killer bees'). Multiple stings can cause haemolysis, rhabdomyolysis, bronchospasm, pneumonitis, and renal failure. No antivenom is commercially available.

Blister beetles ('Spanish fly', 'Nairobi eye')

These beetles exude vesicating fluid containing cantharidin when inadvertently touched or trapped (e.g. antecubital fossa when elbow is flexed), causing erythema, itching, and formation of large, painless, thin-walled blisters. 'Spanish fly' (*Cantharis vesicatoria*, family *Meloidae*) is iridescent green. 'Nairobi eye' and similar blistering conditions in Australia and South East Asia are caused by pederin-containing secretions of rove beetles (*Paederus*, family *Staphylinidae*; Fig. 16.8). Toxin from crushed beetles or blister fluid is easily spread to other sites such as the eye by fingers. Treatment is palliative.

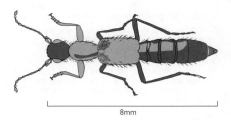

8mm

Fig. 16.8 Nairobi eye beetle.

Moth and caterpillar sting ('lepidopterism', 'erucism')

These insects, in particular brightly coloured, hairy caterpillars, can cause severe problems: local pain, inflammation, nettle rash, blistering, and arthritis on contact and, in Venezuela, Colombia and Brazil, systemic bleeding and incoagulable blood. Treatment is non-specific (anti-histamines, corticosteroids, analgesics) except in the case of the most dangerous genus of moth caterpillars (*Lonomia*), for which a specific antivenom is manufactured in Brazil.

Spider bite

The most dangerous genera of spiders are:

• *Latrodectus*—black/brown widow spiders (Americas: 2500–3000 cases/year the US, southern Europe, Southern Africa, Australia, New Caledonia; Fig. 16.9).
• *Phoneutria*—wandering, armed or banana spiders (Latin America; Fig. 16.10).
• *Atrax* and *Hadronyche*—(Sydney) funnel web spiders (Australia).
• *Loxosceles*—brown recluse spiders (Americas, southern Africa, and Mediterranean).

Many completely innocent (hobo, wolf, white-tailed, sac) spiders have been vilified as causes of 'necrotic arachnidism', the true aetiology of which was chronic ulcerative/granulomatous conditions such as pyoderma vegetans.

Clinical

Bites usually happen when the victim brushes against a spider that has crept into curtains, clothes, or bedding. *Latrodectus*, *Phoneutria*, and *Atrax* are neurotoxic, causing local puncture marks and surrounding erythema, severe pain spreading from the bite site, cramping abdominal or chest pains simulating an acute abdomen or myocardial infarction, muscle spasms, weakness, sweating, salivation, gooseflesh, fever, nausea, vomiting, priapism anxiety and feelings of doom, and alterations in pulse rate and blood pressure. Local pain, sweating, and gooseflesh at the site of bite is a useful sign. *Loxosceles* venom is necrotic, causing evolution over a few hours at the site of bite of pain and a circumscribed lesion (red-white-and-blue sign) (Coloured Plate 12). Rarely, there are systemic effects: fever, scarlatiniform rash, haemoglobinuria, coagulopathy, and renal failure.

Deaths are unusual except among children. Antivenoms are manufactured in countries such as South Africa, Australia, Mexico, and Brazil, where serious spider bites are common.

Scorpion sting

The most dangerous scorpions are:

- *Leiurus quinquestriatus, Androctonus* spp., *Hemiscorpius lepturus,* and *Buthus* spp. in North Africa and the Middle East.
- *Parabuthus* spp. in South Africa.
- *Centruroides* spp. in North America (15000 stings by *C. exilicauda* per year reported in Arizona, USA) and Mexico.
- *Tityus* spp. in Latin America and the Caribbean (Fig. 16.11).
- *Mesobuthus tamulus* in the Indian subcontinent.

All are found in dry desert or hot dusty terrains.

Clinical

Almost all stings (except *H. lepturus*) are excruciatingly painful and fatalities do occur, especially in children. Systemic symptoms reflect release of autonomic neurotransmitters, initially acetylcholine (causing vomiting, abdominal pain, pancreatic secretion, sphincter of Oddi constriction, bradycardia, salivation, nasolacrimal secretion, generalized sweating, priapism etc.) then catecholamines (causing piloerection, palmar sweating, hypertension, tachycardia, pulmonary oedema, ECG abnormalities). *Centruroides* envenoming causes erratic eye movements, fasciculations, muscle spasms simulating tonic–clonic seizures, and respiratory distress. *Hemiscorpius lepturus* (Iran, Iraq, Pakistan, and Yemen) envenoming causes a distinctive syndrome of painless sting, local erythema, bruising, blistering and necrosis, bleeding tendency, myocardial damage, and acute renal failure with high case fatality.

Treatment

The severe local pain is best treated by infiltrating local anaesthetic at the site of the sting (e.g. 1–2% lidocaine), ideally by digital block if the sting is on a finger or toe. Powerful opiate analgesia may be required. In the base hospital, hypertension, acute left ventricular failure, and pulmonary oedema may respond to vasodilators such as prazosin.

Antivenoms are available for dangerous African/Middle Eastern, South African, American, and Australian species. In Arizona, a new antivenom Anascorp™ (Alacramyn™) from Mexico may soon be available.

Prevention

When establishing camp in a scorpion-infested country, first clear the area of rocks, undergrowth, and debris to expose the scorpions. At night, a UV lamp is a useful adjunct as it makes scorpions fluoresce. They hide in cracks, crevices, and under rubbish. Don't walk around in bare feet, be sure to sleep off the ground, and use a permethrin-impregnated bed net. Always shake out your boots and shoes before putting them on (see also above: Prevention of snake bite).

Other venomous invertebrates

Bites by some tropical centipedes can be dangerous as well as painful (e.g. in the Seychelles). Some millipedes can squirt highly irritant defensive secretions, causing blistering and staining of skin and mucosae. No specific treatment is available. Some ticks in North America (e.g. *Dermacentor* spp.), eastern Australia (*Ixodes holocyclus*), and Europe can inject a neurotoxin while sucking blood. If one of your team develops an ascending flaccid paralysis while in these countries, search hairy areas and the external auditory meatus, and detach any ticks as soon as possible using the correct technique (see Skin 📖 p. 268). Paralytic symptoms should then subside.

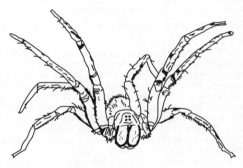

Fig. 16.9 Brazillian wandering spider *Phoneutria*.

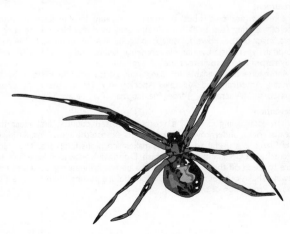

Fig. 16.10 Brown widow spider *Latrodectus geometricus*.

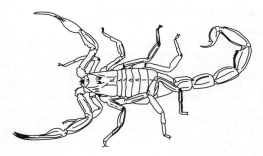

Fig. 16.11 Brazilian scorpion *Tityus serrulatus.*

Venomous marine animals

Sea snake bite

Sea snakes occur in colossal numbers in warmer oceans, estuaries, and rivers but not in the Atlantic or the Red Sea (Fig. 16.12). They are encountered mainly by fishermen in the Indo-Pacific region but bite only if handled incautiously (e.g. while being picked out of hand nets or off fishing lines). Head-end and tail-end may be difficult to distinguish. The principal symptoms of envenoming are progressive myalgia and muscle tenderness with trismus, passing dark (Coca Cola-coloured) urine (myoglobinuria), ptosis, descending paralysis threatening respiratory failure, and acute renal failure. Rhabdomyolysis can be so severe that potassium released from damaged muscles causes cardiac arrest. Hyperkalaemia may be controlled with iv calcium chloride, sodium bicarbonate or insulin and dextrose. Treatment is the same as for other snake bites (see above). Wet suits are protective against the bites of all but the longest-fanged and most aggressive of sea snakes.

Fish sting

More than 1200 species of fresh water and especially marine fish are venomous, but only about 200 species can cause dangerous stings. They inhabit both tropical and temperate waters. Important species include: stingrays, mantas, catfish, weevers, toadfish, stargazers, stone lifters, scorpion fish, stone fish, sharks, and dogfish. Their venomous spines are in the gills, fins, or tail. Beautiful lion, zebra, tiger, turkey, or red fire fish (*Pterois*, *Dendrochirus*; Fig. 16.13) are popular aquarium pets. Stingrays are common in the oceans and in rivers of South America and Equatorial Africa. If trodden upon they lash their tails, impaling the ankle with a venomous spine (Fig. 16.14).

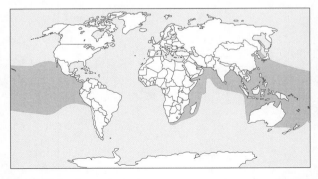

Fig. 16.12 Distribution of sea snakes.

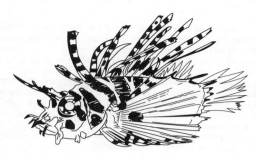

Fig. 16.13 Lion fish Dendrochirus.

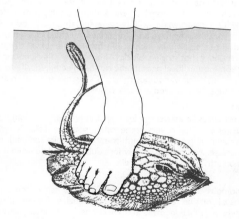

Fig. 16.14 Stinging action of stingray.

Stings occur when fish are:
- Handled by fishermen or tropical aquarium keepers.
- Trodden on or touched by bathers and waders on beaches or by people fording rivers in the Amazon region, especially in the dry season.
- Irritated by swimmers and scuba divers around coral reefs.

Clinical

There is immediate excruciating pain followed by swelling and inflammation at the site of the sting. Rarely, severe systemic effects may develop during the following minutes or hours: vomiting, diarrhoea, sweating, irregular heart beat, fall in blood pressure, spasm or paralysis of muscles, including respiratory muscles, and fits. Stingrays' barbed spines may be large enough to cause fatal trauma (pneumothorax, penetration of thoracic or abdominal organs), as in the case of Steve Irwin who was killed in September 2006 when a stingray's spine punctured his heart. Spines with their venomous integument are often left embedded in the wound and will cause infection unless removed.

Expeditions involving activities in aquatic environments should find out in advance about the local venomous hazards.

First aid

The agonizing local pain is dramatically relieved by immersing the stung limb in hot but not scalding water. Test the temperature with your own elbow. If you have a thermometer, check that the temperature does not exceed 45°C. Hotter water will cause a full thickness scald. Ad hoc methods of local heating have been described: a lighted cigarette, cigar or lighter advanced to within inches of the wound, or a damp towel wrapped round a hot engine block. Alternatively, 1% lignocaine (lidocaine) or some other local anaesthetic can be injected, ideally as a digital block (📖 p. 566). The venomous spines of stingrays and catfish are often barbed but must be removed as soon as possible.

Antivenom

Australia produces an antivenom for stonefish (genus *Synanceja*), the most dangerous genus. This covers some other scorpion fish. Exceptionally, a stung patient might need mouth-to-mouth respiration and external cardiac massage. Atropine (0.6 mg iv for adults) should be given if there is hypotension attributed to bradycardia.

Infection

Both venomous and non-venomous fish wounds can become infected with unusual marine pathogens (e.g. necrotizing fasciitis caused by *Photobacterium* (*Vibrio*) *damsel*, and infections by *Vibrio alginolyticus* and *Fusarium solani* following injuries by stingrays; see Skin 📖 p. 276).

Prevention

Employ a shuffling gait when wading or prod the sand ahead of you with a stick to disturb venomous fish. Avoid handling fish (dead or alive) and keep clear of fish in the water, especially in the vicinity of tropical reefs. Footwear, the thicker the better, protects against most species except stingrays.

Cnidarian (coelenterate) sting: jellyfish, Portuguese man o' war ('blue bottle'), sea nettle, sea wasp, cubomedusoids, sea anemones, stinging corals, etc.

The tentacles of these marine animals are studded with millions of stinging capsules (nematocysts) triggered by contact to fire their venomous stinging hairs into the skin. This produces lines of painful blisters and inflammation.

Hypersensitivity may lead to recurrent urticarial rashes over many months. The venom of some species, such as the notorious box jellyfish (*Chironex fleckeri* and *Chiropsalmus* spp.) of Northern Australian and Indo-Pacific waters, has caused more than 70 deaths since 1883. Severe systemic effects can result in cardiorespiratory arrest within minutes of the stings. 'Irukandji' syndrome is caused by *Carukia barnesi* and other tiny transparent cubomedusoids. There is severe musculoskeletal pain, anxiety, trembling, headache, piloerection, sweating, tachycardia, hypertension, and pulmonary oedema starting within about 30 min of the sting and persisting for hours. Other medically important jellyfish include Portuguese men o' war (*Physalia*) which are worldwide in distribution, and have caused a few fatalities and local gangrene owing to arterial spasm; *Stomalophis nomurai* of the north-west Pacific, China, and Japan which can cause fatal pulmonary oedema; the sea nettle (*Chrysaora quinquecirrha*) which is very widely distributed but is most common in Chesapeake Bay, USA, and the mauve stinger (*Pelagia noctileuca*), which can swarm in enormous numbers causing stinging epidemics in the Adriatic and other parts of the Mediterranean.

Coral cuts are common injuries inflicted by coelenterates in tropical waters. Painful superficial grazes and cuts result when tender areas of the body are inadvertently brushed against coral outcrops. Mechanical injury from the spiky calcified crust is combined with envenoming and the risk of a marine bacterial infection (see Skin 📖 p. 276).

Treatment

- Remove the victim from the water to prevent drowning.
- Prevent further discharge of nematocysts on fragments of tentacles stuck to the skin:
  - For *Chironex* spp. and other cubozoans, including Irukandji (Indo-Pacific region, perhaps Caribbean), apply commercial vinegar or 3–10 % aqueous acetic acid solution. This is not recommended for stings by other jellyfish.
  - For *Chrysaora* spp. apply a slurry of baking soda and water (50% w/v).
  - Tentacles should be removed manually and with a shaving razor.
  - Alcoholic solutions such as methylated spirits and suntan lotion must not be used as they cause massive discharge of nematocysts.
- Relieve agonizing pain:
  - *Chironex* spp. and *Physalia*—hot water treatment (as for fish stings; see above) has proved more effective than ice.
  - Pressure immobilization is not recommended.
- Treat severe envenoming:
  - Cardiopulmonary resuscitation on the beach has saved lives.
  - Antivenom for box jellyfish, 'Sea wasp' (*C. fleckeri*), is manufactured in Australia. It has been given on the beach by surf lifesavers by intramuscular injection.
- Coral cuts: should be cleaned and débrided as far as possible, irrigated, cleaned with antiseptic and dressed. Infection should be treated promptly (see Skin 📖 p. 276).

Sea urchin and starfish injuries (echinoderms)

The sharp venomous spines and grapples of some sea urchins may become deeply embedded in the skin, usually of the sole of the foot when the animal has been trodden upon. Soften the skin with salicylic acid ointment and then pare down the epidermis to a depth at which the spines can be removed with forceps. If the spines are visible, it is tempting to try to remove them immediately, but this may be difficult or impossible. They are absorbed over several days provided they are broken into small pieces in the skin. If they penetrate a joint or cause infection, surgical removal is necessary.

Molluscs: octopus bite and cone shell sting

The blue-ringed octopuses of the Indo-Australasian region rarely exceed 20 cm in diameter but can cause fatal envenoming by biting (Fig. 16.15). Cone shells (Fig. 16.16) are beautiful collectors' items but they can sting by harpooning and implanting a venom-charged arrowhead. Beware of picking up these attractive animals bare-handed. Their stings can be fatal and no antivenoms are available. Treatment of mollusc bites and stings is purely supportive, based on the knowledge that their venoms (tetrodotoxin in the case of the blue-ringed octopus) are ion-channel agonists/antagonists that may cause paraesthesiae, paralysis, and cardiac arrest.

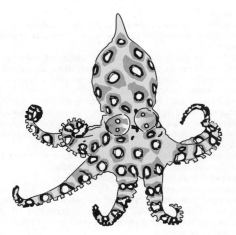

Fig. 16.15 Blue-ringed octopus.

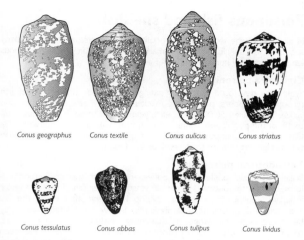

Conus geographus   Conus textile   Conus aulicus   Conus striatus

Conus tessulatus   Conus abbas   Conus tulipus   Conus lividus

Fig. 16.16 Cone shells.

Poisonous fish and shellfish

In all parts of the world, but especially in the tropics, the flesh of many species of fish, shellfish, and other marine animals is dangerously poisonous when ingested by humans and other animals.

Ciguatera poisoning

Symptoms develop 1–6 h after eating warm-water shore or reef fish (groupers, snappers, parrot fish, mackerel, moray eels, barracudas, and jacks). There are >50 000 cases each year and, in some Pacific Islands, up to 1% of the population is affected each year, with a case fatality of 0.1%. Gastrointestinal symptoms resolve within a few hours, but paraesthesiae and myalgia may persist for a week or even months.

Tetrodotoxin poisoning

Scaleless porcupine, file, trigger, puffer, and sun fish (order: Tetraodontiformes) become poisonous at certain seasons. Puffer fish ('fugu') is popular in Japan. Neurotoxic symptoms develop 10–45 min after eating the fish and death from respiratory paralysis may follow 2–6 h later. There may be no gastrointestinal symptoms. Skin changes include erythema, petechiae, blistering, and desquamation. 'Zombification' in Haitian 'ju-ju' has been attributed to the use of this toxin. Tetrodotoxin, ultimately derived from bacteria, accumulates in parrotfish (*Scaridae*), Californian newts (*Taricha*), toads (*Atelopus*), blue-ringed octopuses (see above), starfish, the eggs of horseshoe crabs (*Limulidae*) and in certain species of angelfish, polyclad flatworm, *Chaetognatha* (arrow worm), nemertean (ribbonworm), and xanthid crab.

Scombroid poisoning (histamine-like syndrome)

Bacterial contamination and decomposition of dark-red-fleshed fish (tuna, mackerel, bonito, skipjack), and canned sardines and pilchards generates histamine. *An early warning is immediate tingling or smarting of the lips and tongue at the first mouthful!* A few minutes to a few hours later, there is flushing, burning, sweating, urticaria, pruritis, headache, abdominal colic, nausea, vomiting, diarrhoea, bronchial asthma, giddiness, hypotension, and collapse.

Paralytic shellfish poisoning

Bivalve molluscs (mussels, clams, oysters, cockles, and scallops) become toxic when there is a 'red tide' of algal blooms. Many fish, sea birds, and mammals perish. Within 30 min of ingestion, paralysis begins and may progress to fatal respiratory paralysis within 12 h in 8% of cases. Milder gastrointestinal and neurotoxic symptoms (neurotoxic shellfish poisoning) without paralysis may occur.

Treatment

- In all cases, attempt to eliminate the toxic materials from the gut by gentle gastric lavage and purgatives, and give repeated doses of activated charcoal which is of unproven benefit but is unlikely to do harm.
- Scombroid poisoning responds to antihistamines and bronchodilators.

- Severe cases of paralytic poisoning require assisted ventilation.
- Victims of tetrodotoxin poisoning have recovered despite fulfilling the criteria for brain death.

Prevention
NOTE!
Marine poisons are not destroyed by cooking or boiling.

Do
- Take local advice about what it is safe to eat.

Don't eat
- Seafood if there is an obvious 'die off' of marine life (rows of dead fish and sea birds on the shore).
- Shellfish if there is a 'red tide'.
- Very large reef fish (ciguatera poisoning) and any parts of any fish other than muscle (i.e. no skin, viscera, gonads, roe, etc.).
- Notorious poisonous species such as Moray eels (ciguatera), parrotfish (saxitoxin and others), large sharks (ciguatera, carchatoxin, trimethylamine), marine and fresh water puffer fish (tetrodotoxin/saxitoxin) and, especially, horseshoe crabs' eggs, a delicacy in Thailand (*Carcinoscorpius rotundicauda*—Thai 'mengda tawai' and *Tachypleus gigas*—Thai 'mengda chaan'; tetrodotoxin).
- Livers of any carnivorous polar mammal (polar bear, seals, cetaceans, huskies, etc.) because of the risk of fatal vitamin A toxicity.

Advice on venomous bites and stings
Guy's and St Thomas' Poisons Unit
Tel. (24 h):   +44 (0) 870 2432241
guyspoisons@gstt.nhs.uk
http://www.medtox.org

Centre for Tropical Medicine, University of Oxford
Tel. (24 h): +44 1865 741166
(0900–1700 h Mon–Fri)+44 1865 220968
Fax: +44 1865 220984

Liverpool School of Tropical Medicine
Tel. (0900–1700 h Mon–Fri) +44 (0) 151 708 9393
 (24 h ask for tropical/ID physician on call) +44 (0) 151 706 2000
Fax: +44 (0) 151 705 3368 or +44 (0) 151 708 8733
http://www.liv.ac.uk/lstm/travel_health_services

Useful websites
Snake bite in South and South-East Asia:
http://www.searo.who.int/en/Section10/Section17/Section53/Section1024.htm
Envenoming worldwide:
http://www.toxinology.com/
Antivenoms: general
http://www.afpmb.org/pubs/living_hazards/antiv.html
http://globalcrisis.info/latestantivenom.htm
Protherics: http://www.protherics.com/Products/critical_care.aspx
WHO: http://www.who.int/bloodproducts/animal_sera/en/

European antivenoms:
Zagreb Immunology Institute in Croatia http://www.imz.hr/ZMIJA-eng.pdf
Australian antivenoms:
http://www.csl.com.au/search.asp?qu=antivenom
http://www.toxinology.com/generic_static_files/cslavh_antivenom.html
South African antivenoms:
http://www.savp.co.za/Products.htm
Venomous snake taxonomy updates:
http://sbsweb.bangor.ac.uk/%7Ebss166/update.htm

Plants and fungi

David Warrell

'I wanted to eat of the fruit of all the trees in the garden of the world' (Oscar Wilde). **Please don't do it!**

Dangers of living off the land

The abundant and richly diverse flora of the wilderness environment offers the expeditioner a chance to survive by 'living off the land'. This ideal is enthusiastically encouraged in some military survival exercises and by certain heroic TV personalities! Attractive-looking and -smelling fruits and fungi may tempt the traveller but, without the expert local guidance of indigenous people, mistakes may prove lethal. An essential adjunct to this chapter is a profusely illustrated guide or website covering the poisonous (and edible) plants and fungi of the expedition's location. However, toxic plants and fungi are easily confused with edible ones and it is salutary that even expert botanists and mycologists are occasionally poisoned. You should not be reassured by watching wild animals and birds feeding with apparent impunity. For example, Zanzibar's red colobus monkeys *(Piliocolobus kirkii)* eat charcoal to prevent poisoning by phenolic compounds in Indian almond *(Terminalia catappa)* and mango *(Mangifera indica)* leaves, their staple diet. Sometimes poisoning results from rash experimentation in quest of psychoactive effects (a 'trip'). In South India and Sri Lanka, toxic plants are ingested as a means of suicide (e.g. yellow oleander—*Thevetia peruviana*).

Prevention of plant and fungal poisoning

DO

- Educate expedition members about the local toxic flora
- Rely on your own food supplies
- Confine collection of food from the environment to what you can identify with certainty as being safely edible or what is confidently recommended by local indigenous people
- REMEMBER! Cooking does not destroy fungal toxins!

DON'T

- Experiment
- Eat 'forbidden fruits': those resembling familiar cultivated fruits may be highly poisonous. To a non-expert, the death cap toadstool looks very like an edible mushroom (see below)
- Eat wild fungi and certainly none with white gills (see below)
- Accept invitations to inhale, 'snort', or ingest the local psychedelic brew:
  - a splitting headache, nausea, vomiting, and terrifying hallucinations are more likely than any pleasurable trance or 'out of body' experience

Plant poisoning

Effects on skin

Contact dermatitis is by far the commonest risk posed by plants. Examples include: stinging nettles, euphorbias, and 'dumb cane' (*Dieffenbachia*).

Allergic dermatitis may be caused by a large variety of plants, notably poison ivy (*Rhus radicans*), poison oak (*Toxicodendron diversilobum*), primula (*Primula obconica*), and citrous fruits. Some plant saps are photosensitizing, resulting in erythema, papules, vesicles, bullae, and persistent hyperpigmentation confined to exposed areas.

Treatment is based on identifying the cause and avoiding further contact, reducing solar exposure if there is photosensitization, and the use of systemic antihistamines and topical corticosteroids to control symptoms.

When to suspect plant poisoning

Within minutes to hours (exceptionally 24 h) after ingesting any part of a wild fruit, plant, or fungus (mushroom or toadstool).
- Nausea, vomiting, abdominal colic, diarrhoea
- Confusion, hallucinations, or convulsions
- Atropinic, nicotinic, or muscarinic symptoms
- Cardiac arrhythmias
- Flushing in response to alcohol ingestion
- Oliguria/anuria

Effects on gut

Cuckoo pint/arum lily, dumb cane, and many other plants have an irritant sap. Ingestion causes immediate soreness, reddening, and blistering of buccal mucosa, salivation, and dysphagia. Most poisonous plants cause rapidly evolving nausea, abdominal cramps, vomiting, and diarrhoea (e.g. laburnum, anemone, hellebore, horse chestnut, ivy, privet, pokeweed, and snowberry). Some even more toxic plants cause severe gastrointestinal symptoms after a delay of several hours up to 2 days (e.g. autumn crocus (*Colchicum autumnale*), glory lily (*Gloriosa superba*), jequirity bean (*Abrus precatorius*), and castor oil bean (*Ricinus communis*).

Effects on cardiovascular system

Bradycardia, heart block, other arrhythmias, ECG changes ('digoxin effect'), and gastrointestinal irritation are caused by foxglove (*Digitalis purpurea*), oleander (*Nerium oleander*), yellow oleander (*Thevetia peruviana*), monkshood (*Aconitum napellus*), yew (*Taxus baccata*), and death camas (*Zigadenus*).

Effects on nervous system
- **Hallucinogenic**: e.g. cannabis (*Cannabis sativa*), khat (*Catha edulis*), morning glory (Ipomoea), and peyote (*Lophophora williamsii*).
- **Convulsant**: e.g. cowbane (*Cicuta virosa*), ackee (*Blighia sapida*), and nux vomica (*Strychnos nux-vomica*). Cowbane poisoning causes gastroenteritis, increased secretions, and longlasting intense episodes of generalized tonic–clonic convulsions, resulting in severe metabolic acidosis and multiple organ failure. Consumption of unripe ackee fruit is responsible for 'Jamaican vomiting sickness' associated with hypoglycaemia and fatal encephalopathy.
- **Atropine-like**: e.g. deadly nightshade (*Atropa belladonna*), angels' trumpets (*Brugmansia suaveolens*), and thorn apple (*Datura stramonium*). There is facial flushing, tachycardia, and dilated pupils (mydriasis), and, in serious poisoning, arrhythmias, urinary retention, psychosis, convulsions, coma, and fatal respiratory failure. Some of these plants are also hallucinogenic.
- **Nicotine-like**: e.g. spotted hemlock (*Conium maculatum*), responsible for killing Soctrates and Hamlet's father, first stimulates and then paralyses autonomic ganglia, and can cause convulsions and respiratory arrest.

Effects on liver
Pyrrolizidine alkaloid-containing plants such as comfrey (*Symphytum officinale*) can cause hepatic veno-occlusive disease, which has occurred mainly in Jamaica, India, and Afghanistan. Nausea, abdominal pain and distension, hepatomegaly, and sometimes fever and vomiting develop a few days after ingestion.

Effects on kidneys
Oxalate-rich plants such as rhubarb (*Rheum rhabarbarum*), dock, and sorrel (*Rumex*), and plants containing other nephrotoxicins may damage the kidneys.

Poisonous food plants
Staple food plants in many tropical countries can be poisonous if inadequately soaked, dried, fermented, or cooked:
- Cassava (*Manihot esculenta*), sweet potato, yam, some fruit kernels, pips, and cherry laurel (*Prunus laurocerasus*) can cause acute or chronic cyanide poisoning.
- In Africa, tropical ataxic neuropathy and spastic paraparesis ('konzo') are attributed to cassava poisoning.
- Inadequately cooked beans and pulses (Leguminosae) can cause diarrhoea, while long-term exposure can lead to retarded growth and may even be fatal.
  - Lathyrism is an epidemic paralytic disease (e.g. in the Denbia depression of Ethiopia) caused by a neurotoxic amino acid in chick peas (*Lathyrus sativus*).
  - Favism occurs in some Mediterranean and Middle Eastern countries. Those with congenital glucose-6-phosphate dehydrogenase deficiency may develop intravascular haemolysis after eating broad (fava) beans (*Vicia faba*).

Fungal poisoning

Fungal poisoning is usually sporadic and accidental but occasionally may be homicidal, suicidal, or epidemic. In Europe (especially France, Scandanavia, and Russia), where there are many enthusiastic collectors and connoisseurs of wild mushrooms, poisoning is more common than elsewhere in the world. In 1999, 357 people were poisoned and 39 died from deathcap mushroom (*Amanita phalloides*) poisoning in Voronezh in central Russia. Recently, poisonings and deaths have been reported from Nizhniy Novgorod, Russia (*Boletus luridus*), Rovno, Ukraine, and Kazakhstan. Toxicity of fungi varies with location and season, from year to year, and with individual susceptibility.

The deathcap looks superficially like an edible mushroom (*Agaricus*) but it has white gills (radiating linear structures under the mushroom's cap) and a sac or volva at its base, whereas the edible mushroom has dark brown or black gills and no volva at the base of its stem (Fig. 17.1).

Poisoning with early symptoms (within a few hours)

- **Gastrointestinal symptoms**: vomiting, diarrhea, and abdominal pain are usually transient but sometimes more intense, resulting in fluid and electrolyte disturbances. They may be caused by many species of common fungi, including honey agaric (*Armillaria mellea*) and *Boletus luridus*.
- **Cholinergic effects (muscarinic poisoning)**: abdominal pain and diarrhoea, sweating, lacrimation, salivation, miosis, bronchorrhoea, and sometimes bronchospasm, bradycardia, and hypotension may develop 5–120 min after ingesting *Inocybe* and *Clitocybe* species.

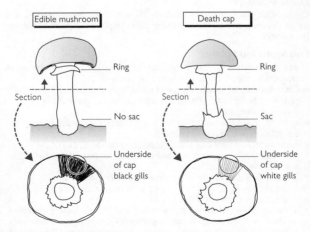

Fig. 17.1 Distinguishing edible mushrooms from deathcap.

- *Confusion (Ibotenic poisoning)*: nausea, vomiting, confusion, disorientation, anxiety, euphoria, hallucinations, visual disturbances, ataxia, muscle cramps, and coma may develop 20–120 min after ingestion of panther cap (*Amanita pantherina*), fly agaric (*Amanita muscaria*), and *Amanita strobiliformis*.
- *Hallucinations (Psilocybin poisoning)*: LSD-like, mainly visual hallucinations are induced by eating 'magic mushrooms' (*Psilocybe, Conocybe, Gymnopilus, Panaeolina, Panaeolus, Pluteus* and *Stropharia* species). Within 30 min, there is mydriasis, tachycardia, euphoria, confusion, dizziness, and vomiting.
- *Antabuse-like reactions (Coprine poisoning)*: eating ink cap (*Coprinus atramentarius*) or club foot (*Clitocybe clavipes*) may produce a reaction similar to that induced by disulfiram (Antabuse). If alcohol is drunk within 72 h of eating the fungi, there is flushing of the skin, metallic taste, sweating, mydriasis, nausea, vomiting, anxiety, confusion, dyspnoea, severe headache, tachycardia, chest pain, and hypotension.

Poisoning with delayed symptoms (6 h to several days)
- *Gastroenteritis with hepatotoxicity and nephrotoxicity (Amatoxin poisoning)*: may result from eating the deathcap (*Amanita phalloides;* Fig. 17.1), destroying angel (*Amanita virosa*), fool's mushroom (*Amanita verna*), *Conocybe filaris*, and some *Galerina* and *Lepiota* species. Abdominal pain and vomiting, but in particularly severe cases, watery or bloody diarrhea, starts 6–24 (usually 12) h after ingestion, leading to dehydration. After a period of apparent recovery, lasting up to 72 h, fatal hepatorenal failure may supervene.
- *Gastroenteritis with neurological symptoms (Gyromitrin poisoning)*: there is gastroenteritis with a feeling of bloating, severe headache, vertigo, pyrexia, sweating, diplopia, nystagmus, ataxia, cramps, delirium, and sometimes coma, lethargy, hypoglycaemia, hepatic damage, haemolysis, and renal damage starting 2–24 h after ingesting false Morel (*Gyromitra esculenta*) or inhaling fumes while it is being cooked.
- *Renal damage (Orellanine poisoning)* may develop 2–17 days after eating *Cortinarius* species. There is fatigue, intense thirst, headache, chills, paraesthesiae, tinnitus, and abdominal, lumbar, and flank pain. After a transient polyuric phase, oliguria and anuria may ensue.
- *Ergotism ('St Anthony's fire')* results from eating cereal crops whose seed heads are infected with the hard, purplish-black fruiting bodies of *Claviceps purpurea*. Symptoms include vasoconstriction, leading to peripheral gangrene and muscular tremors, convulsions, and hallucinations.

Treating plant and fungal poisoning

First aid

- Treat topical irritant effects on skin and mucosae by washing, rinsing, or gargling with generous volumes of water or any other bland fluid.
- Gastric lavage is potentially dangerous because of the risks of aspiration and trauma to pharynx and oesophagus. If performed gently and safely with a few hours of ingestion, it can help to eliminate poisonous gastric contents.
- Give the patient a glass of milk to drink provided they are fully conscious and not vomiting.
- Give oral activated charcoal 50 g immediately, followed by 25 g every 2 h for at least 48 h (this is not evidence based but is very unlikely to be harmful).

At the base hospital

Severe cases will require supportive treatments for organ failure such as mechanical ventilation and renal dialysis, with therapy for hypovolaemia, acid–base disturbances, hypoglycaemia, cardiac arrhythmias, and convulsions.

- For *cholinergic (muscarinic) symptoms*—atropine (adult 0.6–1.8 mg iv).
- For *central and peripheral anticholinergic (atropine-like) effects*—physostigmine (adult 1–2 mg iv) to control hallucinations, delirium, and psychotic behaviour.
- For *confusion or hallucinations*—tranquillizers such as diazepam (adults 5–10 mg).
- For *psychotic behavior*—chlorpromazine or haloperidol may be required.

Specific antidotes:

- For poisoning by yellow oleander, other *Apocynaceae,* and any plant containing cardiac glycosides: digoxin-specific antibodies (ovine Fab fragments such as Digibind™ or DigiTab™).
- For severe autumn crocus (*Colchicum autumnale*) poisoning: colchicine-specific Fab antibodies.
- For amatoxic fungal poisoning: infuse silibinin (silybin, silymarin) 5 mg/kg iv over 1 h, followed by 20 mg/kg/24 h (available in Germany but not in the UK or USA) or large doses (300 000–1 000 000 U/kg/day by continuous iv infusion) of benzylpenicillin. N-acetyl cysteine might reduce liver damage. In severe cases, liver transplantation is life-saving.
- For gyromitrin fungal poisoning: pyridoxine 25 mg/kg over 30 min, glucose iv, and promote diuresis.

Reference

Poisonous plants and fungi in Britain and Ireland. ISBN 1 900347 92 X. Interactive CDRom from Publications Sales, Royal Botanic Gardens, Kew, Richmond, Surrey TW9 3AE, UK.

Advice about plant and fungal poisoning

Guy's and St Thomas' Poisons Unit. Tel. (24 h)+44 (0) 870 2432241. e-mail: guyspoisons@gstt.nhs.uk. Website: http://www.medtox.org WHO International Programme on Chemical Safety World Directory of poisons Centres http://www.who.int/ipcs/poisons/centre/directory/en/

Anaesthesia in remote locations

Joe Silsby

While local anaesthetic infiltration using recommended doses of appropriate drugs is safe, other forms of sedation and anaesthesia described in this section normally demand extensive specialist training. They should only be attempted by untrained personnel in circumstances where life or limb is threatened; for instance, if personnel have been trapped or injured by accident or rock fall.

Introduction

The basic principles that govern 'field' anaesthesia are similar to those governing conventional hospital anaesthesia, but the practical aspects of working safely in remote locations and the adverse conditions under which the operations may be performed can be a formidable challenge even to experienced specialists.

Anaesthesia must be:
- Simple.
- Safe for the patient.
- Adaptable to constraints of the situation.
- Essential for life or limb preservation.

Four types of field anaesthesia can be differentiated:
- *Military*—during conflicts armed forces retrieve casualties to forward bases where sophisticated resuscitation, surgery, and intensive care commence. They then aim to evacuate casualties to secondary treatment facilities within 72 h. Such arrangements involve costly resources and a complex logistic infrastructure, and are inapplicable to the majority of expeditions.
- *Mass casualties*—non-combatants during conflicts, and casualties of natural disasters may present in large numbers to healthcare facilities run by non-governmental organizations (NGOs) such as Medecins sans Frontiers or the International Red Cross. There are often shortages of personnel, equipment, drugs, and disposables. Sophisticated techniques or equipment and back-up facilities are rare, and the principle of the 'best for most' is paramount. Trauma, general surgical, and obstetric emergencies may all require treatment.
- *Surgical camps*—several NGOs now provide planned surgical treatments for people living in very remote areas of developing countries where local facilities are primitive. They establish surgical camps with the objective of taking reasonable standards of care to places where such services are not normally available.
- *Expeditions*—polar expeditions, ships' crews, and oil exploration groups may spend prolonged periods in isolation where accidents and acute surgical conditions can occur. Individuals may require treatment necessitating sedation or anaesthesia prior to, or whilst awaiting, evacuation. Minor ailments might also require treatment using local anaesthesia during such expeditions.

When to give an anaesthetic

Some conditions, usually treated by surgery in advanced healthcare facilities, are more safely dealt with in the field by intravenous fluid resuscitation, analgesia, and antibiotics. Examples include acute surgical conditions such as suspected appendicitis, where conservative management should allow sufficient time to arrange evacuation of the patient.

Sedation or anaesthesia may be required to salvage limb or life before evacuation. An example would be lower limb fracture-dislocation with occlusion of the blood supply or associated haemorrhage. The patient must be evacuated as soon as possible, but the limb will be lost unless the dislocation can be reduced and blood flow restored within a short period. Effective sedation or anaesthesia may be a necessary adjunct to fluid resuscitation and analgesia.

Other situations may not require evacuation, but treatment to prevent further complications. Examples include removal of foreign bodies from soft tissues, incision of abscesses, cleansing and suturing of superficial lacerations and wounds. Often local anaesthetic techniques provide a safe and effective way of relieving discomfort.

Use general anaesthesia in the field only as a last resort when there is no other option.

Know your limits

All anaesthetics are potentially dangerous; an anaesthetic given by inexperienced hands can cause more harm than good. When selecting a technique consider:

- The risks and benefits to the patient—both of operating and of doing nothing.
- The physiological state of the patient, especially if they have lost blood, or if illness has led to dehydration. Pre-anaesthetic resuscitation is essential.
- The drugs and equipment available.
- The effects and side-effects of the chosen anaesthetic technique.
- What help is available; simultaneously trying both to operate and look after the patient is very difficult.
- The capabilities of the anaesthetic administrator, and of the surgeon.
- Local or regional anaesthesia is usually safer than general anaesthesia.
- Airway management requires considerable expertise—ventilating a patient using bag and face mask, or insertion of an endotracheal tube or laryngeal mask airway (LMA) should not be attempted unless you have been trained appropriately.
- The side effects of potent drugs and complications of anaesthesia or surgery can be difficult or even impossible to deal with in remote locations.

Local infiltration anaesthesia

Suitable for minor surface surgery such as:
- Wound suturing.
- Small superficial abscesses—although local anaesthetics are less effective in the presence of infection.
- Digital blocks.
- Dental work (see Chapter 10).
- Pain relief—for instance, following some animal bites or stings.

Local anaesthetics can also be used topically on the surface of the eye or other mucous membranes.

Advantages
- Safe.
- Easy to learn.
- Minimal equipment required.
- Additional monitoring (other than clinical) unnecessary.

Disadvantages
- Not appropriate for large or multiple areas, as safe dose may be exceeded.
- The rare, but serious, side effects of local anaesthetic toxicity are a challenge to treat in remote situations.
- Not always effective, especially if affected area is inflamed or infected.
- Inadvertent intravascular injection, or use in a highly vascular area such as the intercostal space between the ribs, may cause systemic toxicity before reaching 'maximum dose'.

Local anaesthetic agents

Lidocaine, bupivacaine, and prilocaine are the commonly available drugs.
Lidocaine and prilocaine have a higher maximum safe dose if adrenaline is added, but do not use adrenaline-containing local anaesthetic drugs on areas supplied by end-arteries such as fingers, toes, tips of ear, or penis, as the circulation to the area may cease.
Multi-use glass vials of local anaesthetics (as opposed to ampoules) designed for skin infiltration often contain preservatives and their contents should not be used for spinal or epidural anaesthesia.

Lidocaine is the most widely available local anaesthetic drug.
Dose: 3 mg/kg plain, up to maximum of 300 mg; or 7 mg/kg with adrenaline, up to maximum of 500 mg. Main toxic effect is to cause convulsions.

Prilocaine can be used in relatively large volumes and is fairly safe, although relatively short-acting.
Dose: 5 mg/kg plain or 8 mg/kg with adrenaline. Up to maximum of 400 mg.

Bupivacaine has a slower onset, but its long duration of action can be useful. Bupivacaine must never be injected intravascularly as it can cause irreversible cardiac arrest. Its isomer levobupivacaine is more expensive, but may be safer.
Dose: with or without adrenaline 2 mg/kg, up to maximum of 150 mg.

To calculate a drug dose:
Drugs in solution are quoted as percentage concentrations.
1% means that 1 g of drug has been dissolved in 100 ml of solvent.

So:
1% solution = 10 mg/ml, 0.25% solution = 2.5 mg/ml.
10 ml of a 1% solution contains 100 mg drug.
10 ml of a 0.25 % solution contains 25 mg.
If maximum permissible dose of a drug is 3 mg/kg and your casualty weighs 70 kg:
   Then you can use up to $3 \times 70 = 210$ mg of the local anaesthetic.
This is equivalent to 21 ml of a 1% solution or 10.5 ml of a 2% solution.

Symptoms and signs of overdose
Mild
- Perioral paraesthesia.
- Tinnitus.
- Metallic taste.
- Blurred vision.

Moderate
- Restlessness.
- Slurred speech.
- Nystagmus.
- Tremor.

Serious
- Fits.
- Coma.
- Hypotension.
- Dysrhythmias.
- Cardiac arrest.

Treatment
- *Stop* injection.
- Resuscitate using ABC approach.
- Diazepam 10 mg or other benzodiazepine drug can be used to treat fits.

Local infiltration techniques
First calculate the maximum safe dose for your casualty based upon their weight and draw calculated volume into a syringe.

If you think a large volume of local anaesthetic may be required, consider using a local anaesthetic solution containing adrenaline (epinephrine) 1:200 000 provided that it is safe to use this vasoconstrictor on the injured part of the body (see above).

Wound infiltration
- Wearing sterile gloves, cleanse the skin with an antiseptic solution.
- Using a fine gauge needle (23 G or 25 G), inject subcutaneously along both sides of the wound. Aspirate prior to injection to avoid intravascular injection. An alternative technique is to inject around the area in a diamond shape with a single entry point at either end of the wound.

Digital nerve block
- Used for surgery distal to the base of the proximal phalanx of fingers or toes. Never use adrenaline-containing solutions as there is a risk of ischaemia. A 25 mm 25 G needle is ideal.
- At the base of the proximal phalanx place needle in a vertical injection from the dorsal aspect until the needle almost reaches the palmar surface. Inject 2–3 ml of 1% lignocaine or prilocaine, or the same dose of 0.25% bupivacaine on each side of the digit, and then add a small additional dose over the dorsum of the digit.

Other peripheral nerve blocks
Other blocks take more skill and practice to perfect. Techniques such as axillary or femoral nerve blocks can be very useful in field situations if you have the experience and skill to administer them. A simple femoral nerve block is described in Chapter 13, p. 430.

Spinal anaesthesia

Spinal anaesthesia is an excellent technique to use in the field, but is not a technique for the inexperienced. It is very suitable for surgery below the umbilicus, such as lower limb surgery.

Contraindications include:

- Hypovolaemia and uncorrected dehydration.
- Generalized sepsis.
- Suspected or known clotting problems.
- Infection at site of injection.
- Spinal anaesthesia is associated with falls in blood pressure: cannulae, intravenous fluids, and vasopressors are essential to counteract this effect. Resuscitation equipment must be available.
- Antiseptic solution, sterile gloves, syringes, and disposable spinal needles are required.
- Vasopressor, e.g. ephedrine 30 mg ampoules—dilute into 10 ml.

Preparation

- Explanation to patient.
- Obtain iv access, ideally with 14 or 16 G cannula.
- Fluid pre-load: 500–1000 ml of crystalloid.
- Vasopressor available, e.g. 30 mg ephedrine in 10 ml saline.
- Check blood pressure.

Procedure

- Same as for a diagnostic lumbar puncture.
- Sit the patient with their feet supported, back arched forwards, vertebrae pushed backwards, and chin tucked towards chest. Useful to have helper.
- Tuffier's line joins the iliac crests crossing the dorsal spine at the fourth lumbar vertebra. Above this line is the L3/4 interspace, and below is the L4/5 interspace. *Do not go above L3 as the needle may injure the spinal cord.* (Fig. 18.1).
- Using sterile gloves, clean a large area around the planned insertion site with antiseptic.
- Raise a subcutaneous wheal of local anaesthetic (e.g. 1% lidocaine) at L3/4 or L4/5.
- Using a 22–29 G disposable spinal needle (preferably 25–29 G as there is less risk of postdural puncture headache), insert the spinal needle at the chosen interspace in the midline. Advance with 15° cephalad (towards the head) angulation until a click or pop is felt at an approximate depth of 4–6 cm (dura punctured). (Fig. 18.2).
- If bone is hit first, withdraw the needle to just below skin and re-insert, usually with more cephalad angulation, checking that you are in the midline.
- Withdraw stylet and check free flow of cerebrospinal fluid. If blood flows, withdraw the spinal needle completely and try again. If the patient complains of shooting pain on insertion, withdraw needle immediately, check pain settles, and try again.

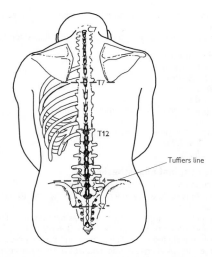

Fig. 18.1 Landmarks for spinal anaesthesia. Reproduced with permission from *Oxford Handbook of Anaesthesia*.

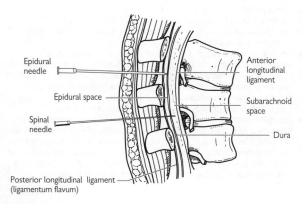

Fig. 18.2 Position for spinal anaesthesia injections. Reproduced with permission from *Oxford Handbook of Anaesthesia*.

- Inject the local, ensuring that the spinal needle is not moved inadvertently.
- Following injection, lie patient on back with legs flexed for 10 min.

Suggested spinal doses

- Heavy 0.5% bupivacaine
  - T6–T10: 2.5–3 ml
  - T11–L1: 2.5 ml
  - L2–L5: 2.0 ml
  - S1–S5 (saddle block): 1.0–1.5 ml (stay sitting)
- Plain 0.5% bupivacaine
  - T6–T10: not reliable
  - T11–L1: 2.5–3.0 ml
  - L2–L5: 2.5 ml.

Monitoring of spinal anaesthesia

- After injection maintain verbal contact with patient.
- Check blood pressure every few minutes for the first 10 min, then every 5 min.
- Nausea is quite common—it often indicates hypotension. Treat with fluids and a vasopressor such as ephedrine 3–6 mg boluses iv.
- Opioids, often included in spinal injections in hospital practice, should not be added to spinal anaesthetic mixtures used in the field as they may cause delayed respiratory depression.
- Before surgery starts, test that the patient has lost their sense of pain in the relevant area.
- A spinal bupivacaine injection should last for 2–4 h.
- Urinary retention may occur.
- Patients can mobilize after the block has completely worn off.
- The spread of blocks is more variable if plain, as opposed to heavy or hyperbaric solution, is used.
- Beware of 'high blocks'. The patient will notice numbness or weakness in their arms and may find it difficult to take a deep breath. High blocks can result in more extreme falls in blood pressure, which require treatment with vasoconstrictors. Supplementary oxygen should be given if available. Monitor the patient carefully to ensure that a high block does not progress to a total spinal block.
- Excessive cephalad spread of a large volume of local anaesthetic can produce a 'total spinal' in which all the muscles of respiration can be involved. Consciousness can be lost. Treatment is with fluids, ephedrine, and resuscitation on an ABC approach. A rare complication and very scary to all concerned, the patient should make a full recovery providing their breathing and circulation are properly managed.

Ketamine anaesthesia

Ketamine is widely used in field and developing world anaesthesia. Its ease of administration should not tempt the inexperienced to use it except in desperate circumstances.

- Produces a dissociative state with profound analgesia and light anaesthesia.
- Ideal sole agent for induction and maintenance of anaesthesia.
- Sympathetic tone is maintained—good for 'shocked patients'.
- A safe airway is usually maintained, although pulmonary aspiration can occasionally occur. Ketamine does not depress respiration, a benefit if anaesthesia is required at altitude.
- Doses can be given as intravenous boluses, intravenous infusions, or intramuscularly.
- Can be used in low 'sedative-analgesic' doses for reduction of fractures, splint application, small abscess drainage, and burns dressings.
- Anaesthetized patients often have involuntary movements; their eyes may remain disconcertingly open.
- Some patients get unpleasant hallucinations following ketamine anaesthesia. Small doses of benzodiazepines (diazepam 2–5 mg or midazolam 2–5 mg) can reduce this problem.
- Resuscitation equipment must be available.
- Administer supplemental oxygen when available.

Monitoring

Clinical and, if available, blood pressure and pulse oximetry.

Doses

- Intravenous bolus for anaesthesia:
  - Induction: 1–2 mg/kg. Onset 1–2 min, lasts 10–15 min.
  - Maintenance: 0.5–1 mg/kg iv every 15–20 min.
- Intramuscular dose for anaesthesia:
  - 8–10 mg/kg im. Onset 5 min, duration 20–30 min.
- Continuous infusion—for longer cases:
  - Add 500 mg of ketamine to a 500 ml bag of crystalloid fluid (=1 mg/ml).
  - Give iv bolus of 1–2 mg/kg, followed by a maintenance dose of 0.5–1 drop/kg/min (2–4 mg/kg/h). May be used with spontaneous ventilation or after intubation for controlled ventilation.
  - Stop infusion 30 min before expected procedure end.
- Sedation–analgesia:
  - 0.3–0.8 mg/kg iv or 2–4 mg/kg im.
- Whenever ketamine is used:
  - Salivation increases. Consider atropine (0.6 mg iv) at induction.
  - 'Emergence phenomenon' can be unpleasant; minimize stimulation to patient whilst waking. Consider iv benzodiazepine, such as diazepam or midazolam 0.1 mg/kg with induction.

Sedation

Defined as a state of reduced consciousness where verbal contact with patient is maintained. It differs from 'anaesthesia' where verbal contact is lost. Sedation can help during uncomfortable procedures, e.g. manipulation of a fracture.

Sedation is produced by use of a benzodiazepine drug, or the combination of a benzodiazepine with an opiate painkiller, but beware that opiate/benzodiazepine combinations are much more potent than either drug given alone and it is very easy to over-sedate.

Best titrated carefully by the intravenous route.

Benefits

- May avoid need for general anaesthesia.
- As an adjunct to a local anaesthetic technique.
- Hypnosis, anxiolysis, anterograde amnesia, and some muscle relaxation.
- Quicker recovery than general anaesthesia.

Hazards

- Risk of cardiorespiratory depression. Must have resuscitation equipment available.
- Side effects of sedating drugs can be difficult to treat in remote areas.
- Ideally should have antidote reversal agents available: naloxone 0.1–0.4 mg iv or im to reverse opiate respiratory depression and flumazenil 0.1–1.0 mg to reverse the effects of benzodiazepines.
- A poorly delivered sedative technique can be more dangerous than a planned general anaesthetic.
- As with general anaesthesia, there is a risk of gastric aspiration when not starved.

Typical sedation drugs

- Midazolam—0.07–0.1 mg/kg iv initially if used as sole sedative; additional doses carefully titrated to response.
- Diazepam—2.5–10 mg iv, initially, carefully titrated to response.
- If opiate painkillers such as morphine, pethidine, or fentanyl have been given previously, or are administered simultaneously, there is a greatly increased risk of respiratory depression. The benzodiazepine should be given in small doses of 1–2 mg, with a gap of at least 3 min between each dose to give time for effects to develop.

Suggested minimum equipment and drugs for field anaesthesia

Airway
- Self-inflating bag and selection of face masks.
- Oral (Guedel) airways and nasal airways.
- Portable, e.g. hand- or foot-powered, suction unit. Suction catheters.
- Laryngoscope and blades plus spare bulbs and batteries.
- Oral endotracheal tubes with 15 mm connectors.
- Gum elastic bougie.

Intravenous
- Selection of cannulae, needles, and syringes.
- Tourniquet, securing tape, or dressings for cannulae.
- Crystalloid, e.g. Hartmanns or 0.9% sodium chloride.
- Colloid such as Gelofusine.
- Giving sets.

Resuscitation
- Adrenaline, atropine.
- Ephedrine.

Local anaesthetic
- Lidocaine/bupivacaine for local anaesthesia.
- Preservative-free 'heavy' bupivacaine 0.5% for spinal anaesthetic.

Anaesthetic/sedation drugs
- Ketamine, benzodiazepine such as midazolam.
- Opioid such as morphine, or other analgesic such as tramadol.
- Naloxone and flumazenil to reverse above.
- If intubation a possibility, muscle relaxant and neostigmine.

Spinal
- Spinal needles: 22, 25, or 27 G needles.

Monitoring
- Portable battery-powered pulse oximeter, stethoscope, sphygmomanometer.

Miscellaneous
- Antiseptic cleaning solution, sterile and non-sterile gloves, sterile swabs.
- Nasogastric tubes, scissors.
- Torch/headlight.

Local facilities
- Will possibly have use of local hospital facilities.
  - Likely to be basic, especially in developing countries.
  - If possible, rely on own equipment and drugs.

Oxygen sources
- Compressed oxygen cylinders may have faulty or pressure gauges, making estimation of remaining supply unreliable.
- May not have reliable labelling or colour coding of cylinders.

- Oxygen concentrators are reliable if serviced and power supply guaranteed; these yield approximately 90% oxygen at flows <4 l. With age the concentration may decrease.
- Ideally use techniques not dependent on oxygen availability.

Drugs

- Drugs sourced in developing countries have less quality assurance.
- Store drugs appropriately, especially muscle relevants such as suxamethonium and atracurium, which should be kept cool, especially in the tropics.
- Be vigilant of 'use by' dates.

Anaesthetic delivery equipment

- Carefully check any anaesthetic equipment if you plan to use it. Is it safe/complete?
- Draw-over vaporizers and Oxford inflating bellows are reliable if well serviced.
- Halothane vaporizer can be cleaned with trilene or ether.
- Ether still used in developing world.
- The use of unfamiliar equipment by the inexperienced is dangerous.

Monitoring

- Equipment may be poorly maintained, incomplete, or faulty.
- Pulse oximeter often available. ECG and automated blood pressure usually absent.
- Clinical observation—mucous membrane colour, capillary refill, central pulses, and precordial stethoscope are all useful.
- Ideally utilize a conscious anaesthetic technique, e.g. spinal or regional/local.

Further reading

Allman KG, Wilson IH (2002). *Oxford Handbook of Anaesthesia*. Oxford, Oxford University Press.
Dobson MB (2000). *Anaesthesia at the District Hospital*. Geneva, World Health Organization.
Vreede E (2001). *Field Anaesthesia—Basic Practice*. Medecins sans Frontieres.
    E-mail: guide.anaesthesia@msf.org

Cold climates

Chris Johnson, and Howard Oakley

The environment

Polar environments surround both poles and extend to lower latitudes during winter. Similar conditions are found at high altitudes anywhere on earth. The predominance of snow in a polar climate disguises the fact that many polar environments have very little precipitation; Antarctica is one of the driest places on earth, but winds move the snow around, regularly generating blizzard conditions. Sub-Arctic continental environments such as the Yukon, Alaska, and Siberia have bitterly cold winters, but their summers can be mild or even hot, with a rich diversity of wildlife, flowers, insects, and even a significant risk of huge forest fires.

The dominant factors in polar climates are air temperature, wind speed, and sunlight. Around freezing point, high humidity (freezing fog) can make conditions feel bitterly cold, but humidity falls at lower temperatures and ceases to be a significant influence.

The windchill index combines temperature and wind speed to estimate the hazard to humans of the environment. Formulated by Siple and Passel in 1945, the original calculations were based upon the rate at which plastic bags of water froze. North American studies in 2003 instead studied the rate of cooling of exposed human faces, and derived a complex mathematical formula[1] to calculate the cooling effect of the climate. In practice it is easier to use tables such as Figs. 19.1 and 19.2 to judge the hazard of the prevailing environmental conditions.

Prevailing meteorological conditions may be modified by local circumstances; for instance, wind speed and therefore windchill are reduced by contour features, trees and clothing, but increased by skiing or travelling on a skidoo. Temperatures may be lower in sheltered valleys, but travel that is safe in the valley can become dangerous when crossing an exposed and windy pass. Bright sunshine raises the apparent temperature considerably. Careless behaviour can lead to frostbite in conditions that should pose a low physical risk.

Websites

http://www.mb.ec.gc.ca/air/wintersevere/windchill.en.html
http://www.nws.noaa.gov/om/windchill/index.shtml

---

1 Windchill $= 13.12 + 0.6215T - 11.37(V^{0.16}) + 0.3965T(V^{0.16})$ where windchill is given as an apparent temperature. T is the air temperature in °C; V is the meteorological windspeed in km/h measured at five foot.

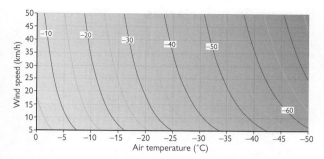

Fig. 19.1 Windchill index. Reproduced with the permission of the Minister of Public Works and Government Services Canada, 2007.

The following are approximate values

Temperature (°C) Wind (km/h)	−15	−20	−25	−30	−35	−40	−45	−50
10	*	*	22	15	10	8	7	2
20	*	30	14	10	5	4	3	2
30	*	18	11	8	5	2	2	1
40	42	14	9	5	5	2	2	1
50	27	12	8	5	2	2	2	1
60	22	10	7	5	2	2	2	1
70	18	9	5	4	2	2	2	1
80	16	8	5	4	2	2	2	1

*Frostbite unlikely.
The wind speed, in km/h, is at the standard anemometer height of 10m (as reported in weather observations).

Frostbite possible in 2 min or less — 2

Frostbite possible in 3–5 min — 5

Frostbite possible in 6–10 min — 10

Fig. 19.2 Windchill—minutes to frostbite. Reproduced with the permission of the Minister of Public Works and Government Services Canada, 2007.

Humans in polar areas

Humans have little physiological ability to acclimatize to cold environments. The only proven response to chronic cold exposure is the Lewis 'hunting response'. Fit, experienced workers who regularly expose their hands to temperatures below 5°C can develop a cyclical vasodilatation of the skin vessels that enables them to maintain higher mean hand temperatures than new arrivals in a cold environment. At a time when hunting and fishing required hand agility at low temperatures, this mechanism had survival benefit. However, most modern polar travellers will not regularly expose their hands to such low temperatures, and those who do run the risk of suffering recurrent minor cold injury instead of acclimatizing. Native peoples in circumpolar areas have a short, stocky build, suggesting that an endomorphic body shape has survival benefits in very cold climates.

Travellers in cold dry climates encounter few problems if the temperature is above −10°C. As temperatures fall further:
- The need to humidify dry air causes the nose to drip.
- Facial and anorak hood encrustation with icicles develops.
- Lips become dry and cracked—a good moisturizing sunscreen is essential. During prolonged arctic journeys travellers can have serious problems with lip ulceration and bleeding.
- Bright sunlight can cause snow blindness, but sunglasses or goggles can be difficult to use in very cold conditions as condensation from forehead or eyes freezes on their surface.
- Strenuous exercise in very low temperatures, below −40°C, can result in chest pain, possibly caused by very cold air reaching the bronchi. Asthma is commoner amongst cross country skiers than in the general population.

Chronic conditions that may be exacerbated by cold dry air include:
- Cold-induced asthma.
- Peripheral circulatory problems, including Raynaud's syndrome, and the presence of cold agglutinins in the blood.
- Angina.
- Sufferers from these conditions should consider whether they will be able to travel and work safely—if in doubt test the effects of the cold by persuading your local butcher to let you into the cold store.

Children

Children can be safely taken into cold climates, but must be properly dressed and closely supervised as they can lose body heat rapidly. Early signs of chilling include grumpiness and a reluctance to move. Young children should not be carried in backpacks in the cold; the parent may slip and fall, while the youngster's legs can become constricted by the base of the pack, resulting in poor circulation and cold injury to the legs. Ski pulks—sledges for towing youngsters in the snow—are popular in Scandinavia; legislation bans their use if the air temperature is below −10°C. Parents or guides should regularly check to ensure that their charges' hands and feet have not become numb.

Preparations for a polar trip

- Dental check-up as problems may be exacerbated by the cold.
- Physical and mental endurance are essential on multi-day trips. Middle-aged participants in 'adventure' holidays that involve long distances skiing, snow-shoeing, or pulling sledges must have prepared properly.
- Consider rabies vaccination if the disease is endemic amongst local sledge dogs.
- Appropriate insurance is essential; it remains difficult, dangerous, and very expensive to evacuate casualties from remote polar areas.
- Tents, skis, and other equipment must be appropriate to the area visited and capable of surviving extreme conditions.

Bases and campsites

Polar expeditions will usually choose a permanent building as a base camp for their work. When the camp involves several buildings, doorways should be linked by hand-lines, as it is easy to become disorientated in dark and in a blizzard. This particularly applies to latrines sited some distance from the base. Fire is a serious threat in areas where water is not available to extinguish flames. Fuel should be stored away from the main base building, and there should be an emergency dump of clothing and food in case of serious conflagration.

Snow holes are warmer than tents in extreme conditions, but more laborious to construct. Tents and snow holes must be positioned away from avalanche runs and trails; both should be well marked so that vehicles and skiers do not accidentally cross them, and they can be re-located in poor weather.

Carbon monoxide poisoning

Carbon monoxide poisoning and dangerously low oxygen levels are both serious risks in closed areas if candles or cooking stoves are used. If a candle flame burns low or goes out, oxygen levels are dangerously low. Carbon monoxide from cooking stoves is odourless and causes insidious poisoning. Headache and nausea usually precede unconsciousness, but the cause may not be apparent to fatigued travellers, or at altitude where such symptoms are common. Tents designed for extreme conditions are very windproof, particularly if they become partially buried in drifting snow; ventilators may block with condensation and must be checked regularly. Deaths have occurred. Supplementary oxygen should be given to a survivor and the victim evacuated. If facilities exist in the area, hyperbaric oxygen is a valuable treatment.

Water, fluids, and personal hygiene

Fresh water can usually be obtained by melting snow, and is safe to drink unless it comes from an area frequented by animals or birds. But large amounts of fuel[2] are needed to melt snow, particularly at very low temperatures, so whenever practical dig or drill through overlying snow to obtain stream water running below. The upper layers of sea ice usually contain little salt and are potable. In the Northern hemisphere, deer and beaver may live close to apparently pristine melt streams and can contaminate the water with *Giardia*. Glacier outwash streams contain fine, highly abrasive rock dust in suspension; this is a powerful laxative. If in doubt, filter water and then boil or sterilize it (📖 p. 106).

Because polar air is very dry, sweat evaporates quickly and fluid losses may be underestimated. Dehydration is a risk during the first days of an expedition; even if people do not feel thirsty, they should drink sufficiently to ensure that they urinate dilute, pale urine. A combination of malaise, headache, and raised body temperature is common when groups first arrive in the cold; this may be a mild form of heat exhaustion. Bathing in cold climates is a masochistic pastime. On shorter expeditions and

---

2 At least double the fuel requirements for your stove if temperature is minus 40°C.

when facilities permit, people and clothes should be washed whenever possible to prevent fungal skin infections and boils. In the field, 'wet wipes' can provide a practical way of maintaining hygiene. However, without washing, the Inuit and members of prolonged field expeditions develop a natural balance with their body oils and the risk of infection reduces. To avoid offence, it is wise to shower shortly after returning to heated accommodation!

Food

Around base camp, or travelling using motorized transport, energy requirements will be similar to those of an outdoor worker in the UK (3000 kcal/12000 kJ per day), but manhauling sledges and cross country skiing are extremely energetic pastimes requiring two to four times this energy intake. A greater proportion of the diet is likely to be made up of fatty foods. In the past, polar expeditions have lived off the land, but nowadays most Arctic species are protected and licences are required before they are hunted. The internal organs of some polar animals contain toxic amounts of Vitamin A and should never be eaten. When travelling in areas where big mammals hunt, you should ensure that food is stored appropriately. Airtight containers in rucksacks and animal-proof food dumps reduce the risk of unwanted visitors.

Sanitation

Polar environments are extremely fragile ecosystems in which organic matter degrades very slowly. Removing waste is your gift to future generations. In Antarctica, expeditions are required to ship out all their waste, including faeces and sanitary materials. National Parks in North America also have specific requirements about waste disposal.

Communications

Satellite beacons (emergency position-indicating beacons; EPIRBs) may be worth taking if there are sophisticated emergency services in the area. Mobile phone coverage extends to fairly remote areas of Scandinavia; satellite phones are valuable, though expensive, when beyond the range of terrestrial equipment. In 2008, only the Iridium system guarantees polar coverage. Avalanche transceivers are essential in mountainous areas. Short wave radio communications are disrupted by auroral activity.

Clothing

Clothing should be adequate to prevent body cooling, but excess clothing leads to a build-up of body heat and sweating, which is undesirable as perspiration condenses in clothes, reducing their insulation. Modern anoraks often incorporate side and underarm zips to improve ventilation and heat dissipation. Although modern breathable synthetic fabrics function adequately in cold dry climates, many experts prefer cotton 'ventile' shell garments. After prolonged use without washing, woollen base layers such as merino are less malodorous than synthetics. Energetic cross country skiers often wear thin garments, but must carry windproofs in case conditions change; the groin area can become painfully cold and requires effective thermal protection, for instance using thermal windproof underpants. If such 'wind-pants' are not worn, the penis is alarmingly vulnerable to frostbite. At any rest or meal break, conserve heat by zipping up anorak vents, and by putting on scarf, hats, and gloves.

Mittens are superior to gloves at retaining peripheral heat in very cold climates. Chemical hand warmers are useful when hands or feet become uncomfortably cold, and are a great morale booster for children in the snow, but should be used with caution if peripheries have become numb, as there is the risk of thermal injury. Loose fitting, well-insulated footwear, with gaiters to prevent snow getting onto socks, are desirable. Battery-powered heated insoles are available if feet are to be exposed to the cold for lengthy periods at low exercise levels; for instance, when travelling by skidoo, or making scientific observations. Whenever possible, boots should be warmed and dried; over a period of days they accumulate moisture and can freeze if taken off in a tent overnight.

Eyes

Eyes must be protected from UV glare by appropriate sunglasses or goggles (see Snow blindness, below). For those with visual defects, contact lenses, prescription sunglasses or spectacles with photochromic lenses all work reasonably well. Wearing ordinary spectacles under goggles is cumbersome. Anyone whose vision is so poor that they always need to wear glasses or contact lenses must plan to avoid the difficulties that would arise from loss or breakage: as a minimum, a spare pair of spectacles should be taken. Below –20°C glasses invariably mist over, and contact lenses may be preferable. However, contact lenses can adhere or even freeze to the eye. Forced or clumsy removal can then result in corneal abrasion, requiring topical treatment with antibiotics and local anaesthetic (📖 p. 309).

Metal spectacle frames can become very cold and cause cold injury if in direct contact with the skin; opticians sell silicone sheaths that cover the side arms. Plastic-framed glasses or snow goggles are preferable, but become brittle at low temperatures. Carry spare filters for goggles as these too can crack after prolonged exposure to the cold.

Infectious disease

In the past, imported infectious diseases such as diphtheria, measles, and tuberculosis tragically decimated circumpolar native populations, but infectious diseases are nowadays uncommon in polar areas. Some sledge dogs carry rabies, and inoculation is advisable if the expedition is visiting an endemic area. Sexually transmitted infections have a worldwide distribution. After prolonged residence in a cold climate—for instance, over-wintering on a polar base—travellers will be particularly susceptible to upper respiratory tract infections.

Risk management

Novice travellers in polar climates encounter many unfamiliar hazards.

Environmental	Medical
Low temperatures	Hypothermia
High winds	Frostnip
Whiteout	Frostbite
Avalanche	Sunburn
Crevasse	Snow blindness
Shifting sea ice	Trench foot
Wildlife (especially bears)	Contaminated water
Thin lake, stream, or marsh ice	Dehydration
Transport (ski and skidoo)	Slips and falls
Insects in summer season	Recreational hazards

Animal hazards (📖 p. 518)

Animal life at the two poles differs considerably. In the south hazards are rare, and can be avoided by watching animals from a sensible distance and keeping away from the sea ice edge. Research scientists are at greater risk. Killer whales and leopard seals are potential threats in or on the water and ice edge. Fur seals bite intruders in their colonies, while bull elephant seals will aggressively guard their territory. At both poles, birds, particularly terns, will attack intruders on nesting sites by flying at their heads; an umbrella or walking pole may prevent collisions.

In northern areas, bears, wolves, elk, and moose pose substantial threats. By far the commonest problem occurs on roads at night. Moose use roads as convenient thoroughfares and frequently collide with cars, sadly often with fatal results to both animal and humans. In Newfoundland there are about 700 moose/vehicle collisions each year, and elk create serious problems for Scandinavian drivers. Away from roads, these large animals can also be a threat. Avoid approaching male moose during the autumn rutting season, and do not stray between a mother and her calf. At other times, the animals are generally placid and can be safely observed from a distance.

Bears are a danger. In North American tourist areas national park rangers monitor bear activity and offer advice about travel, closing campsites and trails if aggressive bears have been reported. Advice on dealing with a bear encounter is widely available (see http://www.canadianrockies.net/backpack.html#bear).

Most bears prefer to keep away from humans and will move on if parties make noisy progress through the wilderness. Brown and grizzly bears usually hibernate in winter and are the greatest threat if early autumn snow forces them down from the mountains into tourist areas. Do not leave food where it is accessible to bears. They become accustomed to this easy source of food, threaten humans, and then have to be culled or transported to very remote areas. Travellers on back-country trails should carry pepper sprays.

Polar bears are a serious danger, particularly in areas such as Northern Canada and Svalbard (Spitzbergen), which are increasingly popular adventure tourism destinations. Campsites can be protected by a perimeter alarm system of ropes, bells, or empty cans; sledge dog teams can be spanned around the periphery, and it may be essential to carry firearms (📖 p. 518).

During the summer huge numbers of biting insects breed in the ponds and marshes of low Arctic regions; clothing with ankle and wrist elastics, and midge hoods will make life bearable.

Recreation hazards

Visitors to snowy areas want to enjoy the recreational opportunities, but the environment is not always accorded the respect it deserves. Icy areas around living accommodation are a common place for injuries—spread grit or ash to improve grip. Skiing, snowboarding, and sledging are hazardous, and an expedition with scientific goals and limited medical back-up must minimize the risk that team members injure themselves during their leisure time. Rocks may be frost-fractured and unstable, while ice climbing is a high-risk pastime.

Tracked vehicles have small turning circles and unprotected machinery. Noise and limited visibility prevents their drivers from being fully aware of their surrounding—skiers and pedestrians must stay well away. Skidoos range from slow load haulers to racing vehicles; keep your legs and arms inboard, follow trail rules, and beware of wire fences.

Cold weather and alcohol don't mix. Drunkenness leads to injuries and the risk of hypothermia. Many circumpolar peoples have exceptionally low alcohol tolerance and should not be encouraged to drink alcohol, particularly when they are in the field.

Supplies

Cold will affect many items, including batteries, contact lens fluids, and drugs. Aqueous drugs freeze, crystallize, and may degrade in the cold; therefore powdered preparations and plastic containers should be selected whenever possible. Critical items can be kept warm by body heat or heat packs used to maintain temperature.

Website

For Antarctic news and information: http://70south.com/home

Hypothermia

Hypothermia

Hypothermia is a fall of the victim's core body temperature to an extent that their ability to function normally is impaired. Normal core temperature is 36.5–37°C. Temperatures below 35°C usually cause symptoms that are similar to drunkenness; the victim is confused, poorly coordinated, and falls frequently. They may shiver uncontrollably, but do not always do so. They may vehemently deny that anything is wrong and reject help. Untreated, they will eventually become comatose and die. Fig. 19.3 indicates the approximate temperatures at which serious malfunction develops.

In the field, diagnosis can be difficult, but anyone whose torso feels 'as cold as marble' should be treated as a cold casualty. Diagnosis can be confirmed by measuring body temperature using a low reading rectal thermometer, preferably a calibrated electronic device with the sensor inserted to 15 cm beyond the anal sphincter. Conventional oral thermometers do not measure low body temperatures, and infrared tympanic membrane thermometers can be inaccurate by several degrees, particularly when the ear has been exposed to cold, heat, or water.

Body core temperature (°C)	Associated symptoms
37	Normal body temperature
36	
35	Judgement may be affected: poor decision–making
	Feels cold, looks cold, shivering
34	Change of personality, usually withdrawn—'switches off/doesn't care'
	Inappropriate behaviour—may shed clothing
	Stumbling, falling, confused
33	Consciousness clouded, incoherent
	Shivering stops
32	Serious risk of cardiac arrest
	Body cannot restore temperature without help
	Limbs stiffen
31	Unconscious
30	Pulse and breathing undetectable
29	
28	Pupils become fixed and dilated
27	
26	
25	
24	Few victims recover from this temperature
23	
22	
21	
20	
19	
18	
17	
16	
15	
14	Lowest recorded temperature of survival

Fig. 19.3 Symptoms of hypothermia.

Prevention

Hypothermia is uncommon in a properly clothed fit person, but develops if someone is injured, lost, short of food and/or water, or if their clothing is inadequate or wet, especially in windy conditions. Typically it develops insidiously over several hours, but death (usually from 'cold shock' or drowning when disabled by hypothermia) can occur within minutes if someone is immersed in cold water.

Field management

Experts disagree about the best treatment for severe hypothermia and this has led to conflicting advice in textbooks. However, the controversies are irrelevant to most expeditions as they are unlikely to carry the advanced resuscitation equipment now available to mountain rescue groups. The aim of treatment is to restore the body heat of the victim.

- Seek shelter—building, tent, snow hole, survival bag, or group shelter.
- Remove damp outer clothing. Wrap casualty in additional dry insulation such as a sleeping bag. If this is impossible, place inside a heavy plastic bag and seal around the neck to eliminate evaporative heat loss. Do not bother using inefficient 'space blankets'.
- Lie down and insulate from the ground using, for instance, rucksacks.
- If conscious:
  - Restore body heat by providing warm drinks (not alcohol), warming the air with a stove, and sharing the body heat of unaffected rescuers.
  - Chemical heat pads can be helpful if they are available, but ensure that they do not cause burns.
  - Do not give alcohol.
  - Ensure casualty rests and is kept under close supervision for at least 24 h.
- If unconscious or body temperature very low:
  - Ensure breathing does not obstruct, try to prevent further heat loss, arrange urgent evacuation if feasible
  - Rewarm using any method that can be improvised
  - Support circulation with warmed iv fluids if available.

It may be very difficult to tell whether a hypothermic casualty is dead or alive. Breathing will be slow and shallow, while the pulse may be slow, thready and palpable only in the neck and groin. If unsure, assume that the casualty is alive. In an isolated base camp, the best than can be done is to keep the victim as warm as possible, ensure that their breathing does not obstruct and, if possible, infuse some warmed intravenous fluid to maintain hydration. The patient needs to be turned regularly to ensure that they are not lying in one position for a prolonged period. Advanced life support measures such as intubation or the insertion of a laryngeal mask airway can precipitate intractable ventricular fibrillation, but may sometimes be a necessary risk. Similarly, starting external cardiac massage may tip the hypothermic heart into ventricular fibrillation. Once started, cardiac massage should be maintained until the patient has been rewarmed or delivered to a hospital: in very remote areas this makes it inadvisable to start massage because evacuation will be impractical.

If you do start CPR, it is clearly difficult to give evidence-based advice on how long to continue. Following immersion in very cold water, there have been cases of full recovery following several hours of external cardiac massage. The most effective form of rewarming from severe hypothermia is extracorporeal circulatory rewarming, but this will require rapid evacuation to a tertiary care hospital. Declaring a victim dead is more confidently done if they are warm, but the difficulty here lies in warming up someone in the wilderness enough to be able to do this.

The Scottish Mountain Safety Forum in 1997 produced guidelines to assist with decision-making (Fig. 19.4).

Sequelae

Recovery from mild hypothermia is usually uneventful, although the victim may feel exhausted for hours or a few days. Although rare, fulminating acute pancreatitis can cause rapid deterioration during or after rewarming. Severe hypothermia, especially if the patient has been unconscious for some time, requires careful monitoring in hospital. Peritoneal lavage, bladder irrigation, and cardiopulmonary bypass can be used to rewarm the casualty. Arrhythmias, muscle damage, and kidney failure can develop. Maintaining the patient at 33°C for 48 h before fully rewarming may reduce complications.

	Criteria	Action
Definitely alive	Conscious	Insulate from heat loss Rewarm Monitor regularly Evacuate
Definitely alive	Unconscious Respiration and/or pulse present	Insulate from heat loss Rewarm only after arrival at hospital Maintain airway Evacuate in recovery position
May be alive	No respiration No circulation (1 min) Clear airway No obvious fatal injury Temperature below 32°C	Radio/phone for medical advice with evacuation plan Rewarm only after arrival at hospital
Definitely dead	No respiration No circulation (1 min) Airway blocked Obvious fatal injury Temperature below 32°C	Evacuate as dead

Fig. 19.4 Recommendations for evacuation of cold-injured.

Cold injury (Fig. 19.5)

Frostnip

Frostnip is a superficial reversible freezing of the skin surface, which resolves completely within 30 min of starting to rewarm the frozen part. In the field, it looks as though pale wax has been dropped on the skin. Typically affecting parts of the body that are exposed to prevailing cold and wind, such as chin, cheeks, and earlobes, frostnip is rare if the environmental temperature is above $-10°C$, but common in conditions below $-25°C$. Strong winds, either natural, or generated by travel (running, skiing, or skidooing), increase the risk. Some experienced cold-weather travellers believe they can feel the onset of frostnip as a sudden burning 'ping' sensation. Once established, the lesions are numb and painless.

Pathophysiology

There is vasoconstriction of the skin blood vessels and freezing of the outermost layers of the skin. Deeper tissues are unaffected.

Prevention

Novice visitors to very cold climates must be constantly aware of the dangers of the environment. Using a system of 'buddy' pairs is sensible if travelling in adverse conditions, with the buddies checking each other regularly for cold injuries. Try to protect your face from high winds using a facemask or the hood of an anorak. If working outdoors, turn your face away from the full force of the wind. Metal in contact with the skin, for instance metal-framed spectacles, earrings, or other facial piercings, makes chilling more likely. For men, the protective value of beards is a hotly debated topic. In some Scandinavian countries, ointments are sold that are claimed to reduce the risk of cold injury. Evidence suggests that these are not effective and some may actually increase the risk of injury.

Treatment

Frostnip should be treated as soon as possible, before permanent tissue injury develops. The skin can be gently warmed by blowing exhaled air across the affected skin, or by contact with a warm ungloved hand. Do not rubbed nipped areas. Once rewarmed, the affected area will look red and may tingle or burn. Frostnip is an indication that weather conditions are hazardous and additional skin protection is required or shelter should be sought. No additional treatment is required.

Sequelae

Initially the area will look red and may be slightly swollen, but the skin will return to normal rapidly. Once frostnipped, the affected areas of skin are susceptible to repeat injury. If the cold injury does not resolve within 30 min, if a zone is repeatedly injured, or if the skin blisters, the condition should be regarded as frostbite, the casualty evacuated, and treated accordingly.

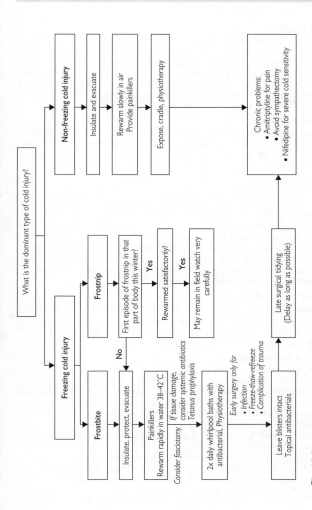

Fig. 19.5 Treatment algorithm for cold injury.

Frostbite

Frostbite is freezing of body tissues, with extensive damage to the affected areas. This type of injury is most likely to occur in novices in polar areas who do not care for themselves properly. Serious frostbite injury is rare in experienced travellers, but develops following serious injury, immersion in cold water, or when extreme weather conditions prevent travel. Dehydration and high altitude substantially increase the risk of frostbite. The affected part will be cold, white, numb, and rigid.

Pathophysiology

Frostbitten tissues are seriously damaged, cell structures being disrupted through the formation of ice crystals and osmotic damage to the cells. Circulation will cease in the affected area with muscles frozen and no nerve conduction.

Prevention

Consider carefully whether travel is necessary in severe weather conditions, dress appropriately, drink sufficient fluids, and pair off using the 'buddy' system. Avoid tight clothing and boots that may restrict circulation. Tape gloves to clothing so that they cannot be lost in a gale, and carry spare hat, gloves, and socks. Do not ignore painfully cold hands and feet; try to rewarm affected parts as soon as possible and seek shelter urgently. Never immerse hands or feet in seawater near freezing: seawater typically freezes at temperatures below the freezing point of tissues, making severe frostbite a common result. Beware of cold fuels.

Field management

Frostbite injuries are always serious and the casualty must be evacuated. Although undesirable, a victim can continue to travel with a frozen limb, but, once the affected area has been thawed, they will be incapacitated. Try to protect the numb area from further damage until shelter is reached.

Initial base management

- Once shelter and safety are reached the limb can be thawed.
- Give the victim painkillers; the rewarming process will be very painful.
- Place the affected part in clean water and warm the water quickly and carefully to 40°C. Ensure that the water never becomes hot enough to cause additional thermal damage. Stir the water constantly to ensure good heat transfer.
- Once warmed, protect the damaged areas from pressure and do not allow them to re-freeze.
- Cover raw areas with sterile dressings and change regularly.
- Wherever possible leave blisters intact. Although some experts suggest removing the tops from white, but not blood blisters, discuss before following this treatment pathway.
- Treat with a simple antibiotic (penicillin, erythromycin); a non-steroidal painkiller such as ibuprofen provides both pain relief and may improve healing.

Severe limb frostbite

The only reason for delaying rapid rewarming is if an arm or leg is very badly frozen. In such cases, the cellular structure of the deep tissues has been seriously damaged. As the tissues thaw, they swell, and pressures in the deep fascial compartments of the limb can exceed arterial pressure, leading to complete ischaemia. Fasciotomy prior to rewarming can prevent this disaster. Appropriate surgical follow up will be required to close wounds and repair skin defects.

Sequelae

In the early phase after rewarming, the affected area will look red, blistered, and severely swollen. Raw areas leak copious amounts of serous fluid. Later, peripheral parts of affected limbs will turn black and mummify. Systemic antibiotics and tetanus prophylaxis should be given to anyone who has significant amounts of dead or dying tissue.

The mainstay of continuing treatment is the whirlpool bath into which affected parts are placed for 30 min twice daily. An appropriate antibacterial should be added to the water. Exposure in a warm environment and early mobilization should be encouraged; smoking should be forbidden.

In temperate climates, where frostbite is very rare, vascular surgeons are familiar only with dry gangrene caused by vascular insufficiency. Such patients have deep-seated, often painful, gangrene, and require amputations. Frostbite injuries can look very similar but the damage is usually more superficial and, unless infection develops, surgical interventions should be avoided until a natural demarcation line becomes obvious between dead and healthy tissue. Better scanning techniques and anti-prostaglandin drugs are improving the outlook for patients with serious frostbite injuries.

Non-freezing cold injury

Non-freezing cold injury is a protean condition that occurs in cold, wet conditions ('trench foot'), shipwreck survivors ('immersion foot'), wet jungle ('paddy foot'), even those with dependent and immobile legs ('shelter limb'). Common to these is a period of relative ischaemia in the feet or hands, during which there is impairment or loss of sensation, followed by hyperaemia when they are rewarmed, often accompanied by lasting and severe pain. Predisposing factors are similar to those of frostbite, but tissues do not freeze. Cold exposure is longer in duration, typically hours or days, although non-freezing cold injury can occur in less than an hour. Individuals of African ethnicity are particularly susceptible to developing the condition.

Pathophysiology

Although less understood than frostbite, current evidence suggests that cold and ischaemia damage nerves and the vascular endothelium in local tissues. Rewarming then results in further damage from free radicals and inflammation.

Prevention

High standards of foot care are essential, with frequent regular replacement of wet socks with dry ones, and wiggling of toes to try to maintain local blood flow. Even assiduous care can only postpone the onset of injury, so periodic removal from cold, wet conditions is also necessary. Footwear that relies on eliminating evaporative heat loss ('vapour barrier') or surrounding the feet with impermeable materials leads to accumulation of sweat next to the skin, resulting in non-freezing cold injury. Foot care routines and drying are even more important when rubberized or impermeable boots are worn.

Management

Cases that present before rewarming must be allowed to rewarm slowly, and thus non-freezing cold injury must be distinguished from frostbite, which should be rapidly rewarmed. Sometimes the only clue is that socks remained wet and did not freeze. Many cases present after rewarming, with florid redness, swelling, and pain. As this is neuropathic in origin, conventional approaches to pain management are futile, but early administration of amitriptyline in a single 25–50 mg dose a couple of hours before sleep normally brings relief. Dosage can be increased to 100 mg or greater if necessary, but patients must be cautioned about drowsiness, and must not drive, operate machinery, etc. Severe cases may develop blistering, sloughing of skin, and gangrene, which should be managed as for severe frostbite once slow rewarming has completed.

Sequelae

Long-term sequelae are more common following non-freezing cold injury, and include chronic pain and sensitization to the cold. Specialist advice is important, and interference with sympathetic innervation, even brief trial blocks, must be avoided, as it worsens the prognosis.

Snow blindness (photokeratitis)

Snow blindness is sunburn of the corneal and conjunctival epithelium covering the front of the eye. Like sunburn, there is a delay between exposure and development of symptoms, usually some 6–12 h. The eye becomes red, swollen, gritty, and very painful. In serious cases victims are incapacitated, as spasm of the eyelids means that they are unable to open their eyes and they develop a severe headache.

Pathophysiology

Ultraviolet light is a component of sunlight. Because light is reflected off snow, levels of ultraviolet radiation in polar areas can be several times greater than in temperate or tropical areas; additionally, in spring, thinning of the ozone layer allows increased amounts of these wavelengths to penetrate the atmosphere. The radiation causes an inflammatory response, with oedema and multiple dry areas over the superficial cornea. The whole surface epithelium of the eye may come away, a process associated with considerable lacrimation. Healing then occurs and subsequent long-term problems are very rare. The retina of the eye is unaffected.

Prevention

Ultraviolet rays can penetrate cloud so good quality sunglasses should be used in both clear and brightly overcast conditions. Both the front and the side of the eye should be shielded, either by suitable side flaps or by wrap-around spectacles. Some experienced polar travellers find that they rarely experience eye problems; their disregard for eye protection should not encourage novices to emulate them. Should proper sunglasses have been lost, damaged, or rendered useless by recurrent condensation, an effective emergency solution is to recreate Eskimo eye protection by cutting two thin eye slits in a piece of wood, paper, plastic, or fabric, use elastic or string to hold it to the head and use this as a shield for the eyes (Fig. 19.6).

Treatment in the field

- Ensure that the patient has no history of foreign bodies entering the eye. Contact lenses should be removed if still in place.
- Rest in a darkened room or tent.
- Give simple painkillers, such as paracetamol 1 g 4-hourly or ibuprofen 400 mg 8-hourly to relieve pain and headache. In severe cases, a more powerful painkiller such as codeine or tramadol may also be needed.
- Flushing the eye with clean water or saline solutions may relieve discomfort.
- Eye drops that relax ciliary muscle spasm of the pupil (e.g. tropicamide 0.5%) can help in moderate to severe cases, but should not be used if the patient suffers from glaucoma.
- If available, one dose of local anaesthetic eye drops such as tetracaine 0.5% (amethocaine) relieves the initial discomfort, but repeated doses of local anaesthetic drugs are no longer recommended as they may delay healing and increase risk of accidental abrasion.
- Chloramphenicol eye ointment 0.5% three to four times daily is soothing and may prevent infection, although there is some evidence that the regular use of eye ointments may actually slow the healing process.
- The eyes can be double-padded (Fig. 19.6) to provide relief from photophobia and blinking.

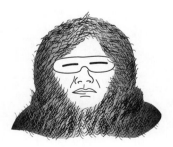

Fig. 19.6 Traditional polar sunshades.

Sequelae

Most cases of snow blindness will recover within 72 h. Seek help and follow up if:
- Infection develops.
- There is evidence of visual loss persisting after eye drops have been discontinued.

Website

Reed Brozen: Ultraviolet keratitis http://www.emedicine.com/EMERG/topic759.htm

Skin problems

Solar energy is intense in polar areas with strong reflections off the snow, and the radiation intensity may exceed that in equatorial regions. High latitude (owing to thinning of the ozone layer) and altitude increase the risk of sunburn, and a high factor (SP30+) suncream should be applied liberally. Sunburn is particularly uncomfortable when rays reflected upwards off the snow burn the eyelids and underside of the chin and nostrils.

When persistently exposed to the cold, lips are particularly vulnerable to severe and painful chapping. They may crack and bleed. It is not certain whether this injury is due to sunburn, cold injury caused by the persistent evaporation of moisture from their surface, or the activation of herpetic cold sores. There is no guaranteed protection, but regular application of a moisturising sunblock may reduce symptoms. The benefits of antiviral cold sore creams are unknown.

Mountains and high altitude

Section editors
Chris Imray, and Chris Johnson

Contributors
Charles Clarke, Chris Imray, Chris Moxon, Andrew Pollard,
George Rodway, Barry Roberts, and Jeremy Windsor

The environment

High altitude environments occur on all the world's continents. The highest peaks are accessible only to well equipped mountaineers, but substantial areas of the American Rockies, the Andes, and the Tibetan plateau lie above 3000 m. High altitude is associated with:
• Reduced atmospheric pressure
• Reduced availability of oxygen to breathe
• Cold—regardless of latitude, the climate may have polar characteristics (see Chapter 19)
• High winds and changeable weather.

Mountains do not have to be high to be dangerous; the Scottish mountains in winter do not exceed 1400 m but claim many lives. Anyone venturing onto the hills at any time of year should have adequate knowledge and equipment.

Specific risks in the mountains include:
• Avalanche
• Ice or rock fall
• Adverse weather
• Steep and slippery surfaces
• Equipment failure
• Human factors.

Climbing and mountaineering have always been high-risk activities associated with significant death and injury rates. This is particularly true when expeditions ascend above 7000 m, where helicopter rescue is impossible and evacuation of a casualty may be impractical, or only remotely feasible if there are large numbers of people on the mountain. Dedicated and experienced climbers accept these risks, but the increase in guided ascents of the great peaks may expose others to hazards that they do not fully appreciate.

Some adventure holiday organizations and charity treks are encouraging people to climb mountains faster than is desirable: this is a particular problem with Kilimanjaro and some Andean mountains where access treks are short.

Mountaineering expeditions need to consider not only high altitude problems, but also the hazards of the journey to the base of the climb.

Avalanches

An avalanche is typically a falling mass of snow which may contain rocks, ice, or other debris. Avalanches are released by either an increase in stress (fresh snow or weight of a climber/skier) or a decrease in strength of the snow pack caused by the heat of the sun. In developed countries, around 150 people die annually in avalanches; estimates suggest that 90% of victims have triggered the avalanche themselves. Death rates in the high mountain ranges are unknown.

In high mountains snow can fall at any time of year, and wilderness travellers will have to evaluate the risks of terrain and snow pack for themselves. Knowledge of avalanche assessment, prudent group management strategies, and the skills and equipment to effect the rescue of avalanche victims are prerequisites to back-country mountainous snow travel both in summer and winter.

Avalanche deaths result from:
• Burial and suffocation: 65% of deaths
• Collision with obstacles: 25% of deaths
• Hypothermia and shock: 10% of deaths.

Overall, only 50% of victims fully buried by an avalanche survive; shallow burial and rapid retrieval significantly improve survival rates.

At up to 15 min buried, survival rates are 90%, but by 35 min the chance of survival is already down to 30% (Fig. 20.1). Burial depth is related to survivability (Fig. 20.2).

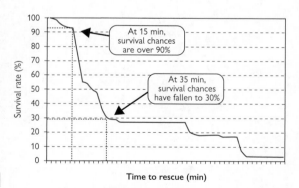

Fig. 20.1 Full burial survival rates.

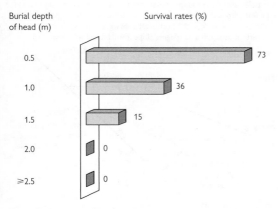

Fig. 20.2 Survival rates by burial depth.

Avalanche classification

Slab avalanche
- Surface layer is densely packed owing to wind redistribution—also called wind pack.
- Blocks of snow are released.
- The fresh snow slab is very poorly bonded to the old snow surface, especially if that surface is icy, smooth, and windblown.
- Slabs release at a fracture line across the slope, sometimes hundreds of metres across, which leaves a visible crown, or step, at the fracture line.

Loose snow avalanche
- Also called powder avalanches.
- Snow is poorly bonded.
- Originates from a specific trigger point such as a human weight, large rock, or base of a cliff.

Wet snow avalanche
- Most common in spring owing to solar radiation and soaking of the snow pack until it loses cohesion.
- Also originate from a trigger point.
- The collapse of seracs (ice towers) on steep glaciated terrain is an associate hazard.

Avalanche hazard

Terrain factors
High risk is associated with:
- Slope angles between 30 and 45°. Slope angles can be estimated using a ski pole technique (Fig. 20.3).
- Smooth ground surface (grass, scree) under snow with nothing to which the snow pack can grip.

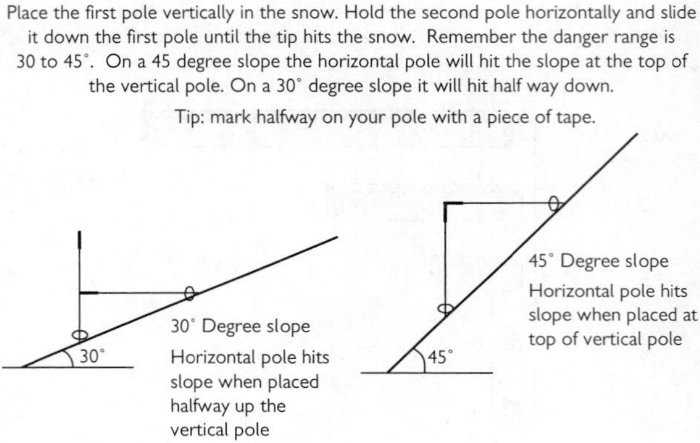

Place the first pole vertically in the snow. Hold the second pole horizontally and slide it down the first pole until the tip hits the snow. Remember the danger range is 30 to 45°. On a 45 degree slope the horizontal pole will hit the slope at the top of the vertical pole. On a 30° degree slope it will hit half way down.

Tip: mark halfway on your pole with a piece of tape.

30° Degree slope
Horizontal pole hits slope when placed halfway up the vertical pole

45° Degree slope
Horizontal pole hits slope when placed at top of vertical pole

Fig. 20.3 Slope angle ski pole test.

- Lee side, high near the ridge line (see wind direction).
- Aspect, taking into consideration:
  - Wind direction—snow accumulates and becomes wind-packed on lee slopes or in gulleys on cross-loaded slopes.
  - Solar radiation—the first sunny day after recent snowfall is particularly dangerous, as is the spring sun in the afternoon.
  - Shade—cold temperatures inhibit snow pack stability and prolong the dangers. Low temperatures, particularly in a shallow snow pack, result in a steep temperature gradient that accelerates the development of faceting of snow grains, resulting in weak, high volume crystals at the base of the snow pack.
- Slopes that terminate in cliffs.
- Terrain traps are topographic funnels, such as V-shaped gullies reaching to ridges, or stream beds. Avalanche from or into these gullies can result in deep burial of a casualty.

Lower risks are associated with:
- Slope angle less than 30°—with no steeper slopes above.
- Densely forested.
- Ridges.
- Tops of knolls and small hills offering 'islands' of safety.
- Wide valleys, away from the run-out zone from surrounding slopes.

Prevailing weather conditions
- The amount and rate of accumulation of fresh snow, together with temperatures and wind speed, affect the risk of avalanche.
- Temperature has a great influence on snow pack stability—rapidly warmer temperatures close to 0°C after snow fall promote instability.
- Intense solar radiation promotes instability.

- Warm temperatures stabilize the snow pack in the long term by encouraging rounding of snow grains which become tightly packed and cohesive.
- Warm/cold cycles accelerate stability.
- Three conditions give rise to the greatest danger level:
  - Fresh snow combined with wind redistribution: 80–90% of alpine avalanches happen within 24 h of fresh snow falls.
  - Rapidly rising temperatures.
  - Weak or poorly bonded layers in the snow pack.

The danger of fresh snow depends upon its depth and whether or not conditions are favourable. Fresh deep snow still represents a significant hazard even when conditions are favourable.

Unfavourable (dangerous) conditions are:
- High rate of precipitation.
- Low temperatures (−5°C to −10°C).
- High winds (>50 km/h).
- Smooth, old snow surface.

Favourable (safer) conditions are:
- Low to moderate winds.
- Air temperature close to 0°C.
- Very irregular old snow surface that acts as a 'key' for new snow.
- Frequently walked or skied slope.

Observation of snow landscapes

'If you don't know, don't go'.

Look for:
- Any obvious avalanche activity (debris, crown lines, avalanche paths).
- Evidence of recent avalanches and past activity; debris, gaps in trees, or piles of snow in run-out zones Obvious snow slabs that break off beneath your feet.
- 'Sun balls' rolling down the slope.
- Evidence of wind redistribution—bare ridges and slopes, snow drifts, deep pockets of snow in hollows and gullies.
- Unmistakable 'whoomf' or cracking sounds underfoot, evidence of the snow pack settling, slabs, or poorly bonded layers.

How to assess snow pack stability
- Dig a snow pit down to the ground and inspect the snow face.
- Note if any slabs spontaneously break away.
- Look for obvious layers:
  - Insert and run a knife down the snow face (like cutting a cake): note any major changes in resistance, which indicates layers you cannot easily see.
  - Ice layers (or lenses) may indicate weak, poorly bonded interfaces.
  - Old slab layers may be buried below the surface.
  - A deep, thick, sugary textured layer of snow which you cannot form into a snowball, is indicative of faceting (also called depth hoar). This layer can collapse with a 'whoomf' or shooting crack sound.

- Note any particularly moist layers which might indicate instability.
- Any layers that differ significantly in hardness and/or grain size are potentially weak boundaries.

For a more advanced test, further isolate a 30-cm square column of snow (dig out the sides of and behind the snow face). Apply graduated pressure to the top of the column with a shovel blade and note any failure point(s) and/or shearing between snow layers in the column.

Any conclusions drawn from the above may be misleading if the site of the test pit is not representative of potentially dangerous terrain with respect to its elevation, slope angle, and aspect. It is normally colder and windier up.

Human factors

- Expert knowledge of snow pack evolution and high risk terrain is worthless if human factors override 'snow science' and objective decision-making.
- Decision-making—have clear, prudent decisions been made or does the group blindly carry on in the face of new information? Groups tend to lend more weight to information that supports their assumptions and pay less attention to information that challenges those assumptions.
- Leadership—who is coordinating decision-making and making unpopular proposals to change the route or plan in light of new information?
- Group size—larger groups equate to a greater load on susceptible snow slopes, are generally less manageable, and more prone to a 'go with the flow' mentality.

Skill level:

- Is the party trained in avalanche search and rescue?
- Do they have the technical skills to alter their route and move on terrain that takes them out of avalanche danger?
- Fitness level—is the group strong enough to turn back to safety or choose a safer route even if it is more physically demanding (longer, uphill)?
- Discipline—will everyone follow safe travel procedures?

Travel in avalanche-prone areas

- Plan your route to follow safe terrain.
- Are you starting early enough and moving fast enough to avoid sun-baked slopes later in the day?
- Avoid terrain traps where deep burial is more likely.
- Avoid areas where there is clear evidence of past avalanche activity—including uprooted vegetation, rocks, soil, and snow and ice debris.
- Beware gaps in the vegetation (past avalanche paths?).

Crossing high risk-terrain

- Ensure that avalanche transceivers are set to send.
- Remove ski pole straps, undo all buckles (ski safety straps, rucksack).
- Zip up your clothes, put on a hat and gloves, cover mouth with a scarf.
- Move gently, one at a time, on a predetermined 'safe' line.

- Don't stop or regroup until you reach an island of safety:
  - A ridge, rock outcrop, hill top, forest, or other area out of all potential avalanche paths.
- Use signals to indicate when it is safe for the next person to cross.

If caught in an avalanche

- Shout to attract attention.
- Jettison poles, rucksacks, and skis—they will drag you down.
- Try to get to the edge of the avalanche and out of its path.
- Fight to stay on the surface using a swimming motion, particularly just before the avalanche settles.
- Cover your mouth as the avalanche settles and fight to create an air pocket around your face.

Avalanche transceivers

- All modern transceivers operate on a frequency of 457 kHz.
- The transceiver must be worn on the body under clothing, so it cannot be ripped off in an avalanche. It should *not* be in a rucksack or pocket.
- Turn it on, put it on, and leave it on all day.
- Test transceivers daily—this ensures they are turned on.
- Transceivers are in SEND mode unless switched to RECEIVE mode to conduct a search.
- Use lithium batteries which operate normally in very low temperatures. As lithium batteries discharge, they do not lose power but they suddenly go flat without any warning, so carry spare batteries.
- Each type of transceiver has specific performance advantages, but all of them require training, education, and practice for maximum proficiency in search situations.
- Transceiver models differ in four significant ways:
  - The range at which they first detect a signal.
  - How distance and direction to the victim is displayed—audible signals, lights, or digital number displays.
  - How the unit deals with more than one buried victim—a multiple burial scenario.
  - Some models incorporate the 'on button' into the harness strap so it is impossible to wear the device without turning it on. Other models can be worn in the 'off' mode and require the user to activate a switch, which introduces scope for human error.

For these reasons it is important for groups to *practise* transceiver searching together to appreciate the differences between transceiver models and the search patterns recommended by the manufacturer.

Shovel

Effective digging requires a proper shovel; skis, hands, trekking poles, ice axes, and skis are slow and ineffective. Strong, light, collapsible shovels are readily purchased in equipment stores.

Probe

For detailed searching—or searching for a victim with no transceiver—a proper avalanche probe is necessary. This is a thin, sectional aluminium pole, like a tent pole, which assembles into a 2–3 m length that can penetrate even dense snow. You cannot probe effectively with ski poles or ice axes.

The RECCO® system (http://www.recco.com)

Some outdoor clothing, boots, helmets, and other equipment is equipped with a RECCO® reflector which 'enables rapid directional pinpointing of a victim's precise location using harmonic radar'. The two-part system consists of a RECCO® detector used by professional rescue groups and RECCO® reflectors. 'The RECCO system is not intended for self-rescue and is not an alternative to transceiver use in the back-country.'

If a party member is caught in an avalanche

- Stop, think, and assess further risk to rescuers before going to help.
- Watch the victim carefully to estimate where they are buried.
- Look for clues as to the path they were swept down—clothing and equipment on the surface—note the last spot seen.
- Count survivors so you know how many victims you are searching for. Multiple burials complicate the transceiver search.
- Make a visual search before starting a transceiver search for any sign of the victim sticking clear of the snow before starting a more complex transceiver search.
- Start a transceiver search; turn rescuers' transceivers to receive.
- Probe search once you have narrowed down the transceiver search.
- Dig the victim out—see Extrication priorities.
- Turn the victim's transceiver off in case of multiple burials.
- Administer medical attention (see below).
- Once all victims have been rescued, switch *all* transceivers back to send.

Extrication priorities

- Burial <35 min: extricate as fast as possible. Clear the airway. If the victim is in a critical condition, suspect acute asphyxia or mechanical trauma. Treat accordingly.
- Burials >35 min: assume hypothermia and extricate as gently as possible. Check carefully for an air pocket around the victim's face and for a clear airway; both are paramount to a favourable outcome.
- Following a complete burial (head and trunk), the victim should be monitored for 24 h to observe for pulmonary complications (aspiration and pulmonary oedema) in a hospital with intensive care facilities.

Conclusion

Assessing the snow, developing a sense of which route to take, and generally getting a feel for the level of risk in a snowy mountain environment is not a science and is hard to learn from a book. Even one day spent in the mountains with a knowledgeable friend or mountain guide practising the techniques outlined and applying the 'science' will substantially raise your understanding of the hazards associated with snow travel and make you a safer, more respectful mountain traveller. Make sure that everyone in the party is properly equipped and trained to respond effectively in an avalanche emergency. There is no point in being the only 'expert' if you are the one buried in an avalanche.

Website

http://www.stayingaliveoffpiste.com

Humans at altitude

While altitude sickness dominates high altitude physiology studies, more mundane problems can cause hazard and accidents. These include:
- Exhaustion and dehydration (📖 p. 696).
- Hypothermia and cold injury (📖 p. 596).
- Ultraviolet keratitis (snow blindness) (📖 p. 604).
- Poor visibility: whiteout or problems with masks and spectacles.
- Communication difficulties in strong winds.
- Disorientation in poor visibility.
- Unstable and slippery terrain.
- Onset of darkness before descent complete.
- Poor decision-making.

Hypoxia and reduced atmospheric pressure

As a climber ascends, barometric pressure falls and there is an associated fall in the partial pressure of oxygen in the inspired air (Table 20.1). Using pulse oximetry, decreases in haemoglobin oxygen saturation can be measured in healthy climbers ascending to over 2500 m. By 5500 m atmospheric pressure has dropped to half that at sea level and an unacclimatized human will be distressed. Significant hypoxia develops—oxygen saturations below 80% are common in travellers among the great ranges (6000–8000 m): they will be breathless and exercise capacity will be significantly reduced.

Humans acclimatize to high altitude; changes include increasing the oxygen-carrying capacity of the bloodstream by raising haemoglobin levels, metabolically altering the binding capacity of that haemoglobin for oxygen, and changing the metabolic characteristics of the blood. Acclimatization develops over several weeks, and most humans are unable to tolerate ascent rates of more than 300 m a day but there is a significant variation in the degree and speed to which individuals are able to acclimatize. A very few climbers have been able to reach the summit of Everest without supplementary oxygen, but such feats are at the extreme limits of human physiology.

Humans spending prolonged periods at high altitude develop long term physiological responses to the environment. In South America, high altitude miners working for prolonged periods over 3000 m develop pathologically high haemoglobin concentrations (>22 g/dl) that may result in pulmonary hypertension and cardiac failure (chronic mountain sickness—Monge's disease). Ethnic Tibetans seem better able to cope at high altitude, with only a small proportion of those living at up to 4000 m affected, but Chinese immigrants living on the Tibetan plateau may experience significant complications and infant mortality is high.

Sleep disorders are common at altitude; see Chapter 10.

Table 20.1 Atmospheric characteristics at high altitude

Altitude (m)	Pressure (mmHg)	Temperature (°C)	Inspired oxygen tension (mm Hg)
Sea level	760	15	148
2500 m (8000 ft)	565	1	108
4500 m (15 000 ft)	430	−15	80
5500 m (18 000 ft)	380	−20	69

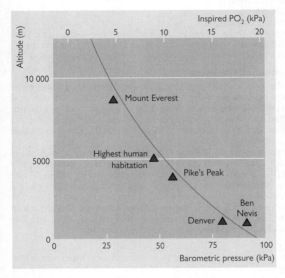

Fig. 20.4 Barometric pressure at altitude.

High altitude illnesses

If ascent is too fast to allow adequate acclimatization, acute mountain sickness (AMS), high altitude pulmonary oedema (HAPE), or high altitude cerebral oedema (HACE) may occur. Of these AMS is much more common and is less severe, but the syndromes overlap considerably.

Risk factors
- Rapidity of arrival at altitude
- Magnitude of altitude gain
- Absolute altitude attained
- Previous history of AMS
- Physical exertion
- Pre-existing lung disease
- It is likely that some individuals are genetically more susceptible than others. However, altitude illness is frequently unpredictable and the reason a person becomes ill at a given time is not fully understood.

Acute mountain sickness

AMS is the most common high altitude illness. It describes a collection of symptoms typically beginning 6–12 h following arrival at altitude. It is common in those who ascend above 2500 m without time for adequate acclimatization and is progressively more frequent at higher altitudes and with higher ascent rates, occurring in approximately 50% of individuals who ascend rapidly to 4500 m.

Since there is no single feature of AMS that is specific, diagnosis is problematic. For research purposes a scale has been used to classify AMS, the Lake Louise acute mountain sickness scoring system (Table 20.2), but it has limited use clinically. From a practical point of view, if a person has a headache and feels unwell at high altitude, without another obvious cause, AMS is a likely diagnosis. Many features of AMS are shared with HACE and HAPE, which are often preceded by AMS, and this should always be considered during assessment and treatment.

Aetiology
The pathogenesis of AMS is poorly understood. One hypothesis is that AMS represents an early form of HACE, caused by brain swelling and pressure symptoms in individuals with insufficient cerebrospinal fluid buffer capacity ('tight fit hypothesis'; see HACE below). However, brain swelling has not been demonstrated as early as 6–10 h after ascent, when symptoms of AMS tend to begin. In addition, mild brain swelling is seen equally in those with and without AMS symptoms. Other possible causes are free radical-mediated damage or derangement in cerebral blood flow autoregulation. Further investigation is required to confirm the mechanism of development of AMS symptoms.

Table 20.2 Lake Louise score

Lake Louise acute mountain sickness scoring system

Self-report questionnaire		Clinical assessment	
1. Headache		**6. Change in mental status**	
0	No headache	0	No change in mental status
1	Mild headache	1	Lethargy/lassitude
2	Moderate headache	2	Disorientated/confused
3	Severe headache, incapacitating	3	Stupor/semi-consciousness
2. Gastrointestinal symptoms		4	Coma
0	No gastrointestinal symptoms	**7. Ataxia (heal-to-toe walking)**	
1	Poor appetite or nausea	0	No ataxia
2	Moderate nausea or vomiting	1	Manoeuvres to maintain balance
3	Severe nausea and vomiting, incapacitating	2	Steps off line
3. Fatigue or weakness		3	Falls down
0	Not tired or weak	4	Can't stand
1	Mild fatigue/weakness	**8. Peripheral oedema**	
2	Moderate fatigue/weakness	0	No peripheral oedema
3	Severe fatigue/weakness, incapacitating	1	Peripheral oedema at one
4. Dizziness/lightheadedness		2	Peripheral oedema at two or more locations
0	Not dizzy		
1	Mild dizziness		
2	Moderate dizziness		
3	Severe dizziness, incapacitating		
5. Difficulty sleeping			
0	Slept as well as usual		
1	Did not sleep as well as usual		
2	Woke many times, poor night's sleep		
3	Could not sleep at all		

Developed at Lake Louise in Canada as a tool to standardize diagnostic criteria for AMS during research, the scoring system consists of a self-reported questionnaire and a, less often used, clinical assessment section. In the context of a recent gain in altitude, a score of 3 or more in the questionnaire alone, or 5 when using a combined score, is deemed to indicate AMS. It is sensitive not specific, as many other illness will result in a score greater than 3.

Symptoms
- Headache
- Anorexia
- Nausea and vomiting
- Fatigue
- Dizziness
- Sleep disturbance.

Symptoms typically evolve gradually and are worse at night. There are no distinct characteristics, but a headache, typically throbbing in nature, and aggravated either by bending down and/or by Valsalva's manoeuvre, is usually present.

Signs
No specific signs. Some common findings are:
- Peripheral oedema
- Tachycardia
- Scattered crackles on auscultation
- Slightly raised basal temperature.

Management
'If in doubt descend'.

Mild
- Do not ascend further
- Rest
- Drug treatment may offer some relief:
  - Simple analgesia, e.g. paracetamol, ibuprofen.
  - Antiemetic.
- Simple measures are usually sufficient to relieve the symptoms, but if symptoms are constant or worsening, descend. Further ascent risks progression to HAPE/HACE.

Moderate–severe
Descent is the main treatment in all serious altitude illness. Ideally, descent is to below the altitude at which the patient was symptom-free. Adjunctive therapy may be used to facilitate descent, but not as an alternative.
- Oxygen
- Acetazolamide 250 mg PO tds
- Dexamethasone 4 mg PO or iv qds
- Hyperbaric chamber
- Give simple analgesia and antiemetic.

High altitude pulmonary oedema

HAPE is a serious form of high altitude illness in which there is movement of fluid from the intravascular to extravascular space in the alveoli. This causes impaired gaseous exchange, initially manifest as increased breathlessness on exertion but progressing to breathlessness at rest and severe compromise. It is reversed by descent to a lower altitude.

HAPE typically occurs 2–4 days after arrival at altitudes >2500 m. Although cases at lower altitudes have been reported, there is a correlation with maximum altitude attained, particularly sleeping height; the incidence is 0.0001% at 2700 m and 2% at 4000 m. It is more common with rapid ascent, particularly when exercise is involved (6% at 4500 m and 15% at 5500 m). AMS is frequently but not always associated.

Aetiology

The condition is incompletely understood. Exaggerated pulmonary hypertension in response to hypoxia may result from an abnormally profound hypoxic pulmonary vasoconstrictive response (HPVR) and lead to transudative capillary leak and mild alveolar haemorrhage. Oedema is patchy, and the HPVR is heterogenous in HAPE. This has led to the proposal that non-constricted vessels become hyperperfused with raised hydrostatic pressure and stretching of the endothelial lining, leading to stress failure. Hypoxia may also cause oedema directly through impairment of fluid and electrolyte transport across the alveolar epithelium. Pre-existing inflammation/infection may play a role in some cases, particularly in children.

Defects in nitric oxide synthesis (which would normally modify the HPVR) and alveolar fluid clearance may be associated with increased susceptibility to HAPE.

Risk factors and susceptibility

- Often preceded by AMS.
- Men > women.
- Cold.
- Fast ascent (including fast re-ascent in a pre-acclimatized individual).
- Hard physical exertion (anecdotal evidence).
- Alcohol and respiratory depressant drugs (anecdotal evidence).
- Possibly viral infection or pneumonia (particularly in children).
- Previous episodes of HAPE.
- Increased pulmonary blood flow/exaggerated hypoxic pulmonary vascular reactivity: occurs commonly in people with structural cardiac defects (e.g. atrial septal defect, absent right pulmonary artery) or in chronic respiratory conditions (e.g. cystic fibrosis, bronchopulmonary dysplasia).
- Possible genetic associations: HLA-DR6, HLA-DQ4, and polymorphisms in pulmonary surfactant protein A, epithelial sodium channel protein, and endothelial nitric oxide synthase genes.

Pre-ascent evaluation

A high proportion (77–93%) of HAPE-susceptible individuals can be identified prior to ascent by measurement of pulmonary artery systolic pressure (PASP) using Doppler. HAPE-prone individuals tend to have an abnormal increase in PASP when compared to non-susceptible individuals, both in response to hypoxia or to exercise. A PASP of >41 mmHg after 2 h of hypoxia or >42 mmHg after vigorous exercise in normoxia strongly correlate with HAPE susceptibility. Changes in BP, saturations, and heart rate do not predict HAPE.

Symptoms

- Decreased exercise tolerance with dyspnoea on exertion, progressing to dyspnoea at rest
- Cough, initially dry, becoming wet
- Haemoptysis
- Chest pain

- Orthopnoea
- Nausea
- Insomnia
- Headache
- Dizziness
- Confusion
- Often accompanied by symptoms of AMS with or without HACE.

Signs
Early
- Mild pyrexia
- Tachypnoea
- Tachycardia
- Accentuated pulmonary second sound
- Right ventricular heave
- Basal crepitations.

Late
- Severe compromise
- Cyanosis
- Coexisting signs of HACE.

Differential diagnosis
- Dry persistent cough is common at altitude, independent of HAPE.
- Clinical features are difficult to distinguish from pneumonia.

Investigations (when available)
- Low peripheral arterial oxygen saturations.
- X-ray: patchy oedematous shadowing, often more densely on the right side and in midzones.
- Arterial blood gas: reduced PO_2 (in comparison with normal PO_2 for that altitude).
- ECG: tachycardia, right axis deviation, and peaked P waves.
- Cardiac catheter studies have shown elevated pulmonary artery pressure.

Management
Descent is the primary treatment; even a few hundred metres may be rapidly beneficial. When prevented by significant compromise or poor conditions, other treatments may be of assistance but should not delay descent:
- Sit patient up.
- High flow O_2 by face mask (6–10 l/min).
- Hyperbaric chamber (if available)—with head elevated if possible.
- Nifedipine: 20 mg PO qds of slow release preparation.
- Treatment for coexistent AMS/HACE with dexamethasone.

Other management strategies that may have some evidence of benefit:
- Other pulmonary vasodilators may also be beneficial although are not usually used (e.g. hydralazine, phentolamine, sildenafil citrate).
- Expiratory positive airways pressure.
- Inhaled nitric oxide (requires extreme care, toxic in raised concentrations).
- Inhaled β_2 agonists.

Prevention
• Adequate acclimatization.
• Slow ascent: 400–600 m height gain per night, resting every 2–3 days.
• Nifedipine 20 mg PO tds of slow release preparation (or Tadalafil 10 mg PO bd which has recently been shown to be equally effective).
• Avoid hard physical exertion for 2–3 days after arrival at altitude (anecdotal evidence).
• Inhaled beta agonists may be beneficial.
• Early descent on any appearance of symptoms (rapidly reversed in early stages).
• Prevention of AMS/HACE may reduce the risk of HAPE.
• Acetazolamide (Diamox) 250 mg bd from 1 day before ascent.
• Dexamethasone 4 mg qds may offer some protection.

Portable hyperbaric chambers (Fig. 20.5)
Now carried by many larger high altitude expeditions, these are capsules constructed from lightweight materials into which a person can be zipped. The capsule is then inflated with a foot or hand pump. This results in a rapid increase in barometric pressure within the chamber and a simulated descent. Manual pumping, with hand or foot pump, must continue inter-mittently, even after inflation, to allow CO_2 clearance.

Single man portable devices weigh 4.8–6.5 kg and cost between US$1400 and 2400. A two-man device is available to allow a medical person to accompany a patient who is seriously ill. Hyperbaric chambers have been shown to treat all forms of altitude illness effectively; however, the effect does not persist long after removal from the chamber and should not replace descent as the primary treatment.

Such bags must be used with care:
• Ensure a constant air supply to casualty.
• Position bag so that casualty lies in head-up position.
• Monitor casualty's condition continuously to ensure that they remain breathing and do not vomit.

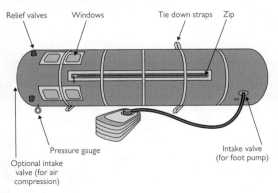

Fig. 20.5 Gamow bag.

High altitude cerebral oedema

HACE is a rare but potentially fatal condition that can occur at altitudes over 2500–3000 m. About 2–3% of people travelling above 5000 m will be affected. Brain oedema typically follows an episode of AMS that fails to recover in the usual 3–4 days and progresses. Hypoxia causes the brain to swell within the fixed confines of the cranium (tight fit hypothesis). Like pulmonary oedema, early cerebral oedema is reversed by descent.

Whilst there is often a prodromal period when the subject exhibits signs and symptoms of AMS and/or HAPE, HACE can develop on its own. Many feel that AMS and HACE are all part of the same continuum of disease, although HACE rarely occurs without HAPE. HACE can also occur suddenly in well-acclimatized climbers at extreme altitudes—there are many recorded cases of this, some without headaches.

Aetiology

The exact pathophysiology of HACE remains to be determined. Cerebral blood flow increases both at altitude and in AMS, and there appears to be a generalized capillary leakage. There also appears to be evidence of impaired cerebral autoregulation on acute exposure to altitude.

The symptoms of AMS and of raised intracranial pressure appear similar, with headaches, nausea, photophobia, and ataxia being features of both conditions. In both severe AMS and HACE, CSF pressures were found to be elevated compared with that after recovery, and subjects dying from AMS have evidence of cerebral oedema on autopsy. Computerized axial tomography demonstrates diffuse low density areas consistent with oedema in subjects with HACE.

Disruption of the blood–brain barrier may be important and is likely to occur in HACE. The blood–brain barrier is influenced by the neuro-transmitters nitric oxide, histamine, substance P, free oxygen radicals, 5-hydroxytryptamine, cytokines, and endothelial growth factors. Local hypoxia triggers a complex cascade of cellular responses resulting in an increase in lactate, altered redox state, capillary basement membrane disruption, and plasma extravasation. Vascular endothelial growth factor (VEGF) may be the most potent agent that causes basement membrane disruption and oedema formation. VEGF has been shown to increase in rats exposed to hypoxic conditions and also in humans after exercise.

Relief of high altitude headache with dexamethasone provides indirect evidence of the importance of cerebral oedema and vascular permeability in high altitude headaches since dexamethasone suppresses lipid peroxidation, blocks VEGF, and reduces endothelial permeability.

Ascent to altitude results in an increase in cerebral blood flow and yet the subjects are known to be hypoxic. Oxygen delivery to the cerebral tissue is likely to be the critical determinant of health and illness at all altitudes.

Risk factors

These are similar to AMS and HAPE. Gradual acclimatization and correct treatment of AMS reduces the risk of brain oedema during the early stages of ascent to high altitudes. Little can be done to prevent sudden brain oedema at extreme altitudes—it is vital to recognize the condition promptly and act swiftly.

No pre-ascent evaluation is helpful, a difference from HAPE.

Symptoms
- Headache
- Nausea
- Hallucination
- Disorientation
- Confusion.

Signs
- Ataxia
- Hypoxia
- Unreasonable behaviour
- Focal neurological deficits
- Cranial nerve palsies (e.g. sixth)
- Papilloedema and retinal haemorrhages
- Confusion, stupor, coma
- Pulmonary oedema may coexist.

Investigations

Few are likely to be available. Oxygen saturation levels and arterial PO_2 levels correlate poorly with the severity of brain oedema. CT or MRI are worthwhile in hospital but will be unavailable in the field.

Management
- Immediate descent (see pulmonary oedema) of 500–1000 m.
- High flow oxygen by mask.
- Dexamethasone. Give 8 mg by mouth or injection, then 4 mg 4-hourly for several days, before reducing the dose over 1 week.
- Whilst a hyperbaric chamber (see above) is potentially beneficial, there are potential dangers if the patient's airway is at risk.
- Evacuate to hospital.
- Do not re-ascend until completely better.

Prevention
- Adequate acclimatization.
- Slow ascent: 400–600 m height gain per night, resting every 2–3 days.
- Avoid hard physical exertion for 2–3 days after arrival at altitude (anecdotal evidence).
- Early descent on any appearance of symptoms (rapidly reversed in early stages).
- Prevention of AMS/HAPE may reduce the risk of HACE.
- Acetazolamide (Diamox) 250 mg bd from 1 day before ascent.
- Dexamethasone 4 mg qds may offer some protection.

High altitude retinal haemorrhages (Fig. 20.6)

Retinal haemorrhages (in the nerve fibre layer) are common >5000 m and are not necessarily related to AMS. They do not predispose to cerebral oedema and rarely interfere with vision unless found over the macula. No treatment is usually necessary but if vision becomes blurred or fails, descent is advisable. Permanent visual loss is exceptional. Haemorrhages not affecting vision are not known to have any clinical significance and do not warrant descent. Haemorrhages have been induced by strenuous exercise, which increases blood pressure and decreases the arterial oxygen saturation levels.

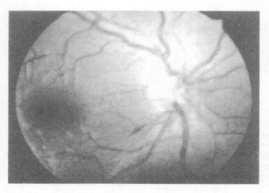

Fig. 20.6 High altitude retinal haemorrhage.

Drugs in altitude illness

Acetazolamide (Diamox)

Acetazolamide is a carbonic anhydrase inhibitor which affects renal bicarbonate excretion to produce a metabolic acidosis and therefore increased respiratory drive.

Uses

- *Prophylaxis:* drug of choice in at-risk individuals. Controversy over dose. While one meta-analysis concluded that a dose of 750 mg/day is required for significant effect, this has been criticized by several authors and does not fit with majority clinical opinion. The widely supported dose of 250 mg bd is supported by several trials and a different meta-analysis. Recommended dose: 250 mg bd or 500 mg od of slow release preparation, beginning 1 day before ascent to altitude; child 2.5 mg/kg bd.
- *Treatment of AMS:* 250 mg tds; child 2.5 mg/kg tds (max 250 mg/dose).

Common side effects

Nausea and vomiting, anorexia, dizziness, tingling in hands, and an odd taste in the mouth. While most people tolerate acetazolamide well, others experience significant side effects and it is recommended that people try it before using it as prophylaxis at altitude.

Dexamethasone

Glucocorticoid steroid.

Uses

- *Prevention and treatment of AMS* (in individuals intolerant to acetazolamide): unknown action. Not as effective as acetazolamide and does not aid acclimatization.
- *Prophylaxis:* 8 mg/day in divided doses (e.g. 4 mg bd).

- *Treatment of AMS:* 4 mg qds; child 0.15 mg/kg/dose qds (maximum 4 mg/dose).
- *Treatment of HACE:* 8 mg initially PO, im or iv then 4 mg qds; child 0.15 mg/kg/dose qds.
- *Treatment of AMS:* 4 mg qds PO or iv; child 0.15 mg/kg/dose PO qds (maximum 4 mg/dose). Relieves symptoms but not physiological abnormalities. May be used in conjunction with acetazolamide.

Common side effects

Usually none with short courses; steroid psychosis occurs rarely.

Nifedipine

Calcium channel blocker. The mechanism that improves HAPE is not known, but it does reverse/prevent pulmonary systolic hypertension.

Uses

- *Prevention of HAPE* in susceptible individuals: has been shown to reduce the incidence significantly in people of known susceptibility.
- 20 mg PO slow release preparation tds.
- *Treatment of HAPE:* drug treatment is secondary to descent and/or supplementary oxygen which address the primary cause.
- 20 mg PO slow release preparation qds. Child 0.5 mg/kg/dose PO tds— ideally slow release preparation (maximum 20 mg/dose).
- Some authors recommend a 10 mg sublingual tablet taken initially but this has been known to cause significant hypotension that may prevent descent for several hours.

Common side effects

Headache, dizziness, and postural hypotension. The latter, which is serious as it may hamper descent, is less likely with a slow release preparation.

Further reading

Bärtsch P, Mairbäurl H, Maggiorini M, Swenson E (2005). Physiological aspects of high-altitude pulmonary edema. *Journal of Applied Physiology* **98**: 1101–10.

Basnyat B, Murdoch DR (2003). High-altitude illness. *Lancet* **361**: 1967–74.

Clarke C (2006). Neurology at high altitude. *Practical Neurology* **6**: 230–7.

Pollard AJ, Murdoch DR (2003). *The High Altitude Medicine Handbook*, 3rd edn. Oxford, Radcliffe: pp. 7–34.

Nutrition at altitude

In mountaineering, as in war, it seldom pays to defer a meal if an opportunity for eating offers; at the best the next opportunity may be long in coming, at the worst it may never come again (H. Tilman 1938).

A 5–20% fall in body weight is typical after time spent at high/extreme altitude. Although fat reserves tend to be metabolized first during an expedition, loss of significant amounts of muscle protein also occurs, leading to dramatic effects upon performance. Weight loss at altitude is due to:
- A rise in basal metabolic rate of 10–30%.
- An increase in energy expenditure (up to 20 000 kJ/5000 kcal per day).
- Symptoms of AMS (lethargy, nausea, vomiting, and anorexia).
- Limited availability of food, water, and fuel.
- Possible changes in the absorption of fat, carbohydrate, and protein.
- Alteration in bowel flora and gastrointestinal infection causing diarrhoea, abdominal pain, and anorexia.

Planning

Dental and medical checks are essential before departure and should identify and treat conditions such as acid reflux, diarrhoea, constipation, and dental problems which can affect eating and absorption. Many experienced mountaineers benefit from deliberately gaining weight to offset later losses; however, this should not be due to lack of exercise! Where possible, the responsibility of choosing menus and purchasing food should be given to an experienced member of the team. Ideally, local cooks and kitchen staff should be employed. If this is impossible, the quartermaster should be responsible for providing:
- A wide variety of safely prepared meals, snacks, and 'packed lunches', together with an abundant supply of clean, cold water.
- A warm, well lit mess tent large enough to accommodate the entire expedition comfortably.
- Adequate cooking utensils and crockery, together with appropriate cooking and storage facilities.
- Careful attention to kitchen and culinary hygiene as well as personal hygiene.

Acclimatization

Any expedition venturing above 3500 m will need a period of acclimatization to ensure appetite and physical performance are optimized. Little, however, is gained from spending long periods of time above 7000 m, where appetites falter, cooking is difficult and weight loss soon becomes apparent.

Hydration

Climbers need to drink 3–4 litres of fluids each day. Dehydration develops quickly at high altitude; a water deficit of as little as 2% has been shown to reduce performance. Water at high altitude is obtained from melting snow, which should be gathered from fresh, uncontaminated sources and added slowly to warm water. Melting large bowls of snow is inefficient and tends to lead to the formation of condensation which can extinguish the stove's flame. Ideally, water should be boiled or treated with 1%

tincture of iodine and left for 4–8 h before drinking; however, this can often prove impractical.

Cooking and eating equipment

Lightweight liquid gas stoves are essential to the success of any expedition. Each set must include spares, cleaning tools, windshield, stove stand, matches (in a waterproof container), and sufficient fuel. The equipment should be designed for high altitude use and will need to be thoroughly tested first. At high altitude all members should carry a minimum of a cooking pot, lightweight plastic bowl (keeps food warmer than metal), and a metal spoon (doesn't break easily), together with a small scrubber and sterilizing 'wipes' for cleaning.

Diet

In recent years carbohydrate-rich diets have been widely used on high altitude expeditions. Theoretically, these not only raise the respiratory exchange ratio (R) and improve the partial pressure of oxygen in the alveoli, but they also reflect the preference tissues have for glucose over free fatty acids at altitude. This results in:

- An increased work tolerance and capacity to produce anaerobic energy.
- Improved mental acuity.
- An increased tolerance to altitude and a decrease in symptoms of AMS.

A combination of simple and complex carbohydrates should be used to provide a sustained source of energy.

Snacks

During expeditions, small snacks eaten every 2–4 h provide invaluable sources of energy. A good mixture of carbohydrates can be found in power gels, muesli bars, nuts, dried fruit, flapjacks, and biscuits. In addition, modest quantities of simple carbohydrate 'treats', such as boiled sweets and chocolate bars, provide a useful boost to morale.

Meals

Noodles, potatoes, rice, pasta, polenta, and cous cous provide ideal sources of carbohydrate. These can be combined with small amounts of meat, fish, eggs, pulses and vegetables, and flavoured with chillis, garlic, pepper, pickles, powdered cheese, butter or olive oil (easily stored in old 35 mm film cases). Breakfasts are essential for both rehydration and food consumption, and should include cereals (porridge or muesli) and breads (chappatis, rotis, etc.) supplemented with spreads (chocolate, peanut butter, etc.) or preserves. At high altitude, foods should be pre-prepared and should only need the addition of hot water (noodles, 'instant' potato). It is vital to sample foods first before taking them to high camps. This provides information on preparation (cooking time, amount of water required) and, most importantly, palatability.

Supplements

In general, additional vitamins and minerals are not necessary during high altitude expeditions. However, those with iron or folate deficiencies may benefit from supplements, as red cell recruitment is an essential feature of acclimatization.

Further reading

H.W. Tilman. The Seven Mountain-Travel Books (Mountaineers' Books) ISBN 0–89886–960–9.

Rivers, lakes, and oceans

Section editor
Chris Johnson

Contributors
Spike Briggs, Campbell MacKenzie,
Patrick Morgan, Andy Pitkin,
and Andy Watt

Aquatic environments

Aquatic environments, whether oceans, rivers or lakes, are very complex, being affected by the flows of water, their interaction with surrounding land, and the interplay with other physical forces such as the wind. Expeditions using rivers or lakes as routes of communication also have to contend with the nature of the surrounding terrain:

- *Wind* affects wave strength and formation. It cools skin, masks sunburn, and increases the risk of hypothermia.
- *Rain* reduces visibility and increases the risk of hypothermia.
- *Ultraviolet light* from the sun reflects off the surface of the water, increasing exposure to radiation. Tropical climates encourage scanty clothing. Sea water washes off protective sunblock creams. Minimize hazards by appropriate behaviour, clothing, and ultraviolet protection. On the plus side, ultraviolet light reduces the bacterial load of waters in coastal areas.

Water

Tides and currents

- Tides, currents, and weather vary unpredictably; information on risks is often difficult to obtain.
- Exposed and inaccessible coastlines are dangerous.
- Incoming tides can isolate people on sandbanks, and at the midpoint of 'flooding' can raise the level of the sea very dramatically in a short period of time. Outgoing tide can pull people and boats out to sea. Both flows can be exacerbated by strong winds or storms.
- Inshore drift: a current lateral to shore. Can displace water users into more dangerous areas.
- Rip current: a body of water moving in a direction other than the general flow (out to sea/across a river). Water will follow the path of least resistance. If it is trapped behind a sandbank as the tide retreats it will flow quickly through channels. Identifying features include:
  - Discoloration of the water from disturbance of silt or sand.
  - Darker water surrounding current.
  - Floating debris or foam on the surface.
  - Surface changes such as rippled water while the surrounding area is calm.
  - Waves breaking behind and either side of the rip.

Rivers

- Risks vary markedly according to height, speed, and volume of water.
- Flash floods are a serious risk in mountain regions.
- Know where hazardous rapids are, and how water level affects them, especially if periods of heavy rainfall such as monsoons are imminent.
- Define the extent and complexity of portage if craft need to be transported around waterfalls and rapids.

Waves

- *Dumping waves* occur if the bottom is steep; they peak rapidly and drop the entire force of the wave into the floor. They commonly pull people off their feet, increasing the chance of spinal injury.

- *Spilling waves* have a gradual slope; white water 'spills' down the front of the wave. The point of breaking is dependent on the wind direction.
- *Surging waves* never break, lose speed, or gain height. They will 'surge' into the beach and retreat as quickly; often dragging people into deep water.

Other issues
- *Depth:* compared to shallow areas, deep water will usually appear darker and be associated with less surface disturbance.
- *Submerged objects:* rocks, sunken vehicles, and outlet pipes are difficult to recognize; in calm areas look for unexpected waves breaking over the obstruction.
- *Plants, reeds, seaweed:* can easily entrap swimmers or waders, use small gentle strokes to escape. Dense vegetation may hide snakes, crocodiles, etc. Floating debris is common after storm weather.
- *Quality:* water may be everywhere, but may not be drinkable as a result of chemical or bacteriological pollutants. Determine local dumping areas and sewage outlets. Smell or coloured algae foam can be an indication of hazardous zones.

Water's edge
Effective risk assessment requires an understanding of the nature of the coastal terrain.

Gradient
- *Vertical:* easy to slip into water of unknown depth, edges often unstable (e.g. canal walls decaying), difficult to extract a casualty.
- *Steeply sloping beaches:* will create dumping waves, prone to creating fast run-offs. Will knock people off their feet.
- *Shallow:* often long tidal range, will run in quickly, stranding people on sandbanks.

Construction
- *Shale/coral:* painful to walk on, sharp pieces can penetrate the skin and establish infections—must be removed completely (may require formal exploration).
- *Sand:* difficult to see animals (e.g. rays) which can be trodden on. May produce inshore holes, sandbanks, and subsequent rip currents.
- *Rock type:* limestone and sandstone beds to rivers will create 'holes' in which feet and equipment can get caught. Strong currents can injure trapped lower limbs.
- *Boat launching areas:* should avoid coral, urchins, dangerous currents, and other water users.

Landscape
- *Sandbanks:* false sense of security as you can stand on them; an incoming tide will produce a deep inshore hole between bather and the shore.
- *Inshore holes:* troughs that run parallel to the shore (can be several feet deep, up to 50 m wide, and several hundred metres long). Often rip currents develop as a wave breaks over a sandbar and then runs out to sea via the inshore hole.

- *Piers, outcrops:* can create rip currents. May be surrounded by submerged objects and waste.
- *Waste:* glass, oil (attracted to fixed structures, often submerged).
- *Flora:* Banyan tree, palm tree—falling coconuts can cause severe head injuries. The Manchineel tree in the Caribbean has caustic sap and fruits.

Humans in the aquatic environment

- *Hypothermia/hyperthermia:* humans are aware of peripheral rather than core temperature. Wet suits, which maintain peripheral temperatures, may disguise drops in core temperature. Regular wave splashes in rough water can lead to insidious loss of heat and serious impairment of judgement (📖 p. 596)
- *Diving:* risk of spinal and head injuries, depending on depth of water and submerged objects.
- *Surfing:* because of the shallow depths that waves break into, increased risk of spinal/head injuries and lacerations on coral/submerged objects.
- *Kite surfing/windsurfing:* similar to surfing with the added risk of joint dislocations. Injuries secondary to line entanglement are a particular hazard for kite surfers.
- *Kayaking:* occasionally craft can be caught between rock and current, or continuous battering by surf prevents 'righting'.
- *Swimming:* swimmers, surfers, and small craft risk being caught in currents and pulled into areas of water they do not want to be in. People often overestimate their ability, risking cramps, hypothermia, and fatigue.

Water-borne infections

- Weil's disease (leptospirosis)—bacterial disease transmitted in the urine of rats and found in stagnant or polluted water (📖 p. 467).
- Cholera (📖 p. 382).
- Onchocerciasis: filarial worm spread by flies, causing 'river blindness' in the tropics (📖 p. 486).
- Schistososmiasis ('bilharzia')—the animal vector is aquatic snails, often found in the tropics in still water or reeds (📖 p. 490).
- Hepatitis A (📖 p. 456).
- Other causes of gastrointestinal upset (📖 p. 380).

Hazardous marine and wildlife (📖 Chapter 16)

- Fish: lionfish, stonefish, weaver fish, candiru, sting ray, sharks.
- Mammals: hippopotamus.
- Reptiles: alligators and crocodiles.
- Coral.
- Jellyfish.
- Anemones.
- Birds.
- Snakes.

Immersion, drowning, and rescue

Definitions (World Health Organization)

- *Drowning* is the process of experiencing respiratory impairment from submersion or immersion in a liquid medium such that normal breathing is prevented. The outcomes of drowning may be death, morbidity, or recovery.
- *Immersion* implies that at least the airway and face are under the water, though the rest of the body may be floating.
- *Submersion* requires that the whole body be below the surface of the fluid.
- *Aspiration* is the process of solids or fluids entering the lungs.

Whether the casualty survives or not, they have been involved in a drowning incident.[1] No significant physiological difference exists between salt water and fresh water aspiration. The terms 'wet drowning', 'dry drowning', 'near drowning', and 'secondary drowning' are no longer in use.

Risk management

All expeditions working on or near water must consider the possibility of immersion and plan rescue procedures.

Drowning often occurs very quickly and unexpectedly.

- A personal flotation device dramatically improves your chances of surviving immersion—so long as you are wearing it. You may not have enough time to react and put it on if not wearing it.
- Accidents often happen out of reach of other party members. Use a buddy system to keep in touch with other team members.
- Many incidents could be avoided with good risk assessment.

Hazards of water

- *Drowning* is the third leading cause of accidental death worldwide (after road traffic injuries and falls) and, after excluding deaths caused by boating accidents and catastrophic floods, causes nearly 450 000 deaths a year[2]. Over 70% of deaths involve alcohol. Serious medical problems such as fits, heart attacks, and strokes may cause a person to collapse into water and then drown as a secondary event.
- *Cardiac arrhythmias* may develop as a result of a fall into cold water. The elderly and anyone with a history of hypertension or ischaemic heart disease are particularly at risk.
- *Swim failure*: very cold water can lead to muscular in-coordination and breathing problems. Shivering may be severe enough to prevent swimming. Wetsuits or drysuits, or habituation to cold water, reduce this effect.

---

1 Idris AH, Berg RA, Bierens J *et al.* (2003). Recommended guidelines for uniform reporting of data from drowning: the "Utstein style". *Resuscitation* **59**: 45–57.

2 Peden MM, McGee K (2003). The epidemiology of drowning worldwide. *Inj Control Saf Promot* **10**: 195–9.

- *Hypothermia* develops during prolonged immersion and is a common cause of death following shipwreck. Survival time in cold water is a matter of minutes for an unsupported, unprotected individual in cold water, but can be extended to hours by use of an immersion suit and buoyancy aid, and days in a covered life raft.
- *Wave splash*: those close to the sea surface can aspirate water following the slap of a wave on the face; turn your face away from waves. Some survival jackets come with face splashguards.

Immersion

There are four phases following immersion: initial response, short-term response, long-term response, and post-immersion response see Table 21.1. In addition, a sudden illness such as epileptic seizure or heart attack may have caused the casualty to fall into the water and must be assessed.

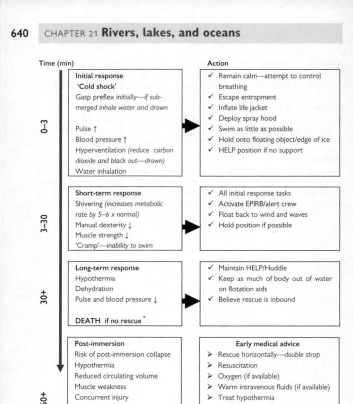

Time (min)

Action

0–3

Initial response
'Cold shock'
Gasp preflex initially—*if sub-merged inhale water and drown*

Pulse ↑
Blood pressure ↑
Hyperventilation *(reduce carbon dioxide and black out—drown)*
Water inhalation

✓ Remain calm—attempt to control breathing
✓ Escape entrapment
✓ Inflate life jacket
✓ Deploy spray hood
✓ Swim as little as possible
✓ Hold onto floating object/edge of ice
✓ HELP position if no support

3–30

Short-term response
Shivering *(increases metabolic rate by 5–6 x normal)*
Manual dexterity ↓
Muscle strength ↓
'Cramp'—*inability to swim*

✓ All initial response tasks
✓ Activate EPIRB/alert crew
✓ Float back to wind and waves
✓ Hold position if possible

30+

Long-term response
Hypothermia
Dehydration
Pulse and blood pressure ↓

DEATH if no rescue*

✓ Maintain HELP/Huddle
✓ Keep as much of body out of water on flotation aids
✓ Believe rescue is inbound

60+

Post-immersion
Risk of post-immersion collapse
Hypothermia
Reduced circulating volume
Muscle weakness
Concurrent injury
Psychological stress

Early medical advice
➢ Rescue horizontally—*double strop*
➢ Resuscitation
➢ Oxygen (if available)
➢ Warm intravenous fluids (if available)
➢ Treat hypothermia
   - Remove wet clothing
   - Handle with care
   - If conscious, give warm sugary drinks *(benefit is from providing fuel for shivering rather than heat)*
   - Prevent further heat loss

*Time to death depends on various factors (weight/water temperature/clothing/wind, etc.).
HELP: <u>H</u>eat <u>E</u>scape <u>L</u>essening <u>P</u>osition.
EPIRB: Emergency Positioning Indicating Rescue Beacon—a satellite rescue beacon.

Fig. 21.1 Responses to immersion.

Survival positions (HELP; Figs 21.2 and 21.3)

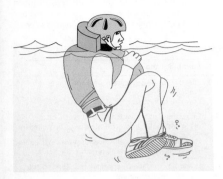

Fig. 21.2 HELP survival position. If alone in the water, assume this position to minimize heat loss from head, neck, sides of body, and groin region.

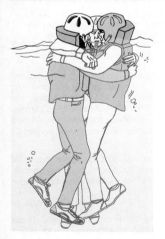

Fig. 21.3 HELP survival position. If two or more people are in water together, form a huddle so that sides of body are close together.

In calm water these positions help to conserve heat, but they are less effective and safe in rough seas, where individuals could be thrown against each other, risking injury.

Website

http://www.tc.gc.ca/MarineSafety

Rescue

However stressful the situation, never add to the death toll; maintain your own and others' safety. Have a realistic view of your own abilities and, unless highly skilled, avoid direct contact with a panicking casualty.

Table 21.1 Rescue techniques

Choice	Intervention	Suitability and risk
1st	Signal and shout	Effective for disorientated, weak, or injured swimmer Low risk to rescuer
2nd	Reach	Casualties that are within physical reach, or in reach with pole/stick, etc. Potential to be pulled in
3rd	Throw	Flotable aids or rope effective for weak/ injured swimmers. Rope throwing requires practice
4th	Boat or dingy	Limited by availability, operator skill, time to set up, and water conditions
5th	Swim with an aid	Swimming with flotable aid, can allow a small distance to be kept from casualty or assist tow
6th	Swim and tow	High risk owing to physical contact with panicking casualty. Energy sapping procedure. Avoid obstructing victim's airway with towing technique

Unconscious casualty

Approach swiftly, turn the casualty into a supine position. Prompt expired air ventilation (EAV) increases survival if the casualty is not breathing properly. Balance difficulties of administering rescue breath against the time taken to exit the water. If there is only a short distance to safety, exit and then resuscitate; if a longer swim is involved, and you have the skill and strength, attempt in-water EAV[3]. Casualties often vomit—be prepared.

Post-immersion collapse syndrome

Prolonged immersion creates dehydration, with blood pressure supported by hydrostatic pressure of water on limbs. Rescue in horizontal position if practical. Vertical extraction carries the risk of cardiovascular collapse and death.

Injuries

Certain aquatic accidents predispose to life-threatening injuries. These include fractures and head injuries from high-velocity impacts such as fast watercraft, cliff diving, or anybody in heavy surf. Surfers and those diving into shallow water are at high risk of cervical spine injuries, which are otherwise relatively uncommon.

Mass rescue
If more than one casualty is present, rescue must be prioritized.

Table 21.2 Priority of rescue

1st	Non-swimmer	Head going under water and unable to maintain a direction
2nd	Weak swimmer	Able to hold position and direction of sight but not move
3rd	Injured swimmer	Holds position, swims slowly, communicates injury
4th	Unconscious	Usually face down. If the casualty seen to go unconscious they are first priority to minimize period of hypoxaemia. But if period of hypoxia is unknown, victim may be dead and extraction of body from water will prevent rescue of other casualties

Basic resuscitation
Follow international guidelines[3] but, as the likely cause is primary respiratory failure, complete five initial breaths and 1 min of CPR before going for help. Approximately two-thirds of drowning victims will vomit, try to keep airway clear by turning head to face downhill. This will allow any fluid or vomit to drain away. Overall, only 0.5% of drowning victims will have associated spinal injury so care of the spinal cord is of secondary importance unless the casualty is known to have head injury or to have dived into shallow water. If spinal injury is suspected, and enough rescuers are present, extract the casualty horizontally from the water with cervical spine control and log-roll to clear the airway if required. Hypothermia and shock are common, even in tropical climates.

Advanced techniques
- An automatic external defibrillator may reveal electrical heart activity if pulses are impalpable.
- All post-drowning victims are hypothermic until proven otherwise. Shivering is a good prognostic sign. Warm appropriately(p. 597).
- Administer high flow oxygen (if available) during resuscitation and recovery.
- Dehydration and acidosis can develop from hypoxia and physiological effects of prolonged immersion. Consider warm intravenous fluids (if available), and monitoring of urine output and respiratory rate.
- Acute respiratory distress syndrome (ARDS) can develop up to 72 h post-immersion. It presents as a non-cardiogenic pulmonary oedema caused by the irritation of water in the lungs and requires hospitalization and ventilatory support[4]. If there is likely to be a delay in getting the patient to hospital and the casualty develops wheeze, consider regular hydrocortisone together with salbutamol inhalers/nebulizers.

3 European Resuscitation Council Guidelines (2005). Chapter 7c, s141–5.

4 Van Berkel M, Bierens J, Lie R et al. (1996) Pulmonary oedema, pneumonia and mortality in submersion victims; a retrospective study in 125 patients. *Intensive Care Medicine* **22**(2): 101–7.

- Aspiration pneumonia can develop later. Give appropriate antibiotics; in remote areas prophylactic antibiotics may be appropriate. It is worth considering other fungal or parasitic pathogens if aspirated water is potentially dirty, e.g. ditches or sewers.

All survivors of an immersion incident who might have inhaled water should, wherever practicable, be sent to a hospital capable of offering advanced respiratory support.

Discontinuing resuscitation

Good quality survival following prolonged immersion occurs, particularly in low temperature waters. Attempt basic resuscitation wherever practical and, if possible, evacuate to a hospital capable of advanced rewarming techniques such as cardiopulmonary bypass. After prolonged hypothermia or cardiac arrest, the core temperature should be re-stabilized at 33°C for 72 h before returning to normothermia. Expeditions in remote areas should attempt to resuscitate and rewarm a casualty, but will have to adopt a pragmatic approach to ceasing resuscitation attempts (see also Chapter 19).

Websites

http://www.surflifesaving.org.uk—Surf Lifesaving Association (GB).
http://www.lifesavers.org.uk—Royal Lifesaving Society (UK).

Kayaking, boating, and rafting

Preparation

Fitness: appropriate to the challenge is vital, especially for multiday trips.

Immunizations: consider hepatitis A, polio, and rabies for remote areas.

Shoulder and back injuries: avoid by developing good paddling and rafting technique. Learn to lift weights safely and efficiently.

Team working: your approach to interaction with the rest of the group is vital. Disputes about goals are a major factor in expedition 'failures'. Before you go, it is important to establish what you are all in it for—a challenging paddle, a holiday, or something in between?

Risk management

Environment: is wet, salty, and humid, leading to skin troubles.

Cold: either from wind or water chill. Hypothermia is a potential risk even in summer, chilblains, and trench foot a risk during prolonged cold water travel. Paddlers who have rolled a lot in a kayak or been immersed on a raft are particularly at risk and, as chilling develops, the likelihood of further capsize increases. The least capable and experienced are at greatest risk. Stop for day as soon as possible if anyone complains of fatigue or is perceived to be lagging behind. The victim will be unable to make this decision for themselves.

Sun glare: reflected off water increases risk of facial sunburn, eye strain, and UV keratitis (□ p. 604).

Insects: on shore and banks can irritate, bite, and carry disease.

Clothing: in semi-tropical and tropical regions wear comfortable warm weather kit with reduced chaff, and ensure warm and waterproof gear is easily accessible. For colder weather the choice of waterproof gear includes dry cagoules and the more comfortable, but less watertight options, like jackets and trousers with stretchy, lined neoprene or velcro at wrists and neck. During the day have easy access to warm clothes, food, and water. In case your boat gets separated from you, carry on your person: iodine, money, passport photocopy, matches, and whistle. Consider carrying a knife.

Footwear: should grip well on slippery rocks or when carrying a loaded boat. A trade off is between a firm sole for safety and a flexible sole that fits in a cramped cockpit.

Headgear: use a helmet in hazardous conditions or a peaked cap in calmer waters. Secure sunglasses with a safety cord around head. Many proprietary cords don't grip the spectacles leg strongly if you capsize—a thin, strong, knotted string may be best.

Shelter: tents are bulky to carry in kayaks. In a warm environment, in the absence of animal or insect hazards, you can reduce weight by taking bivouac bags or, for several people, a lightweight (2-ounce) tarpaulin using paddles as tent poles.

Attitude: mentally you have to remain positive throughout the journey; experience and fitness is important.

Gear: limited space for gear in rafts and kayaks requires careful selection of safety and first aid equipment and restricts options for palatable and nutritious food.

Rescue and evacuation: can be problematical from remote valleys, canyon walls, or inaccessible coastline.

Nutrition: drink only clean, filtered or purified water; at sea you must know the location of your next fresh water source. Rivers receive untreated sewage (especially in monsoon) but splashes encountered in normal paddling are not usually a health risk. The weight, bulk, and risk of mechanical failure or leakage with water filters encourages a lot of river paddlers to use iodine. You need to balance the need to reduce space by using expensive, ready made meals against the benefits carrying of fresh bulky food.

Alcohol: 70% of drowning incidents are associated with alcohol.

Safety
- Work as a team and know where everyone is.
- Use a buddy system; in bigger groups appoint front and rear paddlers. Split large groups into smaller units.
- Agree hand signals and methods of communication that will work despite wind or water noise.
- When scouting rapids, agree routes and running order with safety crafts or lines positioned below rapids.
- Helmets, paddles, and cagoules should be brightly coloured, perhaps even using fluorescent tape on dark-coloured gear.
- If travelling with a guiding company using their equipment, check the experience, qualifications, and first aid training of the guides and the age and serviceability of the vessels.
- Use good quality buoyancy aids and helmets where appropriate.
- Wherever possible in difficult water, ensure there are back-up or rescue craft.

Medical problems in small craft
- *Anterior shoulder dislocation* (📖 p. 414) is the most common serious injury for kayakers. Intermediate kayakers, especially those unfamiliar with the power of big water rivers, should be especially careful. Dislocations occur when the arm is extended and higher than the shoulder. Good paddling technique prevents shoulder dislocation; keep arms below the levels of your shoulders, and don't reach too far out to the side. Think of a box between spraydeck and shoulders, and 'keep your hands in the box'.
- *Diarrhoea* (📖 p. 380).
- *Cuts,* especially on the legs, may not heal until the trip is finished. Even the smallest cut can become infected, so at the end of each day wash the cut, apply antiseptics, and cover with a small plaster. On water trips, Steri-Strips™ don't stick well even with the use of tincture of benzoin. So-called waterproof dressings are not, although some people

use Opsite or similar successfully. Old hands use the ubiquitous duct tape; it isn't stretchy but it sticks well and most paddlers carry some for boat repair. If you have the training, suturing the cut gives better healing, reduces the risk of infection, and makes the cut waterproof after a day; tissue superglue is less effective, as it is not waterproof (📖 p. 284).

- **Paddle blisters** are fairly common on multiday trips, especially with water-softened skin, even amongst experienced paddlers. Strap tape or moleskin over 'hot spots'. If blisters burst, treat as a simple cut.
- **Burns.** Wood fires are often used on river trips, so burns are common. If the burn is severe enough to need sulphadiazine dressing, then keeping it dry is important but difficult.
- **Piles** are common in kayakers and can paradoxically be precipitated by both diarrhoea or constipation associated with dehydrated foods. If you suffer from piles, consider getting them treated before departure—they will only get worse (📖 p. 379).
- **Ear symptoms.** A common complaint amongst kayakers is 'water in the ear', typically resulting from a blocked Eustachian tube secondary to an upper respiratory tract infection and water immersion, after rolling a kayak. In the blocked inner ear, pressure reduces thereby pulling in the tympanic membrane and giving the sensation. Unblocking the Eustachian tube is often not successful, but try inhaling steam or a decongestant like Actifed before swallowing hard or using a Valsalva manoeuvre. You are unlikely to persuade an enthusiastic kayaker to avoid rolling so it is likely that the symptom will not clear up until after the trip ends. Air travel can be painful if ears are blocked.
- **External ear infections** are common in the tropics. Good aural toilet is important; use antibiotic, antifungal, or steroid ear drops. On the water try an ear plug of cotton wool and petroleum gel.
- **Bony exostoses** of the external ear canal are associated with frequent cold water impact from years of kayak rolling. When ear canal obstruction exceeds 50%, the risk of infection increases and hearing is impaired. Many experienced kayakers have over 80% obstruction. Operations to excise the exostoses don't always give symptom-free recovery. Prevent by using custom ear plugs and a neoprene hood (which does reduce hearing ability on the water). Plugs are especially important for athletic youngsters in play boats who are at an increasingly younger age being exposed to frequent immersion in cold water.
- **Dehydration** is a problem, especially when rafting in the heat. You may need to drink over 4 l a day. Early signs are vague symptoms such as headache, light-headedness, and lethargy, and are difficult to recognize unless you are on the look-out for them.

Tenosynovitis

- Tenosynovitis of the wrist tendon is a repetitive strain injury (RSI) owing to flexion and extension of the wrist while using a feathered paddle; that is, one with its blades set at an angle to each other.
- Pain can be severe and crepitus dramatic.
- Point tenderness distinguishes this from a non-specific sprain.

- Treatment is complete rest, which you may not be able to persuade your paddler to take.
- Wrist splint or neoprene support off (?and on) the water.
- Take an NSAID painkiller such as ibuprofen or diclofenac.
- Although value is uncertain, try changing paddle feather.

Back and muscle problems
- Stiff and knotted muscles, especially in the neck and between shoulder blades, are common on multiday trips and after moving heavy craft.
- Stretching exercises before and after paddling are worthwhile, as is evening massages of 'knots'.
- Sea paddlers can get leg strain through constant sitting in the same position.
- Lower back trouble is common in kayakers, especially as the kayaking posture flexes the lower lumbar spine against its natural lordosis.
- If you have back trouble you should remember proper lifting techniques, review your flexibility exercises before departure, fit a good backrest, and consider lifting aids like straps and even portable trolleys.
- Back, pelvis, and thigh strains are a risk in today's tightly strapped play boats. On the flatter river sections, you need to be able to release your legs easily.

Burn out and stress
- Rushed itineraries lead to chronic mild exhaustion.
- On challenging sea trips, safe landings can be hours away, but all team members have to be able to the face consequent fatigue and fear.
- Don't push weaker members into challenging coastlines/rapids.

Additional sea trip issues
- Sea sickness can be debilitating:
  - Risk factors include fatigue, cold, fear, watching compass.
  - Take a break, eat, provide psychological support for members.
  - Take anti-motion sickness drugs (📖 p. 651).
- Sunburn: use sunscreen, wear a cap, and cover exposed areas.
- Fungal infection is common in groins and feet.

Essential medical kit items for water-based expeditions
Often lack of space restricts choice of supplies.
- Plastic dropper bottle for iodine solution (1 per paddler).
- 1 large bandage (cut to size required).
- Suitable painkillers (📖 p. 48).
- Ziplock plastic bags and waterproof container/dry bags.
- Antibiotic ear drops (e.g. Betnesol-N), cotton wool, and petroleum gel.
- Hand cream, lip salve.
- Calamine lotion for sunburn.
- Seasickness tablets.
- Tape—duct tape sticks best, but doesn't stretch.

Offshore yachting and boating

'They who go down to the sea in ships and take their leisure
in deep waters'
(Psalm 107 verse 23)

Environmental factors

- *Isolation* from assistance is a major factor when assessing the fitness
  of crew and planning both medical kits and medical shore support.
- *Exposure* to extreme conditions (high winds, wave impact, motion,
  salt water, humidity, heat, cold, immersion) may cause a multiplicity of
  problems; anticipation and prevention are essential.
- *Trauma, illness, and physical danger* are medical and mental
  challenges, and are common occurrences; pre-existing medical
  conditions may relapse.
- *Seasickness* is a common and frequently disabling condition that is
  treatable in the majority.
- *Living conditions* are enclosed, cramped, and often difficult to maintain
  in clean condition, leading to community infection risks. Regular and
  well planned watch-keeping schedules are essential in avoiding fatigue.
- *Nutrition and hydration* are essential factors in maintaining team health
  and performance.
- *Team dynamics* are central to every facet of boat performance; a
  happy and healthy boat performs well.

Risk assessment

Both yacht racing and cruising involve significant risk:[5]

- 1 death per 200 000 miles or 60 man-years of sailing.
- 1 major incident per 10 000 miles.
- 1 minor incident per 2750 miles.

Specific risk factors

- Crew composition and fitness.
- Proposed route:
  - Distance from land (in/out of helicopter range of 200 miles).
  - Distance from frequented shipping routes.
  - Special obstacles, e.g. ice, fog, other shipping.
- Length of time at sea.
- On-board medical skill.
- Shore support.
- Medical kit contents.
- Communication availability.

Crew selection and preparation

Sailing in remote areas is no longer the preserve of the young and fit.

- Crew should be generally physically fit prior to the expedition, with
  particular attention paid to cardiopulmonary fitness and lower limb
  strength, which will decline when confined on board a yacht.

5 Osborne T (1990). First aid, illness and accidents on board: a Cruising Committee survey.
Cruising Summer Ed. Cruising Association, pp.12–15.

- Generally, there is greater risk taking crew who are dependent on oral medication for life-threatening conditions, such as organ transplant, epilepsy, or severe heart disease. Seasickness may prevent absorption of the medication. Conditions such as insulin-dependent diabetes mellitus and severe asthma also confer greater risk offshore.
- More stringent exclusion criteria should be applied to expeditions beyond helicopter range, probably excluding sailors with those conditions mentioned above.
- The Maritime and Coastguard Agency (MCA) guidelines[6] provide a structure for assessing potential crew with pre-existing medical conditions.
- Crew should be reviewed by a dentist prior to expedition departure.
- Immunizations should be up-to-date for tetanus, diphtheria, meningitis A and C, hepatitis A and B, and typhoid. Other immunizations and chemoprophylaxis (for malaria) may be required depending on the ports-of-call.
- Medical insurance is advisable for all crew.
- Ideally, a suitable crew member should be identified as being responsible for medical care on-board.

Communication and medical shore support

- Ocean sailing may put a yacht crew over 2 weeks from useful medical help. Expectation of self-reliance is the norm, and a realistic consideration of what can be treated offshore should be communicated to the crew.
- Helicopter range is approximately 200 nautical miles from the nearest base, and expeditions beyond this range should be planned more stringently.
- Means of communication must be reliable, and may be via VHF radio when within range. More distant communication may be via satellite telephone system (email or voice) or Inmarsat Standard C. Telemedicine is increasingly common but requires video transmission and reception, and the medical expertise to interpret the images.
- Shore support for medical emergencies is possible via international maritime rescue coordination centres such as MRCC Falmouth (a Maritime and Coastguard Agency service). There are various other organizations that provide support for expeditions to remote places, such as the Remote Health Unit, based at the Accident and Emergency Department, Derriford Hospital in Plymouth.
- Larger expeditions may organize their own shore medical support team that can then be tailored to the crew's specific requirements.

Specific medical problems

Seasickness

The three stages of mal de mer:

'I feel sick'

'I think I'm going to die'

'I'm worried I'm not going to die'

6 Maritime and Coastguard Agency (2002). Seafarer Medical Examination System and Medical and Eyesight Standards. Merchant Shipping Notice 1765(M).

- A common and disabling condition; untreatable in less than 20%.
- Prevention is better than a cure; commencing medication 24 h before leaving port is likely to be most effective.
- Behavioural adaptations may lessen the effects of motion: staying on deck, focusing on the horizon, helming, avoiding chart work down below, avoiding unpleasant smells, eating small meals regularly.
- Drug therapy may be effective in over 80% of sufferers; however, each individual varies in their response and it is worth finding the best drug or combination of drugs for each person.
- There is a wealth of evidence for and against most common remedies.
- Common remedies are cinnarizine (Stugeron), scopolamine, domperidone, and prochlorperazine (Stemetil). Drug delivery may be cutaneous, buccal, oral, rectal, intramuscular, or intravenous.
- Most remedies have side effects such as dry mouth, blurred vision, drowsiness, and urinary hesitancy.
- Dehydration and hypothermia may occur in severe seasickness, requiring active treatment.
- Seasickness susceptibility in females is linked to the menstrual cycle.
- Sickness usually improves after 48 h but may return if rough weather follows a period of relative calm.
- Being sick over the side carries the real risk of following the vomit. Use a bucket.

Immersion and drowning

- Prevention is better than cure.
- The man-overboard drill should be clearly understood and practised by all on board, to facilitate rapid recovery.
- The routine use of harnesses, life jackets with spray hoods, immersion-activated lights, and personal EPIRBs (emergency radio beacons) should be part of the ethos of the boat.
- Concurrent injury is common in the process of being swept over the side.
- Immersion in cold water causes uncontrolled rapid breathing and tachycardia.
- Initial action in the water should be to stay still, trying to minimize aspiration during initial gasps, then limit physical exertion, and heat loss by facing away from the weather. Adopt HELP position if practicable (Figs 21.2 and 21.3).
- Recovery should be in the horizontal position as far as possible to prevent circulatory collapse.
- Victims may require full resuscitation, rewarming, and supportive therapy for a prolonged period.

See 📖 p. 638 for more details.

Trauma

All types of sport and impact injuries may be encountered. Half of all injuries occur below decks[7]. The susceptibility to injury does not seem to be related to age of crew, but may be affected by work pattern on-board.

7 Price CJS, Spalding TJW, McKenzie C (2002). Patterns of illness and injury encountered in amateur ocean yacht racing: an analysis of the British Telecom Round the World Yacht Race 1996–1997. *Br J Sports Med* **36**: 457–62.

- Injuries may be life-threatening and include:
  - Head injuries (📖 p. 292).
  - Long bone fractures (📖 p. 410).
  - Blunt chest and abdominal trauma (📖 Chapter 6).
- Therapeutic manoeuvres that may be required include:
  - Chest drains.
  - Limb splints and cervical spine immobilizers.
  - Reduction of fractures and dislocations.
  - Simple local anaesthetic nerve blocks.
  - Intravenous access and fluid resuscitation.
  - Nasogastric tubes and urinary catheters.
  - Skin suturing or stapling (Steri-Strips™ and tissue glue are of limited use in the marine environment).

Skin
Sun, salt water, heat, cold, damp, and friction have a deleterious effect on the skin. Common complaints include:
- Salt water boils (📖 p. 276).
- Gunwhale bum.
- Prickly heat.
- Cockpit foot (non-freezing cold injury; 📖 p. 603).
- Rope burns.
- Sunburn.

Skin infections (such as impetigo and fungal infections of groin and foot) in the close yacht environment are also common. Personal hygiene is essential, and regular below-decks cleaning should occur. Skin and wound infections should be treated with antibiotics which include activity against the bacterium *Staphylococcus aureus*. Hypertrophy of the skin leads to the development of 'sausage fingers' and a dangerous reduction in dexterity. Barrier cream, moisturizers, and protective clothing such as gloves may reduce this process. Skin and lips must be protected against the sun.

Dehydration
A serious and potentially life-threatening condition, which can have many causes, including:
- Seasickness.
- Hot weather.
- Hard physical work in heavy clothing.
- Inadequately rehydrated freeze-dried food.
- Distraction from the process of regular rehydration.
- Unwillingness to undress to pass water regularly, so intentionally limiting fluid intake.
- Rehydration may be undertaken orally (with Dioralyte, for instance), rectally, or intravenously, which requires special medical training.
- Adequate personal hydration has to be part of the team ethos.

Medical kit

Contents and quantities

The contents and quantities of the medical kit are similar for any expedition to a remote location, and must take into account:

- Duration of expedition.
- Number of crew.
- Type of voyage—racing is obviously inherently more dangerous than cruising.
- Proposed route.
- Medical expertise on-board.
- Medical history of the crew members.
- Opportunities for re-supply in ports of call: generally English-speaking countries are easier for replenishment—drug availability, dosages, and names vary widely in other countries.

Kit format

- Arranged by body system to separate transparent bags or boxes
- In addition, separate bags containing:
  - Emergency/resuscitation drugs.
  - Hardware.
  - Intravenous/intramuscular drugs, needles, syringes.
  - Intravenous fluid (if carried).
- Grab bag (to be taken to the life raft if abandoning ship; may also double as emergency treatment bag):
  - Emergency analgesics (oral and intramuscular).
  - Seasickness medications (a large stock).
  - Antibiotics.
  - Rehydration salts.
  - Suturing kit.
  - SAM splints, strapping, bandages.
- Controlled drugs (e.g. morphine) must be kept secure and usage fully documented.
- First aid books, medical reference manuals, and the *British National Formulary* should be included.
- Oxygen cylinders and concentrators, and marine defibrillators for use on smaller yachts should be kept under review.
- The MCA have formulated a recommended kit list[8] for various classes of commercial vessel and yachts, with proposed quantities of medications.

---

8 Maritime and Coastguard Agency. Ships' Medical Stores (2003). Merchant Shipping Notice 1768 (M&F).

Emergency procedures

Helicopter evacuation

- A very costly resource to be used wisely. Not without risk to boat and helicopter crew. Training exercises are invaluable.
- Good communication with shore and helicopter crew is essential to ensure coordination and convey medical information regarding the victim.
- The normal range for helicopter rescue is within 200 nautical miles, occasionally using a fixed wing plane to locate the boat initially.

Method

- Brief your crew beforehand—it will be too noisy later.
- Communicate with the helicopter on VHF.
- The boat should steer a straight course close hauled on port, with the helicopter hovering off to port (avoids downdraft hitting yacht).
- Rescue will take place from the starboard door of the helicopter and the port side of the boat.
- Be prepared:
  - Clear the deck of loose objects.
  - Do as the helicopter crew tell you; they are the experts!
  - Use gloves.
  - The victim should be dressed and ready, with medical record attached.
  - All crew should be clipped to the boat.
- Initially, a weighted 'hi-line' is dropped from the helicopter. Do not touch until it has earthed in water or on the boat.
- *Do not attach the line to the boat and avoid it getting snagged.* For safety, coil it into a bucket.
- A diver descends on the main lifting wire; pull him in to the boat.
- Follow his directions.
- A single or double strop or stretcher may be used.
- In rough weather, recovery may be from a life raft trailed astern, or directly from the water.

Life raft evacuation

(Always ensure regular life raft servicing.)
- Only abandon a boat if it is sinking under your feet.
- Anticipate the possibility and be prepared. Each crewman should have a pre-assigned abandonment task.
- All crew get very seasick in a life raft; take medications beforehand.
- Take the grab bag (see medical contents above).
- Other essential items (see ISAF recommended list[9]).
- Water (as much as possible) and portable water maker if carried.
- Weatherproof clothing and life jackets (put on before entering raft).
- VHF radio.
- Satellite/mobile phones (the latter if inshore).

9 ISAF (International Sailing Federation) Offshore Special Regulations Appendix A Part 1 and 2 (2003). http://www.sailing.org

- Flares.
- EPIRB(s).
- Polythene or waterproof bags for vomit, faeces, urine.
- Toilet paper.
- Torches.
- Handheld GPS.
- Food.
- Crew get very sick, dehydrated, may be injured, and mentally traumatized by losing their boat.

Sources of further information
The Maritime and Coastguard Agency: http://www.mcga.gov.uk
The Royal Yachting Association: http://www.rya.org.uk
Cruising Association: http://www.cruising.org.uk
Royal Ocean Racing Club (RORC): http://www.rorc.org
Ships Captain's Medical Guide (2003) 22nd edn, HMSO. http://www.hmso.gov.uk

Maritime medical training courses
Sea Survival Course, Elementary First Aid: The Royal Yachting Association.
First Aid at Sea: The Maritime and Coastguard Agency.
Medical Care at Sea: The Maritime and Coastguard Agency.

References

Golden F, Tipton M (2002). *Essentials of Sea Survival.* Human Kinetics, Leeds. ISBN 0736002154.

Howarth F, Howarth M (2002). *The Grab Bag—Your Ultimate Guide to Liferaft Survival.* Adlard Coles Nautical. ISBN 978–0713662214.

International Medical Guide for Ships, 2nd edn. (1997). World Health Organization. ISBN 92 4 154 231 4.

Weiss EA, Jacobs M. *A Comprehensive Guide to Marine Medicine.* Adventure Medical Kits, Oakland, USA. ISBN 0965976823.

Cold Water Casualty Video (1990). British Defence Library A3788. Institute of Naval Medicine.

Website
http://adventuremedicalkits.com

Diving

Fitness to dive

Participants in a diving expedition may have diving qualifications from any of a number of training organizations, which have varying requirements for fitness to dive. Some general standards apply, which may be modified according to the diving activity. The basic principle is that any condition that may unexpectedly impair the diver's ability to exert themselves physically or that may cause a sudden alteration in conscious level will usually mean the candidate is unfit to dive.

Category	Condition	Notes
Absolute	Epilepsy	Ischaemia or dysrhythmias
	Cardiac disease	COPD/emphysema, asthma
	Obstructive airway disease	
	Pregnancy	
	Chronic middle ear disease	
	Insulin-dependent diabetes	
Relative	Obesity	BMI>35 kg/m^2
	Lack of physical fitness	For expedition demands
	Psychiatric disease	Requiring medication
	Penetrating chest injury	Unless medically cleared
Temporary	Acute upper respiratory tract infection	Until resolved
	Tympanic membrane barotrauma	Tympanic membrane perforation 4 weeks, otherwise 24–48 h
	Decompression illness	Review by diving physician

Notes

- Well controlled asthma (i.e. rare requirement for inhaled bronchodilators) may be permissible, but many serious diving incidents have been associated with acute asthma attacks.
- Well controlled insulin-dependent diabetes mellitus may not contraindicate sport diving in controlled circumstances, but the risk of hypoglycaemia is usually incompatible with expedition level diving.
- Any expedition where the diver is receiving monetary or other recompense for diving may bring them within the scope of commercial diving regulations and their (stringent) medical requirements.
- There is insufficient evidence that a fetus is not harmed by diving; pregnancy should therefore be regarded as a contraindication to diving.
- The standard of physical fitness applied should be appropriate for the type of diving that will occur. Various methods of assessment exist (such as the Harvard step test) but may not be appropriate for the underwater environment.
- If in doubt, advice should be sought from an experienced diving physician (contact the Institute of Naval Medicine, *vide infra*).

Decompression illness

Decompression sickness, often known as 'the bends', includes clinical syndromes caused by intravascular or extravascular gas bubbles generated during ascent. At depth, nitrogen (or helium) becomes dissolved in blood and body tissues. If the diver ascends too rapidly, supersaturation of dissolved gas causes bubble formation which may generate a wide variety of clinical effects, or none. A different mechanism of injury is expansion of gas in the diver's lungs into the pulmonary veins during a very rapid ascent, which is then carried through the left side of the heart to the brain, causing cerebral arterial gas embolism (CAGE). In practice, a distinction between this and the effects of dissolved inert gas (DCS) may be clinically difficult and therefore both entities are commonly encompassed within the term decompression illness (DCI). This is classified descriptively according to its manifestations (see below), but the older division of decompression sickness into type 1 (minor) and type 2 (major) is still used in many parts of the world.

Descriptive classification of decompression illness

Manifestations:	Neurological	Evolution:	Progressive
	Limb pain		Relapsing
	Girdle pain		Static
	Pulmonary		Spontaneously improving
	Cutaneous		
	Lymphatic		Resolved
	Constitutional		
Inert gas load:	Depth/time profile	Evidence of barotrauma:	Lung
	Decompression obligation		Sinus
			Ear
	Gas mixture(s) used		Dental

Typical presentations of decompression illness

- Limb pain: typically dull but severe (like toothache), improved or not worsened by movement, relieved by direct pressure, may mask subtle neurological abnormalities in the same limb (type 1).
- Cutaneous: bluish 'marbling' itchy rash of 'cutis marmorata', typically on torso (type 1).
- Constitutional: extreme fatigue, malaise (type 1).
- Rapid loss of consciousness, seizures, hemiparesis: suggests cerebral arterial gas embolism.
- Paraplegia: acute spinal syndrome with girdle pain, lower limb paralysis, sensory level and bladder dysfunction (type 2).
- Other neurological symptoms: paraesthesiae, numbness, weakness, especially of upper limbs (type 2).
- Cognitive dysfunction: subtle cognitive and memory impairment, personality changes (type 2).

- Vertigo ('the staggers'): distinguish from vague 'dizziness'; may also result from inner ear barotrauma (type 2).
- Dyspnoea ('the chokes'): suggests significant venous gas embolism (type 2). Pneumothorax should be excluded.

First aid treatment

First aid treatment of decompression illness is simple, but recognizing that there is a problem often is not. Concealment and denial are common amongst divers because of the perceived stigma attached to decompression illness.

- Resuscitation: ABC.
- Administer 100% oxygen with a demand regulator; constant-flow systems rarely deliver more than 75% even with a reservoir bag.
- Keep lying flat if there is any concern for cerebral gas embolism.
- Give fluids: oral if the diver is alert, otherwise intravenous.
- Keep comfortably cool, but not to the point of shivering.
- Seek expert advice and consider evacuation to recompression facility.

NB. Symptoms may resolve during treatment with oxygen, but (especially with neurological presentations) relapse is common without hyperbaric therapy.

Evacuation

- Recompression becomes less effective as each hour passes. Most benefit is obtained within 6 h of onset, but some cases respond even after several days.
- First aid (oxygen, fluids) should continue during transport.
- Unpressurized aircraft should be flown at the lowest safe altitude.

Recompression treatment

Recompression protocols typically start with compression to 2.8 atmospheres (18 m/60 feet) on 100% oxygen, with subsequent treatment based on clinical response. Most cases are treatable using US Navy Table 6 (RN Table 62) with extensions if necessary. In remote areas, hyperbaric facilities may be limited and unable to sustain a treatment longer than this, even if it is required. Further treatments may then be used to improve any residual manifestations. Recompression treatment (and evacuation) is very expensive and divers should be adequately insured.

Expert advice

The Royal Navy's Institute of Naval Medicine in Alverstoke, Hampshire can give 24-h impartial advice to divers in England and Wales or those travelling abroad. The contact number is: +44 7831 151523 (Duty Diving Medical Officer, INM).

For incidents in Scotland call: +44 845 408 6008 (On-call hyperbaric consultant, Aberdeen).

In the USA/Caribbean: +1 919 684 8111 (Divers Alert Network, USA).

Barotrauma

The volume of an enclosed gas-filled space varies inversely with pressure (Boyle's Law). If rigid air-containing spaces within the body are not 'equalized' with the pressurized breathing gas on descent (or rarely ascent) they will be compressed ('squeezed').

Middle ear (tympanic membrane) barotrauma

- Pressure/pain on ascent or descent.
- 'Muffled' hearing post-dive owing to middle ear effusion.
- Vertigo under water with sudden relief of pain suggests perforation.
- Tympanic membrane may appear inflamed and retracted.
- Return to diving: 24–48 h if no perforation has occurred. If perforation is present, diving should be avoided for at least 28 days and full otolaryngological review should be sought to avoid the disabling complication of chronic non-healing tympanic membrane perforation.

Inner ear barotrauma

- Rupture of the round window of the cochlea caused by pressure differential between inner and middle ear, usually because of excessive Valsalva manoeuvres.
- Severe persistent vertigo associated with a sensorineural hearing loss. It should be distinguished from alternobaric vertigo (transient vertigo on ascent), decompression sickness, and caloric vertigo from tympanic membrane perforation.
- Decompression illness affecting the inner ear may cause severe vertigo; differentiating it from inner ear barotrauma is difficult and may rest on the response to hyperbaric oxygen therapy, which is safe and occasionally therapeutic in inner ear barotraumas.

Pulmonary barotrauma

Rapid expansion of alveolar gas during a rapid ascent must be vented through the airways; if this cannot occur it may rupture into surrounding structures or pulmonary blood vessels. Air can escape into:

- The pleural cavity, causing a pneumothorax (chest pain, breathlessness, cardiovascular collapse).
- The mediastinum, causing pneumomediastinum (central chest pain, voice change, neck swelling, subcutaneous emphysema).
- Pulmonary capillaries, causing arterial gas embolism (see above, Decompression illness). Typical presentation is with rapid loss of consciousness, convulsions, and/or neurological deficits such as hemiparesis and dysphasia.

Alternobaric facial paresis

Some divers have an anatomical variation that may allow air to enter the facial nerve canal during forceful equalization manoeuvres. Expansion of the air bubble on ascent compresses the facial nerve, resulting in painless ipsilateral lower facial weakness. It resolves within a few hours or immediately with recompression and has no long-term significance.

Gas problems

Nitrogen narcosis

- High partial pressures of nitrogen have anaesthetic-like effects.
- Typical symptoms (with increasing depth):
  - Tunnel vision, euphoria, apprehension.
  - Inability to manage complex tasks.
  - Tinnitus, drowsiness.
  - Eventual loss of consciousness.
- Exacerbated by hypercapnia, exertion, cold water, and darkness.
- Large variation in diver susceptibility.
- Resolves rapidly on ascent.
- Main danger is impairment of diver's performance.

Hypercapnia (carbon dioxide retention)

Multiple causes

- Learned diver behaviour: hypoventilation, e.g. by 'skip-breathing'.
- High gas density (excessive depth for gas mixture used).
- High oxygen partial pressure (reduces ventilatory drive).
- Excessive exertion.
- Scrubber 'breakthrough' (rebreather divers).

Symptoms

- Headache, flushing, palpitations.
- Breathlessness (often does not occur in the diving context).
- Eventual loss of consciousness.

Acute (CNS) oxygen toxicity

Aetiology

- Exposure to high partial pressure of oxygen (PO_2).
  - Depth too great for gas mix being breathed (open circuit).
  - Rebreather malfunction or misuse (semi- or closed-circuit).
- Both PO_2 and duration are important.
- Toxicity rare at $PO_2 < 1.6$ bar.
- Threshold for toxicity lowered by immersion, exertion, hypercapnia.

Manifestations

- Facial (especially lip), diaphragmatic, and other muscle twitching.
- Visual disturbances (e.g. central and peripheral visual field defects).
- Nausea, vertigo, tinnitus.
- Dysphoria ('sensation of impending doom').
- Convulsions (may be the first manifestation).

Management

- Reduce the PO_2 as soon as possible (e.g. ascend, switch gas mix).
- Convulsions occurring under water are difficult to deal with:
  - Maintain diver's depth during initial tonic phase of the seizure, to prevent severe barotraumas caused by uncontrolled ascent.
  - Attempt to keep mouthpiece in casualty's mouth if possible.
  - Recover to the surface once the clonic (jerking) phase has started but do not compromise any other diver's safety.
  - Resuscitate on surface and evacuate urgently to a medical facility.
  - Casualty may need recompression or treatment for effects of aspiration.

Hypoxia

- Caused by breathing gas mix with PO_2<0.1–0.12 bar.
- Rare in open-circuit diving as most gas mixes exceed this PO_2 at only a few metres depth.
- Rebreather divers are at greater risk owing to equipment malfunction or misuse (e.g. oxygen injector solenoid failure).
- Cognitive function is insidiously impaired up to loss of consciousness.
- Treatment is administration of oxygen, but emphasis is on prevention.

Carbon monoxide poisoning

- Caused by contamination of gas supply (e.g. compressor intake downwind of petrol/diesel engine exhaust); fortunately now very rare.
- Manifestations are in-coordination, weakness, headache, nausea, and malaise.
- Symptoms appear at depth owing to higher partial pressure of carbon monoxide, offset by higher PO_2 in breathing gas.

Treatment

- Remove cause (surface or breathe alternative gas).
- 100% oxygen; severe poisoning may require hyperbaric oxygen therapy.
- Other defects with breathing air compressors (even electric) may result in contamination with other toxic compounds (such as lubricating oil breakdown products) that may produce similar or other bizarre symptoms at depth.

Non diving-specific hazards

Other medical problems encountered in the diving environment but not specific to it include:

- Trauma.
- Working with heavy equipment on a small boat in a heavy sea.
- Propeller injuries from small surface craft.
- Hypothermia (see 🕮 p. 596).
- Near drowning (see 🕮 p. 638).
- Dangerous marine life (see Chapter 16).

Useful items for an expedition diving medical kit

- 100% oxygen with appropriate delivery system.
- Intravenous fluids and cannulas.
- Sutures and/or adhesive strips for lacerations.
- Bandages and splints.
- Seasickness prophylaxis.
- Simple analgesics (paracetamol, NSAIDs).
- Antibiotics (oral and/or parenteral), antibiotic eardrops.
- Auroscope.

Caving expeditions

Paul Cooper

The environment

Deep, tight caves are found both near to civilization and in very remote areas, the latter adding to the logistic difficulties. In some parts of the world, especially South East Asia, accessing cave entrances may be hazardous because of landmines and other munitions from previous conflicts. When searching for entrances in heavy undergrowth there may be risks from snakes and other venomous animals. Cave expeditions often involve diving (see Chapter 21).

Caves usually have a fairly constant low temperature of 5–8°C. Hypothermia (📖 p. 596) is a significant risk especially where running or falling water creates high humidity, spray, and cave draughts, so intensifying the chilling effect. This is a particular risk if you have to wait for any time, or if you have an unanticipated bivouac—a space blanket in a pocket or kept in your helmet could be a life-saver.

Types of caving expedition

Caving expeditions may be:
- Large expeditions, based at one site, often for several weeks. These are usually exploring a large cave system, will have many members, and will often have a specified medical officer. Deep cave exploration requires major logistic support.
- Smaller lightweight expeditions, with fewer members, often reconnaissance, the caving may be less challenging, but may be more remote.

Humans in the cave environment

Clothing

Typical cave clothing is impermeable and traps perspiration, so a prolonged wait at a pitch head after a vigorous climb can be very cold; the combination of a wet shell garment with damp undergarments leads to rapid heat loss. Up to half the heat loss from an otherwise well insulated person is from the head, so keep a silk or fleece balaclava in your pocket and put it on when stationary. Cold injury, either hypothermia (📖 p. 596) or non-freezing peripheral cold injury (trench foot; 📖 p. 603), is a risk during prolonged trips, especially in wet caves.

Hygiene

Strict food handling and sanitation arrangements are essential underground. Underground latrine arrangements vary depending on the nature of the cave; many modern underground camping expeditions will bring out solid matter in plastic bags. Alcohol gel hand lotion should be available at the camp. When washing is impractical, baby wipes are useful for personal hygiene.

Minor injuries (📖 Chapter 8)

'Crutch rot', split fingers, and minor foot injuries, blisters and the like are common. Experienced cavers have their own views on how to deal with what are usually just minor irritations. Tissue superglue, used to repair skin splits on fingers and feet, is a useful addition to the underground first aid kit.

Risk management

Rescue

Caving has a fatal accident rate twice that of climbing accidents in the UK (although the risk is still much lower than climbing in the Greater Ranges) but a relatively low non-fatal accident rate.[1] Some accidents, for instance those caused by rock falls, may be unavoidable, but others are preventable. Be careful 'pushing the cave' when tired or cold. The low non-fatal accident rate indicates that there is a low margin for error and that death is common if something goes wrong. A relatively minor injury is likely to be fatal if the victim is unable to assist during the extraction. Small independent expeditions are usually incapable of mounting a major rescue without outside help.

An excellent cave rescue ropework manual is presently available at: http://www.draftlight.net/lifeonaline/. An updated edition will be found at: http://www.lifeonaline.com/. If planning to explore vertical caves, download the manual and practise the techniques before departure.

Harness hang (also known as suspension trauma)

If someone is immobile upright in a harness for some time, the usual muscle pump in the legs ceases and venous return to the heart is impeded. This can lead to syncope with loss of consciousness. Usually when someone faints, they fall to the ground, venous return is restored, and cerebral perfusion resumes. However, in a harness this correction cannot occur, and the resultant loss of cerebral blood flow may be rapidly fatal. Cavers are particularly at risk when they are immobile in a harness on a rope, especially if unconscious. The first priority if you have an unconscious companion hanging on a rope, maybe knocked out from a falling rock, is to swing them horizontal, so that their legs, heart, and head are all at the same level. This will probable mean moving the point of suspension down to their waist, obviously taking suitable precautions to ensure that they don't come off the rope. You may only have a few minutes, so act quickly, but get them off the rope as soon as possible.

Bad air

Bad air is an issue in some caves, although you should usually be aware of the risks beforehand. The gases in question result from decaying organic matter, including guano, in caves with poor ventilation.

Important gases are:
- Methane
  - Odourless, lighter than air, disperses
  - Formed from organic matter, common in coalmines
  - Potential asphyxiation hazard
  - Highly explosive, so avoid any naked flames, such as carbide lights
- Hydrogen sulphide
  - Smells of rotten eggs; any such smell should prompt a rapid exit from the cave
  - Early symptoms include headache, dizziness, numbness, and tingling

---

1 Mohr PD (2000). Gauging risk. *Descent* **153**: 20–24.

- May inactivate the olfactory nerves, rapidly reducing ability to sense scent
- Heavier than air, accumulates in caves with poor ventilation
- Present in volcanic areas
- Highly toxic, combining with haemoglobin and with cytochromes in a manner similar to cyanide to block cellular metabolism rapidly.

Specific medical problems for cavers

There are a number of specific diseases that can be a particular risk in caves. If you consider that any of them might be a risk in the area that you are visiting then seek expert advice before you go. Consult the Cave-Associated Disease Database: http://www.latech.edu/tech/education/cavedis/cave-disease-table2_1.html.

American trypanosomiasis (Chagas disease; 📖 p. 483)

Protozoan infection transmitted by faeces of tritomine bugs; widespread in South America. Infection develops through contamination of skin.

Histoplasmosis (📖 p. 53)

Fungal infection from infected bats' droppings. It results in chronic malaise and, as it is usually diagnosed following chest X-ray (which may resemble sarcoid), it is not readily diagnosed in the field. Although it may resolve spontaneously, specialist treatment with antifungals is likely to be required.

Leishmaniasis (📖 p. 482)

Transmitted by sand flies, especially in China.

Leptospirosis (📖 p. 467)

Transmitted by exposure to water contaminated by rodent urine. It presents with an acute generalized febrile illness, usually with jaundice, and specialist investigation may be needed to distinguish it from other febrile illnesses in the tropics.

Rabies (📖 p. 458)

Transmitted by cave bats. If visiting caves in areas where it is prevalent, ensure the party has been immunized pre-departure.

Relapsing fever (📖 p. 467)

Caused by a *Borrelia* spirochaete and transmitted by tick or louse. Tick-borne relapsing fever is prevalent on the west coast of North America and is common in caves, with an intermediate animal host. It results in a relapsing fever(!), together with headaches, abdominal pains, and myalgia. Treatment is with tetracycline, but this can result in a Jarisch–Herxheimer reaction.

St Louis encephalitis

Occurs in epidemics in the southern United States, and may be of particular risk to cavers as the intermediate host includes bats.

Conclusions

Caves are dangerous places, and they can be cold and wet. You are unlikely to survive a significant accident, and therefore *take care*, as rescue is likely to be limited to helping out the 'walking wounded'. However, caves are amongst the last unexplored areas on Earth and there are some great places to find!

Hot environments— deserts and tropical forests

Section editor
Chris Johnson

Contributors
Jon Dallimore, Sundeep Dhillon, Paul Richards, and Shane Winser

The environment

Two of the most popular expedition destinations, deserts and tropical forests, seem very different. Deserts appear barren, arid, and have a very limited range of highly adapted plants and animals, while in contrast the hot and humid tropical forests offer the world's richest ecosystem. Yet the physiological challenge to humans, that of living and working in persistently high temperatures, is the same and so both environments are discussed in this chapter.

Deserts

A desert is a region with little vegetation and much exposed bare soil, where average annual rainfall is less than 20% of the amount needed to support optimum plant growth, and where plants and animals show clear adaptations for survival during long droughts. Covering almost 20% of the earth's land mass, deserts are mainly found between 25° and 35° north and south of the equator, and are home to around 1 billion people.

Some deserts consist of the sand dunes of popular imagination, but others are rocky wastelands or semi-arid grasslands. Diurnal and seasonal temperature ranges can be considerable, with the landscape sculpted by freeze/thaw cycles and by powerful winds driving sand, soil or snow.

Website

http://www.unep.org/geo/GDOutlook/016.asp

Clothing and footwear

Wear light, loose-fitting clothes made of natural materials that allow air to circulate and sweat to evaporate. Protect the head with a hat, scarf, or khaffieh. Shorts and T-shirts are also convenient and usually perfectly adequate, but be conscious that such dress, particularly if worn by women, may cause offence in some countries. Exposed skin must be properly protected by sunblock while both sunglasses and goggles are essential.

Footwear needs to be light, comfortable, and tough; boots, shoes, and trainers all have disadvantages. Enclosed feet become sweaty, smelly, soft, and prone to fungal infections. On the other hand, bare feet or light shoes expose the feet to heat from the ground, injury by rock or thorns, and bites from snakes or scorpions. In sand and gravel deserts, walking sandals, trainers or desert boots suffice; heavier footwear is required in stony and volcanic areas.

Bases and campsites

It is possible to travel for months in deserts without the need for formal shelter. A camp bed off the ground is protection against snakes and scorpions (but remember to shake your shoes out in the morning). A tent or impregnated mosquito net will protect against insects. Guard the area against human or large animal invasion. Beware of making camps in dry riverbeds or wadis which can be susceptible to flash flooding from rainfall miles away.

Travel

Most desert expeditions use vehicles. These must be well maintained and have adequate tyres, tool kits, and spares to cope with the stresses of travel. Ensure the party knows how to extricate a bogged vehicle, and do not lose the keys. Travellers relying on more traditional travel methods require suitable skills in animal husbandry to keep pack animals healthy, content, and tethered at night.

Navigation

Journey times are often very long. Maps can be unreliable and roads may be little more than parallel tracks on the ground, invisible if the wind is blowing. GPS is invaluable but ensure suitable back-up.

Risk management

Difficult travel

Considerable reserves of fuel, food, and water are essential to ensure safety in the event of bad weather, mechanical failure or navigational problems.

Dust storms

Dust storms can develop with little warning in any arid or semi-arid environment. These take the form of an advancing wall of dust and debris that may be miles long and several thousand feet high; they can appear from any direction though generally follow the prevailing winds. Most storms pass within an hour, but some may persist for several hours. High winds can destroy tents and strip campsites bare. Health risks include suffocation from dust inhalation and extremely low visibility both on roads and in the air, leading to disorientation and the possibility of serious accident.

Flora and fauna

Snakes and scorpions (see Chapter 16) live in deserts and may enter discarded footwear or containers. Plants in arid areas can have thorns, tough spiny surfaces, or serrated leaves.

Survival strategies in a dust storm

- Don't panic!
- Avoid travelling in dust storms if at all possible.
- If caught in a dust storm while driving, get off the road. Turn off driving lights and turn on emergency flashers.
- If out in the open with a dust storm coming your way, sit down with your back to the wind, and cover your head with your clothes to keep dust out of your eyes, nose, mouth, and ears (a dry shemagh or bandana is ideal—wet clothing will quickly become clogged up).

Tropical forests

Tropical rain forests cover a dwindling 6% of the Earth's land mass, and are defined by their location (between the Tropic of Cancer 23° 27′ N and the Tropic of Capricorn 23° 27′ S) and their high rainfall, which can be several metres a year. During the day the forests are hot and humid, often with little breeze to give respite, but at night they become much cooler, and travellers in upland forests may require a blanket or lightweight sleeping bag. The forest floor may be under water for much of the year. Primary rain forest, where the high tree canopy suppresses ground growth, is more open than secondary forest. Here, previous felling allows light to reach the forest floor and promote growth of dense jungle.

Clothing and footwear

- Accept daytime wetness. Rinse kit in camp and re-wear wet next day. Keep a dry set of clothing in a plastic bag for evening and bedtime use to preserve comfort and skin.
- Never go barefoot or wear sandals; you risk cuts, insect or snake bites, larva migrans, jiggers, etc.
- Use boots with good treads that dry quickly. De-roofed blisters could develop into ulcers, so ensure that boots are properly worn-in before entering the jungle.
- Cover up—long sleeves and trousers protect you from irritant plants and insect bites.
- Gloves protect against sawgrass cuts, especially when using a machete.
- Hats protect against sun, rain, and barbed leaves.

Bases and campsites

Choose with care:

- Avoid river banks which can flash flood from distant rains upstream. Low river banks are access points to and from the water for wild animals. Check potential campsite for animal spoor and droppings.
- Abandoned native shelters may be structurally unsound and can harbour spiders, ants, rodents, and snakes which feed off them. Even when the fauna have left, there is a potential source of infections such as histoplasmosis and Chagas' disease.
- Look up: site shelters away from rotting trees or branches that could crash down (so-called 'deadfall').
- Sleep off the ground to avoid snakes, scorpions, etc. Construct a raised sleeping platform or sling a hammock. Use a mosquito net and, if outside, protect yourself from rain using plastic sheeting or tarpaulin (Fig. 23.1).
- Clearing enough ground for tents can take a lot of energy and it can be difficult to remove stumps effectively. If used, tents should have a midge mesh, sewn-in bucket-type groundsheet and zips that seal the entrance. They can be stiflingly hot and are heavy when wet.
- Leaf litter can hide snakes and scorpions, so this is best cleared from the ground beneath hammocks and around tent entrances.
- Protect group areas from rain by tarpaulins.

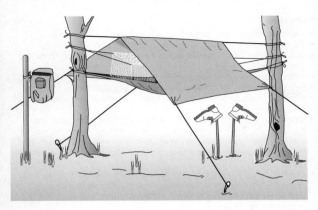

Fig. 23.1 Jungle shelter.

Behaviour

- Minimize risk of insect bites (📖 p. 69, 478 and Table 14.1).
- Be wary of snakes (📖 p. 526) and scorpions (📖 p. 539).
- Avoid trauma. Learn correct use of machete—sheathed when carried and not in use.
- Wear footwear with good grips for muddy ground or log travel.
- Practise crossing rivers safely, but avoid where possible.
- On log bridges, balance is aided by fixing eyes ahead and use of a walking pole.
- Drink only sterilized water and maintain appropriate personal and food hygiene. Beware water contamination with heavy metals such as mercury from gold mining in the Amazon. This will not be removed by boiling, but filters using activated carbon should reduce the risk (📖 p. 106).
- Learn to navigate using map and compass. GPS is useful but may require wide clearings as the canopy impedes the signal. Use trails, walk in file keeping neighbours in sight, use guides, and place one at the back of the group.
- Make sure that you have a survival kit when moving out of camp in jungle, which should include everything you will need to survive for some days if lost. A good aphorism is 'never get separated from your kit'.
- Rise at dawn, eat and drink, and make a camp an hour before nightfall, as it will take at least an hour to put up bashas or hammocks, and get a fire lit before the sudden arrival of the tropical night.
- Respect local customs, including those of dress (📖 p. 26).
- Avoid ingesting hallucinogenic plants or other native drugs.

Psychological stress

Unfamiliar sounds, smells, fear of animals, disease, the intense darkness of night, or the isolation of sleeping exposed in a hammock in a strange place may contribute to anxiety (Fig. 23.1). Learn about the environment, listen to the local guides, become informed. Fear arises from unfamiliarity and uncertainty; knowledge helps you to find the forest accommodating rather than intimidating. Prolonged exposure to wet discomfort saps morale, so regular return to a comfortable environment such as a well constructed base camp is important. 'Social time', particularly for sharing the evening meal and general relaxed chat, is important for team integrity and morale.

Serious heat-related illnesses

In hot weather a major environmental risk is that of developing some form of heat illness. Humans originated in tropical regions and retain the capability to acclimatize physiologically to living and working in hot climates. Yet many people fall victim to the effects of heat, not only in the tropics, but also whilst exercising in temperate latitudes. Various terms have been used to describe heat-related conditions.

Acute heat stress

In areas of extreme heat stress such as the Gulf States where daytime WBGT (📖 p. 693) may exceed 36°, acute heat stress may develop. Over a 2–24 h period a victim may show the symptoms of heatstroke (see box below), but there may be no measurable fever and no biochemical abnormalities. Victims treated immediately will recover rapidly on cooling, although they may be left with a headache that is refractory to analgesics. Untreated the condition will progress to heatstroke with tissue damage.

Heatstroke

Heatstroke is differentiated from acute heat stress and heat exhaustion by the onset of clinically significant tissue damage. The extent of injury relates both to the duration of exposure and the severity of the rise in core temperature, but the seriousness of the condition cannot be predicted from these two parameters alone and requires laboratory confirmation.

Unfortunately these symptoms are non-specific. Anyone looking unwell or behaving abnormally in a hot (and/or humid) environment, or during vigorous exercise in a temperate environment, should be treated as a victim of heat illness until proven otherwise. Typically sufferers from heatstroke will have more than two-thirds of the symptoms (see Box), while someone who has a febrile illness instead of a heat-related disease will show one-third or less. The box may be used as a prompt and all symptoms and signs should be sought.

Heat exhaustion and heatstroke present with the following features

Weakness	Fatigue	Collapse
Lethargy	Hysteria	Convulsions
Headache	Anxiety	Loss of consciousness
Dizziness	Confusion	Muscle cramps
Nausea	Staggering	
Vomiting	Impaired judgement	
Diarrhoea	Hyperventilation/tachypnoea	

Epidemiology

Classical heatstroke affects humans trapped in hot, unventilated environments; for instance, workers in mines, prisoners, stowaways in freight containers, or children left in cars during heat waves. Individuals with impaired thermoregulation such as infants, the elderly, people with underlying medical conditions, or those taking drugs known to interfere with thermoregulation are at greater risk (see 📖 p. 693). Increasing summer temperatures in normally temperate areas, exacerbated by urban environments where buildings can store heat and so raise night-time temperatures by 5°C, are producing urban heat waves and deaths amongst the frail and elderly. Heat waves in Chicago in 1995 and Paris in 2003 caused hundreds of deaths.

The constant heat of jungles and urban environments is a greater physiological stress than that found in deserts, where the nights are often cool.

Exertional heatstroke occurs as a result of physical exercise, and cases may develop even in otherwise temperate conditions if someone becomes dehydrated or overexerts themselves in inappropriate clothing. It typically occurs during military training or during endurance sporting events. This is the variety of heatstroke most likely to be encountered on expeditions.

Hyperthermia is also associated with stimulant recreational drugs such as cocaine, ecstasy, and amphetamines (📖 p. 512).

Incidence

Heatstroke is responsible for about 240 deaths per year in the US; in the UK there are over 200 cases of heatstroke per year. In Singapore's hot, humid climate the incidence in the military may be as high as 3.5 cases per 1000 soldiers. Deaths and serious incidents caused by heat illnesses have occurred on expeditions both in desert areas and in tropical forests. Problems arise most often if newcomers to an area overexert themselves soon after arrival, a particular risk amongst youth groups.

Differential diagnosis of heatstroke in a previously fit person

- Hypoglycaemia—especially if diabetic.
- Hyponatraemia—excess rehydration with plain water.
- Drug toxicity—including alcohol.
- Ischaemic heart disease.
- Cerebrovascular event.
- Epilepsy.
- Head injury.
- Acute onset of fever, especially malaria.
- Inability to reduce core temperature below 39°C with evaporative cooling suggests that a febrile co-morbid condition may be present.

Heat exhaustion (heat prostration)

Heat exhaustion is the most commonly encountered form of he'
Its onset is gradual over several days or weeks. Significant h
disturbances to sodium and potassium may develop with
symptoms. It occurs when the cardiac output is insufficie
demands of increased blood flow to the skin, muscles.
This is compounded by a decrease in effective plasma
of redistribution of blood, dehydration, and salt
Correctly treated, heat exhaustion does not resul'

Pathophysiology of heat illness

Core temperature is the temperature of the vital organs such as brain, heart, liver, and kidneys. Normally it should remain relatively constant regardless of environmental conditions and at rest should be between 35.5°C and 37°C, with a measurement above 37.5°C being abnormal. However, during vigorous and prolonged exercise, such as long distance running on a hot day, core temperature rises and measurements up to 41°C have been recorded without apparent harm coming to the subject. Temperatures above 41°C are definitely abnormal and harmful.

Surrounding the body core is a shell of tissues at a lower temperature, the size of which depends upon the balance between heat generation and heat loss. In hot conditions, metabolic heat generated in the core has to be transferred to the skin, a process that involves substantial increases in skin blood flow.

The most critical factor in predicting the severity of injury is the duration of heat exposure following collapse. An elevated core temperature of 42–43°C can be tolerated for short periods (5–10 min) with little damage. For example, heatstroke in military training usually involves short exposures and rapid treatment; there may be large numbers of casualties, but the mortality rate is relatively low. During the papal visit to Denver, Colorado in 1993, there were 18 000 symptomatic victims among the crowd but no deaths, as the organizers ensured that immediate help was available. If body temperature remains persistently elevated, body metabolism becomes deranged and enzymes denature. The destructive processes are listed in Box 23.1.

Physics of heat transfer

Heat transfer and hence changes in body temperature take place as a result of radiation, conduction, convection, and evaporation.

- *Radiation*: the direct transfer of heat between the body surface and all other sources of radiant energy. The main source of radiant energy in hot climates is the sun. Under clear daytime desert skies the sun can cause great heat stress, but at night heat radiates away from warm bodies.
- *Conduction*: the direct transfer of heat between the body and any solid in contact with it, particularly the ground. Conduction ceases when the two solids in contact reach thermal equilibrium.
- *Convection*: the removal of heat through the flow of one substance over another. Convection augments conductive heat transfer and prevents thermal equilibrium developing by constantly replacing one of the materials so heat transfer can continue.

The rate of heat transfer by conduction, convection, and radiation is dependent on the difference in temperature between the body surface and the materials or radiating surfaces in the environment. If the body surface is warmer than the environment, the body will lose energy to the environment. However, very warm air or surfaces will transfer heat to the body by conduction/convection, and sunlit surfaces or sky will transfer heat to the body by radiation.

Box 23.1 Pathophysiology of Heat Stroke

Cellular oxidative phosphorylation becomes uncoupled at temperatures >42°C.

Cellular damage is directly proportional to the temperature and exposure time.

Compensatory mechanisms for heat dissipation fail.

Dehydration increases the sodium/potassium pump activity and increases metabolic rate.

Complications may arise in multiple organ systems.

Heat stroke should be suspected in anyone who collapses during or after exercise or in conditions of high ambient temperature and high humidity. There is multiple organ damage, especially to the CNS.

- CNS   Oedema and petechial haemorrhages cause focal and generalised damage.
- Muscle   Skeletal muscles show widespread degeneration of fibres. Rhabdomyolysis releases myoglobin, potassium, creatinine phosphokinase and purines (which are metabolised into uric acid) into the circulation.
- Lungs   Non-cardiogenic pulmonary oedema.
- Kidneys   Oliguric acute renal failure due to renal ischaemia, muscle breakdown products, DIC, hyperuricaemia and hypovolaemia. Renal failure occurs in up to 35%.
- Blood   DIC (poor prognosis), thrombocytopaenia, leucocytosis. Thermal injury to endothelium releases thromboplastins which result in intravascular thrombosis and secondary fibrinolysis.
- Metabolic   Metabolic acidosis, respiratory alkalosis, hypoglycaemia, hyper- or hypo-kalaemia.

- *Evaporation*: heat can be lost indirectly by evaporation of sweat. Each litre of sweat evaporated from the body surface at 30°C removes approximately 580 kcal (140 kJ) of heat energy. If sweat drips off the body, it has not been allowed to evaporate, and therefore no heat is lost. Sweating (and therefore evaporative heat loss) occurs when internal heat production exceeds the capacity of direct routes of heat transfer to dissipate it. Importantly, when the environment is sufficiently hot to cause heat gain by the direct transfer routes, evaporative cooling is the only thermoregulatory mechanism available to control body temperature.

Biology of heat transfer

Heat is produced in muscles—by normal metabolism, durin[...] and through shivering—and is conducted to the skin, where [...] the environment. The circulation of the blood augments [...] this heat transfer by varying superficial blood flow. Cloth[...] fies heat loss by acting either as a conductor or an ir [...] 20°C conduction and convection account for only a[...] loss, the majority occurring by radiation.

Once environmental temperature rises above 35°C it is impossible to lose heat through conduction, convection, or radiation. Our ability to survive and function in higher temperatures depends upon the ability to sweat.

Sweating allows the body to lose heat at any environmental temperature through evaporation, but evaporative heat loss can only occur if the air is not saturated with water vapour. So sweating is most efficient in hot dry deserts and is less effective in hot humid rain forests. Humidity has a greater effect on the ability to lose heat than the absolute temperature.[1]

Mode of heat transfer	Contribution		
	25°C	30°C	35°C
Radiation	67%	41%	4%
Conduction and convection	10%	33%	6%
Evaporation	23%	26%	90%

The body's response to thermal stress

Changes in temperature are detected by both sensory nerve endings in the skin and by direct sensing of blood temperature in the hypothalamus of the brain. At rest, the skin receives around 9% of the total circulating blood flow. A rise in core temperature of as little as 0.1°C will increase skin blood flow to dissipate the heat, and under high heat stress skin blood flow can increase fourfold. Heat energy is then lost directly to the environment by a combination of radiation, conduction, convection, and by evaporation of sweat. High environmental temperatures also lead to behavioural changes such as reduced activity, seeking shade, and drinking more.

During physical work blood flow is directed to the working muscles and away from the intestines. This limits the ability of the gut to absorb water to around 1200 ml/h. If the rate of fluid lost in sweat exceeds this amount, then dehydration will occur. Anyone working in these conditions must be allowed adequate rest periods with fluid replacement. If blood flow is further distributed to the skin to allow evaporative heat loss, then the effective circulating volume is further decreased. An adequate blood volume is therefore required to ensure that thermoregulatory blood flow can occur.

Measurement of core temperature

Measuring body temperature accurately is difficult and medics need to be aware of the limitations of the various techniques. In hospital the best ways to measure core temperature are by the use of central venous or oesophageal sensors but neither is practical outside a well equipped medical expedition.

Rectal temperature can be measured using simple portable equipment, there is poor correlation between the rectal temperature and the severity of symptoms; fatalities have been reported with rectal temperature of 39.5°C, while victims have survived core temperatures of 47°C.

noto T (1998) Heat loss mechanisms. In: Blatteis CM (ed.) *Physiology and Pathophysiology rature Regulation*. Singapore, World Scientific Publishing: 81.

During active cooling, there may be rapid changes in temperature of the blood as demonstrated by the sudden onset of shivering, but there is a significant lag before the body temperature change is seen rectally.

In the field, two further methods may be available that more closely reflect the current vascular temperature, but again each method has limitations. Both are subject to environmental error, particularly during treatment of heatstroke with external methods (ice water and evaporative cooling). Oral temperature measurement requires a conscious, cooperative patient and accurate placement of the bulb underneath the tongue for sufficient time to ensure thermal equilibrium. The patient should not breathe through the mouth during temperature measurement.

The tympanic membrane shares its blood supply with the hypothalamus (the body's thermostat). Changes in body temperature are seen sooner at the tympanic membrane than at other sites. For ease of use, most infrared ear thermometers are calibrated to read the mid-canal temperature, rather than the temperature of the tympanic membrane. This region is more susceptible to error than the tympanic membrane. The error is reduced by some thermometers, which take eight measurements within a second and display the highest (e.g. Braun Thermoscan Pro 3000). Proper technique is important—a clean probe cover should be used each time, the ear must be free of wax and water, and the ear canal should be straightened (pull the ear up and back). Nevertheless, ear temperature may offer the best compromise between the lag associated with rectal temperature measurement and the impracticalities and inaccuracies of oral temperature measurement.

Acclimatization to heat

Full acclimatization to heat develops at different rates in different individuals; typically 2–3 weeks are required for all the physiological changes to develop. The rate of acclimatization depends upon factors, including body shape, the severity of the heat stress, and pre-existing physical fitness.

Benefits of acclimatization:
- Reduced resting heart rate.
- Reduced core and skin temperature.
- Decreased salt loss in sweat (may drop from 60 mmol/l to 5 mmol/l).
- Increased sweat production (at lower core temperatures).
- Increased blood flow to skin.
- Improved renal sodium and water retention (aldosterone-mediated).
- Increased plasma proteins maintain extracellular fluid volume and reduce tachycardias.
- Improved ability to exercise (Fig. 23.2).

Physiological acclimatization enhances evaporative heat loss while reducing cardiovascular strain. Exercise becomes easier and exercise syncope, common on day 1, rapidly declines to zero by day 5. The increased sweat rate (0.5 l/h to 2 l/h), coupled with the increased blood flow, can increase heat loss by a factor of 20, but requires a significant increase in water consumption before, during, and after activity.

Some degree of acclimatization can be obtained in temperate climates before departure. Hot baths twice a day, saunas, and exercising while wearing more clothing than normal are all effective. In a hot dry climate, rapid acclimatization requires about 2 h of exercise per day sufficient to raise heart rate to around two-thirds of maximum, which should be conducted during the cooler hours of the morning or evening. Acclimatization may be delayed if substantial portions of the day are spent in air-conditioned environments. In comparison to dry heat, acclimatizing to hot humid climates, especially if the heat is unremitting, is much harder, and initial exercise tolerance will be substantially lower.

Sweating can only remove heat if there is sufficient fluid to spare. Sweat production rates can reach 2 l an hour for short periods and can be up to 15 l a day. In low humidity environments such as deserts where evaporation is rapid, the daily cooling capacity of the sweating mechanism is adequate to maintain body temperature even during vigorous work, but in humid environments such as tropical forest, evaporation is ineffective and slow, so exercise must be limited to avoid overheating.

Sweat is a hypotonic (dilute) solution of sodium chloride. The concentration of sodium chloride in sweat depends on the sweat rate and the degree of acclimatization. Higher sweating rates reduce the opportunity to conserve salt, and the sweat salt concentration rises, but acclimatized sweat glands conserve salt more effectively by producing more hypotonic sweat. In addition to conserving salt in sweat, humans acclimatized to start sweating at lower body temperatures and their kidneys conserve more effectively. As a consequence, an acclimatized person in a hot environment requires no more salt than an unacclimatized individual in temperate conditions, and can maintain lower body temperatures for any degree of heat stress.

Jungle acclimatization readily transfers to desert climates (hot and dry) but the reverse journey requires further acclimatization to humidity. The benefits of acclimatization are lost over 20–40 days after returning to a temperate environment.

Prevention of heat illnesses

Heat stress is the product of the interaction between:
• The individual.
• The environment: temperature, wind, sun, and humidity.
• The workload of the task being undertaken.

Prevention of heat illness

• Identify individuals at risk.
• Monitor environmental heat stress (ideally WBGT see below).
• Adjust the daily aims of the expedition accordingly.
• Educate everyone about the nature of heat illness: prevention, early
  recognition, and treatment.
• Provide adequate clean drinking water, shade, and latrines.
• Ensure that a robust medical evacuation system is in place.

Assessment of risk must consider each of these factors.

The individual

An individual is best able to cope with heat stress when:
• Fully hydrated.
• Physically fit.
• Acclimatized.
• Well nourished.
• Well rested.

Dehydration reduces both blood flow and sweating, so that a dehydrated person has reduced ability to maintain a constant body temperature in the heat. Acclimatization and physical fitness enable high temperatures to be tolerated better, but do not reduce water requirements; indeed, a fit acclimatized person will usually drink more than a new arrival to a hot environment.

Thermoregulation can be impaired by:
• Lack of sleep.
• Missed meals.
• Fever or recent pyrexial illness.
• Sunburn.
• Recent air travel.
• Use of therapeutic medications (see box).
• Other causes of relative dehydration such as diarrhoea and
  menstruation.

People with any of these conditions should be watched closely for signs of heat distress and should avoid excessive exertion. If one member of a team is adversely affected by the heat, then leaders and medics should assume that all other members of the expedition exposed to the same conditions are potential heat casualties.

A few individuals appear to have a genetic predisposition to developing heat illness. Previous heat illness should alert one to a recurrence.

Medications that increase risk of heat illness

Alcohol	ACE inhibitors
Amphetamines	Anticholinergics
Antihistamines	Atropine
Beta-blockers	Cocaine
Diuretics	Major tranquillizers
Phenothiazines	Scopolamine
SSRI antidepressants	Theophylline
Tricyclic antidepressants	

Evaluating environmental heat stress

Four environmental characteristics influence perceived heat stress:
- Air temperature.
- Solar (or radiant heat) load.
- Absolute humidity.
- Wind speed.

Environmental heat stress can vary greatly and unpredictably over short periods of time and space. On a calm, sunny day an open field may present a greater heat stress than an adjacent forest, but on a windy, cloudy day the forest may present the greater heat stress.

Three of these four factors are combined into an internationally accepted measure of heat stress, the Wet Bulb Globe Temperature (WBGT) index:
- Dry bulb (Tamb)—measures ambient air temperature in the shade.
- Black globe (Tg)—measures solar load.
- Wet bulb (Tw)—measures absolute humidity.

$$WBGT = 0.7Tw + 0.2Tg + 0.1Tamb$$

Organizers of endurance races and large outside gatherings should consider investigating the value of WBGT measurements. Further details of this and other temperature indices, including calculation tables are available at: http://www.bom.gov.au/info/thermal_stress/

Table 23.1 Recommended maximum workloads in various conditions

	Workload			Work-rest cycle (per hour)
	Light	Medium	Heavy	
WGBT	30.0	26.7	25.0	Continuous work
	30.6	28.0	25.9	45 min work/15 min rest
	31.4	29.4	27.9	30 min work/30 min rest
	32.2	31.1	30.0	15 min work/45 min rest

Although WBGT is the accepted international standard for estimating the heat stress affecting active individuals (ISO 7243:1989) and has been used to derive workload recommendations (Table 23.1), the measurement of the black globe temperature requires special equipment, is inconvenient, and will be beyond the scope of most expeditions. However, a reasonable estimate of heat stress may be made by adding 1°C to the wet bulb temperature. A (robust) Mason's Wet and Dry Bulb Thermometer with detailed instructions and a chart to calculate humidity is available.[2]

The wet bulb temperature is the most important component of the WBGT index, which reflects the thermoregulatory importance of evaporation in hot environments, but the index does not include wind speed, another important environmental modifier, within its calculation. Air movement increases convective heat transfer and will assist evaporation; cool winds reduce heat stress, but hot winds increase it.

Workload

For expeditions lacking meteorological facilities, an alternative method of judging a safe workload pattern has been suggested:

• Each individual should work out their maximum heart rate (220 minus their age in years) (e.g. a 40-year-old will have a maximum heart rate of 220−40 = 180 beats/min).
• The group should all work to the lowest figure obtained.
• Multiply the age-adjusted maximum heart rate by 0.75 (e.g. 75% age-adjusted maximum = 180 × 0.75=135 beats/min).
• The group should undertake the proposed activity for one work period (e.g. 30 minutes) under close supervision.
• Immediately after this initial work period all should recheck their heart rates.
• If anyone's heart rate exceeds the 75% age-adjusted maximum, the next working period should be reduced by one third (e.g. to 20 min with 40 min rest).
• The group should rest in the shade and rehydrate for the remainder of the hour.
• Repeat the process until the 75% age-adjusted maximum is not exceeded.
• Unless they are lean, athletic, and very fit, women tend to tolerate heat less well than men, and their exercise rates should be adjusted accordingly.
• Fig. 23.2 indicates the rapid improvements in exercise tolerance that develop with acclimatization.

2 Mason's Wet And Dry Thermometer, Philip Harris Educational, Novara House, Excelsior Road, Ashby Park, Ashby de la Zouch, LE65 1NG, UK. Tel: 0970 6000193.

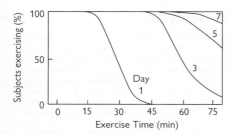

Fig. 23.2 Improved exercise duration with acclimatization during a standard exercise regime in hot conditions. Reproduced from Piantadosi CA (2003). *The Biology of Human Survival*. Oxford University Press.

Fluids and electrolytes

Fluids must be drunk before, during, and after exercise in a hot environment. Dehydration by as little as 1% affects heat tolerance and thermoregulation. Acute mild dehydration (2–3% of body weight) significantly impairs exercise tolerance (overcoming any advantage conferred by acclimatization), but does not initiate thirst. As dehydration progresses, cognitive function deteriorates and both thermoregulation and physical capacity become seriously compromised. A level of 6% dehydration is incompatible with further functioning in a hot environment. Even when a person is significantly dehydrated, urine is still produced and the volume of fluid required to return to full hydration must be at least 1.5 times that lost in sweat (assuming the individual was fully hydrated before the onset of activity). Women have a lower proportion of water in their bodies and may be at greater risk of dehydration than men.

Voluntary dehydration

Thirst is only stimulated when more than 2–3% dehydration has occurred. If an individual drinks only enough to satisfy their thirst they will be chronically dehydrated, particularly if they drink substantial amounts of caffeine-containing drinks, which act as diuretics. It is essential that personnel working hard in any environment are made aware of the need to drink water despite not feeling thirsty. Expedition leaders must enforce water-drinking discipline, permit rest, and provide adequate shade. If toilet facilities are unpleasant or lack privacy, travellers may seek to avoid visits by drinking less. Clean and screened facilities will encourage proper drinking habits—especially if the party consists of easily embarrassed youngsters.

> Thirsty = Dehydrated. Dehydrated *does not* = thirsty

Hydration can be monitored by the colour and quantity of urine along with how often one needs to pass urine. Dark yellow urine is a sure indicator that the individual is dehydrated, as is the need to urinate less than twice a day. Changes in body weight offer a less useful guide, as weight loss is common and caused not only by dehydration, but also by increased workload, gastrointestinal upset, and decreased appetite due to heat and unfamiliar food. Medical officers can check lying and standing blood pressures; a difference of >15 mmHg in the systolic pressure suggests dehydration.

Diabetics need to maintain good glucose control as blood glucose >10 mmol/l will result in glucose in the urine and consequent osmotic diuresis producing lighter urine. This could be mistaken as indicating adequate hydration whereas in reality it would be masking, and at the same time, worsening dehydration.

Water supplies

In hot environments water losses can reach 15 l per day per person. Complete replacement requires realistic estimates of potable water requirements, adequate water logistics, and individuals who understand and act on their water requirement. Water for hygiene will be needed in addition to water for drinking.

Where water supplies are unsafe, expedition leaders must ensure that adequate provision exists to purify sufficient water for the group's requirements. This may be flavoured to increase palatability. If chlorine or iodine is used, there should be a method of removing the taste at the point of use (see Water purification 📖 p. 106). Bottled water supplies purchased in local markets may be contaminated, discarded bottles having been recycled by being refilled from the nearest water source. Aerated water may be preferable as it is harder to tamper with. Carbonated water and soft drinks will fill the stomach with carbon dioxide before sufficient water has been ingested to combat dehydration, and should not be relied upon as the only source of fluid.

Choice of replacement fluid

New arrivals in a hot climate will lose more salt in their sweat than normal and should supplement their salt intake until they become acclimatized. Salt tablets are best avoided as they contain an unknown amount of sodium and may irritate the stomach. Table salt should be readily available at meal times. Salt can be added to fluids in sensible amounts. Soups are an excellent source of both fluid and electrolytes.

Sports drinks manufacturers have heavily promoted their products as the ideal way for active adults to replace the water and salt lost in sweat. To increase water absorption from the gut and prevent this water from being lost as urine, drinks should contain a sodium concentration of at least 50 mmol/l. The contents of sports drinks vary, and athletes relying on these drinks to replace significant fluid losses should pay attention to what they are drinking.

The oral rehydration solution recommended by the World Health Organization has a sodium content of 60–90 mmol/l, but the high sodium content of this significantly reduces palatability, resulting in reduced consumption. Whilst life-saving for diarrhoeal illnesses, its use cannot be recommended for fluid replacement in healthy people in the heat.

Problems with fluid balance

In the absence of serious heat illness or renal failure, dehydration by itself does not cause unconsciousness. Competitors participating in endurance races such as ultramarathons and ironman triathlons can develop symptomatic hyponatraemia if they drink excessive amounts of plain water or hypotonic fluids. Stomach bloating, weakness, and collapse may be followed by unconsciousness.
- Hospitalization is necessary.
- Cerebral oedema can develop.
- Avoid giving further water.
- The bladder should be catheterized and urine output monitored.
- Avoid oral fluids. Salt-containing foods may be given during recovery.
- Hypertonic saline (3%) can be infused slowly intravenously.

Some sports drinks are sold as powders. Dissolving excessive amounts of powder in the hope of increasing absorbed energy produces hypertonic fluids that do not quench thirst and enhance the effects of dehydration. Unless you know exactly what you are doing, always mix such powders according to instructions.

Treatment of heat illnesses

Remove the casualty from the source of heat and place them in the shade. Lying down maximizes heat loss, but only if the ground or mattress is no warmer than the surrounding environment. A hammock is ideal for encouraging heat loss as it enables air to circulate over the whole body.

Evaporative cooling is the mainstay of treatment. The patient should be continuously sprayed with cold water and fanned to encourage evaporation. A wet sheet may be wrapped around the casualty instead and kept moist. In some countries a simple solution to heat exhaustion is to lie the victim in a tepid running stream, but beware that they could become unconscious, that the stream could be polluted, or that aggressive animals could be attracted. It is neither necessary nor desirable to chill using ice cold water, nor to immerse the casualty in cold water, as these techniques cause constriction of the surface blood vessels and a reduction in blood flow to the skin.

Oral or intravenous fluids may be given, the latter being more effective in serious cases. At the Hajj pilgrimage cold intravenous infusions of up to 1 litre of normal saline or dextrose saline at 5°C for heatstroke and 12°C for heat exhaustion have been used successfully. Frequently casualties also suffer from hypoglycaemia, and glucose should be administered orally or intravenously to all casualties. No more than 2 l of intravenous fluids are normally required.

A heat-injured casualty who has not been cooled and yet is shivering is seriously ill. They may complain bitterly of feeling cold. They will not feel hot or thirsty. They will look pale and have cold skin. They will want to be wrapped in warm clothing, which only increases their core temperature further, as does shivering. This is not normal and they must have their core temperature measured to exclude heat illness or a febrile illness such as malaria.

During cooling, the return to a normal temperature is often associated with shivering. It is important to continue to monitor core temperature, as the casualty's thermoregulatory capacity has been damaged and these individuals are at continued risk of either hyperthermia or hypothermia.

Some of the effects of heatstroke, for instance renal or hepatic failure, only develop after 24–72 h. As it is impossible to distinguish accurately between heat exhaustion and heatstroke, all casualties should be evacuated to a hospital with intensive care facilities.

Advanced medical care

- Airway—unconscious patients require support and may need intubation and ventilation.
- Cardiorespiratory collapse—intravenous fluids and blood pressure monitoring required.
- Fitting—may require intravenous or rectal diazepam.
- Renal failure—may require catheterization to monitor urine output.

Table 23.2 The Seven Rs of Managing Heat Illness

Recognise signs and symptoms	if in doubt-treat as heat injury.
Rest casualty in shade	get rest of group under cover and drinking water.
Remove all clothing	strip to underwear.
Resuscitate	maintain ABC.
Reduce temperature ASAP	evaporative cooling and iv fluids.
Rehydrate	oral or intravenous fluids.
Rush to hospital	evacuate all heat casualties.

Other heat-related problems

Heat syncope

Fainting on standing in the heat is thought to occur because of blood pooling in the legs and increased blood flow to the skin. When standing, the blood supply to the brain is temporarily interrupted, causing loss of consciousness. Although most cases of heat syncope are harmless, the potential for heat illness should be considered, especially following physical work in the heat, or after the acclimatization period. Treat with rest in the cool and oral fluids.

Heat oedema

Mild swelling of the limbs may be experienced during the first few days of exposure to heat, during the time when the plasma volume increases to allow for the increased blood flow to the skin.

Heat cramps

The precise mechanism behind heat cramps is unknown. Heat cramps may occur in salt-depleted individuals recovering after a period of work in the heat, but also with any unaccustomed exercise, even in cool conditions such as swimming. Salt supplementation has been found to reduce the incidence of heat cramps. The cramps are painful and usually recur but do not have any long-term effects. If the individual is otherwise well, there is no association with heat illness. Treatment is supportive, with salt supplementation of food for a few days. Intravenous fluids are rarely required.

Miliaria rubra ('prickly heat')

An intensely itchy prickly or burning rash that arises in skin waterlogged from excess perspiration. The sweat pores become blocked with debris and inflamed, producing a large number of tiny blisters on a background of red skin. Commonly affected sites are the waist, upper trunk, neck, axillae, scalp, and flexures. It is often worst where clothing is tight or restrictive or rubs, or where skin rubs against skin. Sleep is disturbed and general mood irritability is common.

Prevent if practicable by wearing loose airy cotton clothing and taking regular cool showers. Treatment consists of frequent bathing in cool water, gently dabbing dry to prevent further damage, and application of talcum powder or calamine lotion. Air conditioning can help if available. Sedative antihistamines such as chlorphenamine (Piriton) may help to relieve symptoms and promote sleep at night, but sedative drugs should be avoided during the daytime as they may increase risk of accidents with machetes, etc.

NB. Many general travellers who claim to have had 'prickly heat' may actually be describing polymorphic light eruption.

Sunburn

Sunburn reduces the thermoregulatory capacity of skin and also affects central thermoregulation; prevent by insisting on the use of adequate sun protection. Sunburnt individuals should be protected from significant heat stress until the burn has healed (see also Skin 📖 p. 246).

Wound infections

In a hot and humid environment, minor skin breaches, including bites, can quickly become secondarily infected. Sawgrass inflicts razor-like cuts which may initially go unnoticed but which take a week to heal. The skin, especially of the hands, forearms, feet, and legs, should be inspected each evening in camp. Wounds should be washed with soap and water as soon as possible, and an antiseptic (e.g. iodine) applied. Apply a dressing if necessary. Healing is more likely if skin can be kept dry. Treat cellulitis with antibiotics such as amoxicillin, flucloxacillin, or erythromycin (📖 p. 48).

Fungal infections

Fungal infections (📖 p. 278) are common in moist skin folds such as the groin (tinea cruris), beneath breasts (intertrigo), and in hot damp feet (tinea pedis). Clean the skin and take every opportunity to dry it.

   Don't sleep in wet clothing or socks. Apply antifungal powder to the feet and skin folds. (See also Tropical ulcer 📖 p. 272, Skin infestations 📖 p. 268, Leeches 📖 p. 270.)

Websites

http://www.graduateresearch.com/thermometry/
Useful discussion about the measurement of body temperature and the pros and cons of various devices and sites.

http://www.nlm.nih.gov/medlineplus/heatillness.html
Information for the public on the prevention, recognition, and treatment of heat illness.

http://www.mindef.gov.sg/joint/smti/downloads/healthfacts/heatdisorder.pdf
Singapore Army guidelines for prevention of heat illness—incorporates UK and USA military perspectives.

Further reading

Gaffin SL, Moran DS (2001). Pathophysiology of heat-related illnesses. In: Auerbach P (ed.). *Wilderness medicine*, 4th edn, Mosby.

Walden J (2001). *Jungle travel and survival*. Guilford connecticut, USA: The Lyons Press.

Wound infections

Fungal infections

Wounds

Further reading

Index

continued . . .

"Victoria (V. I.) Warshawski is one of fiction's toughest an[d] sassiest female private eyes and one of the most beloved and re[silient. . . . This is not your everyday detective story. Paretsky [is] a skilled writer who has something to say and couches her mes[sage] in a compelling page-turner." —*Pittsburgh Post-Gazett[e]*

"[A] riveting exploration of guilt and fear . . . top-notch."
—*Publishers Week[ly]*

"A stellar entry in a celebrated series, which offers a provocativ[e] history lesson along with very contemporary commentary on loy[alty] and betrayal and how the past shapes the present. . . . A tightl[y] woven and thoughtful thriller, this enticing mix of history an[d] mystery showcases sharp, clever, vulnerable V. I. at her best."
—*Booklist* (starred review[)]

"A compelling tale of secrets that can't stay buried."
—*Kirkus Review[s]*

"This may be Paretsky's most complex novel to date. Highly rec[ommended]." —*Library Journal* (starred review[)]

"Sheer brilliant storytelling. . . . Sara Paretsky's best tale in sev[eral] years . . . a political thriller wrapped around a fast-paced who[dunit] . . . well written, exquisitely exciting." —BookBrowse

"Gripping . . . a surprising ending."
—*The Daily Telegraph* (Sydney, Australia[)]

"A crime-busting treat." —*The Independent* (London[)]

"Disparate parts come together seamlessly under the hand o[f] Paretsky, an old-school crime-writing pro." —*The Boston Glob[e]*

Praise for Sara Paretsky
and her bestselling novels

"Paretsky still writes with the kind of dazzling, diamond-hard clarity that can break your heart on every other page."
—*Chicago Tribune*

"Paretsky is still the best. . . . She doesn't pull punches."
—*The Washington Post Book World*

"Paretsky's books are beautifully paced and plotted, and the dialogue is fresh and smart. . . . V. I. Warshawski is the most engaging woman in detective fiction."
—*Newsweek*

"A wrenching tale that closes with surprise revelations."
—*USA Today*

"[V. I.] returns in great form. . . . Defiant, sardonic, ostentatious, she stirs every hornet's nest and breasts the murkiest currents to emerge vindicated and triumphant in the end."
—*Los Angeles Times*

"No one, male or female, writes better P.I. books than Paretsky."
—*The Denver Post*

"The plot [is] fast-moving, the dialogue is snappy, the premise for murder persuasive. The novel hasn't a single snag in its springs."
—*Chicago Sun-Times*

"Terrific . . . expertly plotted."
—*The New York Times Book Review*

"Articulate and independent . . . Warshawski never wears thin."
—*San Francisco Chronicle*

"Complex, satisfying . . . Paretsky's V. I. is a rare literary entity, a woman quick to anger and action, yet sympathetic and credible."
—*Publishers Weekly*

ALSO BY SARA PARETSKY

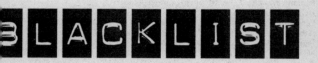

BLACKLIST

A V. I. WARSHAWSKI NOVEL

SARA PARETSKY

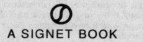

A SIGNET BOOK

SIGNET
Published by New American Library, a division of
Penguin Group (USA) Inc., 375 Hudson Street,
New York, New York 10014, USA
Penguin Group (Canada), 90 Eglinton Avenue East, Suite 700, Toronto,
Ontario M4P 2Y3, Canada (a division of Pearson Penguin Canada Inc.)
Penguin Books Ltd., 80 Strand, London WC2R 0RL, England
Penguin Ireland, 25 St. Stephen's Green, Dublin 2,
Ireland (a division of Penguin Books Ltd.)
Penguin Group (Australia), 250 Camberwell Road, Camberwell, Victoria 3124,
Australia (a division of Pearson Australia Group Pty. Ltd.)
Penguin Books India Pvt. Ltd., 11 Community Centre, Panchsheel Park,
New Delhi - 110 017, India
Penguin Group (NZ), 67 Apollo Drive, Rosedale, North Shore 0632,
New Zealand (a division of Pearson New Zealand Ltd.)
Penguin Books (South Africa) (Pty.) Ltd., 24 Sturdee Avenue,
Rosebank, Johannesburg 2196, South Africa

Penguin Books Ltd., Registered Offices:
80 Strand, London WC2R 0RL, England

Published by Signet, an imprint of New American Library, a division of Pen,
Group (USA) Inc. Previously published in a G. P. Putnam's Sons edition.

First Signet Printing, September 2004
10 9 8

Printed in the United States of America

PUBLISHER'S NOTE
This is a work of fiction. Names, characters, places, and incidents either are
product of the author's imagination or are used fictitiously, and any resembla
to actual persons, living or dead, business establishments, events, or locale
entirely coincidental.

The publisher does not have any control over and does not assume any resp
sibility for author or third-party Web sites or their content.

Geraldine Courtney Wright, artist and writer—valiant, witty and formidable—a true grande dame:

I cannot rest from travel; I will drink life to the lees . . .

THANKS

Dr. Sarah Neely provided valuable medical advice. Jill Koniecsko made it possible for me to navigate Lexis-Nexis. Judi Phillips knew exactly how a robber baron would have constructed an ornamental pond in 1903. Jesus Mata helped V. I. with her neighborhood Mexican restaurant. Sandy Weiss was a demon on technology topics and Jolynn Parker's Fact Factory as always turned up amazing results. Eva Kuhn advised me on Catherine Bayard's music tastes. The senior C-Dog did his usual witty riff on chapter titles; chapter titles, as always, are provided in loving memory of Don Sandstrom, who cherished them.

Michael Flug, archivist at the Vivian Harsh Collection, was immensely helpful in directing me to documents about the Federal Negro Theater Project. Margaret Kinsman introduced me to this great resource in my backyard.

The great forensic pathologist Dr. Robert Kirschner died in the summer of 2002. His presence in prisons and at mass graves from Nigeria to Bosnia, from El Salvador to Chicago's South Side, brought a measure of justice to victims of torture and mass murder, and his loss is a grievous one. Despite the nature and importance of his work, Dr. Kirschner also took pleasure in V. I.'s adventures. For the last sixteen years, he found time to advise me on the ways and means her adversaries used to murder. During his final illness, we talked about the unpleasant ends the characters in *Blacklist* were meeting. I miss him as an adviser, a friend, and a great humanitarian.

This is a work of fiction. I do mention historical events, such as the Federal Theater Project, the Dies Committee, HUAC, and some figures active in the arts in the nineteen-thirties, like Shirley Graham, as part of the background of the novel. All characters who actually play a role in the story, as well as events like the destruction of the Fourth Amendment, are solely the fabrication of a brain made frenzied by chronic insomnia. Any resemblance to any real person, institution, government or legislation is purely coincidental.

CHAPTERS

1

A Walk on the Wild Side

The clouds across the face of the moon made it hard for me to find my way. I'd been over the grounds yesterday morning, but in the dark everything is different. I kept stumbling on tree roots and chunks of brick from the crumbling walks.

I was trying not to make any noise, on the chance that someone really was lurking about, but I was more concerned about my safety: I didn't want to sprain an ankle and have to crawl all the way back to the road. At one point I tripped on a loose brick and landed smack on my tailbone. My eyes teared with pain; I sucked in air to keep from crying out. As I rubbed the sore spot, I wondered whether Geraldine Graham had seen me fall. Her eyes weren't that good, but her binoculars held both image stabilizers and night-vision enablers.

Fatigue was making it hard for me to concentrate. It was midnight, usually not late on my clock, but I was sleeping badly these days—I was anxious, and feeling alone.

Right after the Trade Center, I'd been as numbed and fearful as everyone else in America. After a while, when we'd driven the Taliban into hiding and the anthrax looked like the work of some homegrown maniac, most people seemed to wrap themselves in red-white-and-blue and return to normal. I couldn't, though, while Morrell remained in Afghanistan—

even though he seemed ecstatic to be sleeping in caves as he
trailed after warlords-turned-diplomats-turned-warlords.

When the medical group Humane Medicine went to Kabul
in the summer of 2001, Morrell tagged along with a contract for
a book about daily life under the Taliban. I've survived so
much worse, he would say when I worried that he might run
afoul of the Taliban's notorious Bureau for the Prevention of
Vice.

That was before September 11. Afterward, Morrell disappeared for ten days. I stopped sleeping then, although someone
with Humane Medicine called me from Peshawar to say Morrell was simply in an area without access to phone hookups.
Most of the team had fled to Pakistan immediately after the
Trade Center attack, but Morrell had wangled a ride with an old
friend heading to Uzbekistan so he could cover the refugees
fleeing north. A chance of a lifetime, my caller told me Morrell
had said—the same thing he'd said about Kosovo. Perhaps that
had been the chance of a different lifetime.

When we started bombing in October, Morrell first stayed
on in Afghanistan to cover the war up close and personal, and
then to follow the new coalition government. *Margent.Online,*
the Web version of the old Philadelphia monthly *Margent,* was
paying him for field reports, which he was scrambling to turn
into a book. The *Guardian* newspaper also occasionally bought
his stories. I'd even watched him on CNN a few times. Strange
to see your lover's face beamed from twelve thousand miles
away, strange to know that a hundred million people are listening to the voice that whispers endearments into your hair. That
used to whisper endearments.

When he resurfaced in Kandahar, I first sobbed in relief,
then shrieked at him across the satellites. "But, darling," he
protested, "I'm in a war zone, I'm in a place without electricity
or cell phone towers. Didn't Rudy call you from Peshawar?"

In the following months, he kept on the move, so I never
really knew where he was. At least he stayed in better touch,
mostly when he needed help: (V. I., can you check on why

Ahmed Hazziz was put in isolation out at Coolis prison? V. I., can you find out whether the FBI told Hazziz's family where they'd sent him? I'm running now—hot interview with local chief's third wife's oldest son. Fill you in later.)

I was a little miffed at being treated like a free research station. I'd never thought of Morrell as an adrenaline junkie—one of those journalists who lives on the high of being in the middle of disaster—but I sent him a snappish e-mail asking him what he was trying to prove.

"Over a dozen Western journalists have been murdered since the war began," I wrote at one point. "Every time I turn on the television, I brace myself for the worst."

His e-response zipped back within minutes: "Victoria, my beloved detective, if I come home tomorrow, will you faithfully promise to withdraw from every investigation where I worry about your safety?"

A message which made me angrier because I knew he was right—I was being manipulative, not playing fair. I needed to see him, though, touch him, hear him—live, not in cyberspace.

I took to wearing myself out running. I certainly wore out the two dogs I share with my downstairs neighbor: they started retreating to Mr. Contreras's bedroom when they saw me arrive in my sweats.

Despite my long runs—I'd go ten miles most days, instead of my usual five or six—I couldn't wear myself out enough to sleep. I lost ten pounds in the six months after the Trade Center, which worried my downstairs neighbor: Mr. Contreras took to frying up French toast and bacon when I came in from my runs, and finally bullied me into going to Lotty Herschel for a complete physical. Lotty said I was fine physically, just suffering as so many were from exhaustion of the spirit.

Whatever name you gave it, I only had half a mind for my work these days. I specialize in financial and industrial crime. It used to be that I spent a lot of time on foot, going to government buildings to look at records, doing physical surveillance and so on. But in the days of the Internet, you traipse from website to website. You need to be able to concentrate in front of a computer for long hours, and concentration wasn't something I was good at right now.

Which is why I was wandering around Larchmont Hall in the dark. When my most important client asked me to look for intruders who might be breaking in there at night, I was so eager to do something physical that I would even have scrubbed the crumbling stone benches around the house's ornamental pond.

Darraugh Graham has been with me almost since the day I opened my agency. The New York office of his company, Continental United, had lost three people in the Trade Center disaster. Darraugh had taken it hard, but he was flinty, chalklike in grief, more moving than the bluster we were hearing from too many mouths these days. He wouldn't dwell on his loss or the aftermath but took me to his conference room, where he unrolled a detail map of the western suburbs.

"I asked you here for personal reasons, not business." He snapped his middle finger onto a green splodge northwest of Naperville, in unincorporated New Solway. "All this is private land. Big mansions belonging to old families out here, you know, the Ebbersleys, Felittis, and so on. They've been able to keep the land intact—like a private forest preserve. This brown finger is where Taverner sold ten acres to a developer back in 'seventy-two. There was an uproar at the time, but he was within his rights. He had to meet his legal fees, I think." I followed Darraugh's long index finger as he traced a brown patch that cut into the green like a carrot.

"East is a golf course. South, the complex where my mother lives." At the best of times, Darraugh is a wintry, distant man. It was hard to picture him in normal situations, like being born.

"Mother's ninety-one. She manages on her own with help, and, anyway, I don't want—she doesn't want to live with me. She lives in a development here—Anodyne Park. Town houses, apartments, little shopping center, nursing home if she needs medical help. She seems to like it. She's gregarious. Like my son—sociability skips generations in my family." His bleak smile appeared briefly. "Ridiculous name for a development, Anodyne Park, offensive when you think about the Alzheimer's wing at the nursing home—Mother tells me the word means something like 'soothing' or 'healing.'

"Her condo overlooks the grounds of Larchmont Hall. One of the grand mansions, big grounds. It's been empty for a year—the original owners were the Drummond family. The heirs sold the place three years ago, but the new buyers went bankrupt. Felitti was talking about buying, so he could keep more developers out of the area, but so far that's fallen through."

He stopped. I waited for him to get to the point, which he is never shy about, but when a minute went by I said, "You want me to find a plutocrat to buy the place so it doesn't get divided up for the merely affluent?"

He scowled. "I didn't call you in for ridicule. Mother thinks she sees people going in and out of the place at night."

"She doesn't want to call the police?"

"The police came out a couple of times, but found no one. The agent that manages the place for the holding company has a security system in place. It hasn't been breached."

"Any of the neighbors seen anything?"

"Point of the area, Vic: neighbors don't see each other. Here are the houses, and all this is hundred years' worth of trees, gardens, so forth. You could talk to the neighbors, of course." He snapped his finger on the map again, showing me the distances, but his tone was uncertain—most unlike him.

"What's your interest in this, Darraugh? Are you thinking of buying the place yourself?"

"Good God, no."

He didn't say anything else, but walked to the windows to look down at the construction on Wacker Drive. I stared in bewilderment. Even when he'd asked me to help his son beat a hacking rap several years ago, he hadn't danced around the floor like this.

"Mother's always been a law unto herself," he muttered to the window. "Of course people in her—in our—milieu always get better attention from the law than people like—well, than others. But she's affronted that the police aren't taking her seriously. Of course, it's possible that she might be imagining—she's over ninety, after all—but she's taken to calling me every day to complain about lack of police attention."

"I'll see if I can uncover something the police aren't seeing," I said gently.

His shoulders relaxed and he turned back to me. "Your usual fee, Vic. See Caroline about your contract. She'll give you Mother's details as well." He took me out to his personal assistant, who told him his conference call with Kuala Lumpur was waiting.

We'd talked on a Friday afternoon, the dreary first day of March. On Saturday morning, I made the first of what turned into many long treks to New Solway. Before driving out, I stopped in my office for my ordnance maps of the western suburbs. I looked at my computer and then resolutely turned my back to it: I'd already logged on three times since ten last night without word from Morrell. I felt like an alcoholic with the bottle in reach, but I locked my office without checking my e-mail and began the forty-five-mile haul to the land of the rich and powerful.

That westward drive always makes me feel like I'm following the ascent into heaven, at least into capitalist heaven. It starts along Chicago's smoky industrial corridor, passing old blue-collar neighborhoods that resemble the one where I grew up—tiny bungalows where women look old at forty and men work and eat themselves to early heart attacks. You move past them to the hardscrabble towns on the city's edge—Cicero, Berwyn, places where you can still get pretty well beat up for a dollar. Then the air begins to clear and the affluence rises. By the time I reached New Solway, I was practically hydroplaning on waves of stock certificates.

I pulled off at the tollway exit to examine my maps.

Coverdale Lane was the main road that meandered through New Solway. It started at the northwest corner of the township and made a giant kind of quarter circle, opening on Dirksen Road at the southeast end. At Dirksen, you could go south to Powell Road, which divided New Solway from Anodyne Park, where Geraldine Graham was living. I followed the route to the northwest entrance, since that looked like the main one on the map.

I hadn't traveled fifty feet down Coverdale Lane before getting Darraugh's point: neighbors couldn't spy on each other here. Horses grazed in paddocks; orchards held a few desiccated apples from last fall. With the trees bare, a few mansions were visible from the road, but most were set far behind imposing carriageways. Poorer folk might actually see each other's driveways from their side windows, but most of the houses sat on substantial property, perhaps ten or twelve acres. And most were old. No new money here. No McMansions, flashing their thirty thousand square feet on tiny lots.

After going south about a mile and a half, Coverdale Lane bent into a hook that pointed east. I followed the hook almost to its end before a discreet sign on a stone pillar announced Larchmont Hall.

I drove on past the gates to Dirksen Road at the east end of Coverdale and made a loop south and west so I could look at the complex where Darraugh's mother was living. I wanted to know if she really could see into the Larchmont estate. A hedge blocked any view into the New Solway mansions from street level, but Ms. Graham was on the fourth floor of a small apartment building. From that vantage, she might be able to see into the property.

I returned to Coverdale Lane and drove up a winding carriageway to Larchmont Hall. Leaving the car where anyone could see it if they came onto the land, I armed myself with that most perfect disguise: a hard hat and a clipboard. A hard hat makes people assume you're doing something with the air-conditioning or the foundations. They're used to service in places like this; they don't ask for credentials. I hoped.

As I got my bearings, I whistled under my breath: the original owners had done things on a grand scale. Besides the mansion itself, the property held a garage, stables, greenhouse, even a cottage, which I assumed was for the staff who tended the grounds—or would tend the grounds if someone could afford to have the work done. The estate agent wasn't putting much into maintenance—an ornamental pond, which lay between the mansion and the outbuildings, was clogged with leaves and dead lilies. I even saw a carp floating belly-up in the middle. A series of formal gardens was overgrown with weeds, while no one had mowed the meadows for some time.

The neglect, and the number of buildings, was oppressive. If you were grandiose enough to buy such a place, how could you possibly take care of it? Circling each building, trying to see if there were holes in foundations or windows, looked overwhelming. I squared my shoulders. Whining doubles the job, my mother used to say when I balked at washing dishes. I decided to work from smallest to largest, which meant inspecting the cottage first.

By the time I'd finished prying at windows, balancing on fence posts to see if any of the roof glass of the greenhouse was broken, and making sure that the doors to the stables and garage were not just secure, but showed no recent signs of tampering, it was past noon. I was hungry and thirsty, but dark still comes early the first week in March. I didn't want to waste daylight searching for food, so I grimly set about circling the house.

It was an enormous building. From a distance it looked graceful, vaguely Federal in design, with its slender columns and square façades, but all I cared about was four floors' worth of windows, doors at ground level on all four sides, doors leading off upper-level balconies—a burglar's paradise.

Still, all the windows on the two lower floors held the telltale markers of a security system. I checked some on the ground floor with a meter, but didn't see anyplace where the current was interrupted.

People did come onto the land: beer bottles, the silver foil from potato chip bags, crumpled cigarette packs, the inevitable condom, told their tales. Maybe Ms. Graham was only seeing local kids looking for privacy.

I was debating whether to shinny up the pillars to check the balcony doors when a squad car pulled up. A middle-aged cop came over to me at an unhurried gait.

"You got some reason to be out here?"

"Probably the same one you do." I waved my meter toward the house. "I'm with Florey and Kapper, the mechanical engineers. We heard some woman thinks little green men are hovering around here in the night. I'm just checking the circuits."

"You set something off in the garage," the cop said.

I smiled. "Oh, dear: I was trying brute force. They warned us against that at IIT, but I wanted to see if someone could actually lift those doors. Sorry to bring you out here for nothing."

"Not to worry: you saved me from our eighty-third call to look at suspicious mail."

"It's a hassle, isn't it," I said, hoping he wouldn't ask for my ID. "I've got friends in the Chicago PD who feel stretched to the limit these days."

"Same out here. We've got the reservoir and a bunch of power stations we have to keep an eye on. It's about time the FBI nailed this anthrax bastard—we waste an unbelievable amount of manpower, responding to hysterical calls about letters from old Aunt Madge who forgot to put her return address on the envelope."

We hashed over the current situation the way everyone did these days. Police forces were badly affected, because they had to gear up for incalculable terror attacks and couldn't keep up with their local crime loads. Drive-by shootings, which had dropped to their lowest level in decades, had jumped in the last six months.

The cop's cell phone rang. He grunted into it. "I'd better be going. You okay out here?"

"Yeah. I'm taking off, too. Place looks clean to me, except for the usual garbage—" I pointed a toe at an empty cigarette wrapper near the foundation. "I don't see how anyone could be using the place."

"You find Osama bin Laden in the attic, give me a call: I could use the extra credit." He waved good-bye and got back into his squad car.

I couldn't think of anything else to look for, and, anyway, it was getting too dark to see clearly. I walked to the edge of the gardens, where they faded into a substantial woods, and looked up at the house. From here I could see the attic windows, but they presented a blank face to the sky.

The Iron Dowager

I had to go through various security checkpoints to reach Geraldine Graham. Anodyne Park was a well-gated community, with a guard at the entrance who wrote down my license plate number and asked my business before phoning Ms. Graham for permission to let me enter. As I snaked along the curved road that suburban developers relish, I saw that the complex was bigger than it appeared from the outside. Besides the town houses, apartment buildings and a nursing home the size of a small hospital, it held a little row of shops. Several golfing quartets, undeterred by the dreary weather, were leaving their carts outside a bar at the edge of the shops. I ran into a grocery store designed like an Alpine chalet for a bottle of overpriced water and a banana. Getting my blood sugar up would help me interview my client's mother.

When she opened the door, I was disconcerted: Geraldine Graham looked so much like her son that I could almost believe it was Darraugh in the doorway dressed in rose silk. She had his long face and prominent nose and eyes of the same frosty blue, although hers were clouded now with age. The only real difference was her hair: over the years Darraugh's blond has bleached to white; hers was dark, a white-streaked nut-brown that owed nothing to a bottle. She held herself as ramrod straight as her son. I pictured her mother tying her to a Victorian backboard which she passed in turn on to Darraugh.

It was only when Geraldine Graham moved away from the doorway and the light caught her face that I saw how deeply lined it was. "You're the young woman my son sent out to see who is breaking into Larchmont Hall, eh?" She had the high fluting voice of deep age. "I wondered whether that policeman was going to arrest you, but you seemed to talk your way out of it. What made him arrive?"

"You were watching me, ma'am?"

"The hobbies of the elderly. Peeping through windows, prying into locks. Although I suppose my hobby is your livelihood. I'm making a cup of tea. I can offer you one. Or I have bourbon: I know detectives are used to stronger beverages than tea."

I laughed. "That's only Philip Marlowe. We modern detectives can't drink in the middle of the day: it puts us to sleep."

She moved down the short hallway to her kitchen. I followed and felt a stab of envy when I saw the double-door refrigerator and the porcelain cooktop. My own kitchen was last remodeled two tenants back. I wondered what it would cost to install an island cooktop like this one, with sleek electrical burners that looked painted into the surface. Probably two years of mortgage payments.

Ms. Graham saw me staring and said, "Those are designed to keep the old from burning down the house. They turn off automatically if there's no pan on them, or after some minutes if you haven't set a special timer. Although we're told the old should burn and rave at the end of day."

When she slowly pushed a small stepladder into position to reach her tea bags, I moved forward to help. She waved me off with a brusqueness like her son's.

"Just because I'm old and slow doesn't mean the young and swift need muscle me away. My son keeps wanting to install a housekeeper here so I can vegetate in front of the television or behind my binoculars. As you can see, we'd be tripping over each other all day in this tiny space. I was glad to give up all that nonsense when I moved out of the big house. Housekeepers, gardeners, you can't take a step without consulting someone else's feelings and timetables. One of my old maids comes every day to tidy and prepare meals—and to make sure I haven't died in the night. That's enough intrusion."

She poured hot water over tea bags into slender porcelain mugs. "My mother would be shocked to see me use tea bags, or to drink my tea out of a great mug. Even when she was ninety herself, we had to get down the Crown Derby every afternoon. Mugs and tea bags feel like freedom, but I'm never sure whether it's freedom or laxity."

These cups, with their gold-leaf rims and intricate stencils, weren't exactly Pacific Gardens Mission service. When Ms. Graham nodded at me to pick them up, I could hardly get my fingers into their slender handles. The tea scalded my fingers through the eggshell-thin china. Following her slow tread down the hall to her sitting room felt like some kind of biblical ordeal involving furnaces.

If Geraldine Graham had been living in a mansion like those across the street, the apartment might seem like tiny space, but the sitting room alone was about the size of my whole apartment in Chicago. Pale Chinese rugs floated on the polished wood floor. Armchairs covered in straw satin straddled a fireplace in the middle of the wall, but Ms. Graham led me to an alcove facing Larchmont Hall, where an upholstered chair stood next to a piecrust table. This seemed to be where she lived: books, reading glasses, her binoculars, a phone, covered most of the tabletop. An oil painting of a woman in Edwardian dress hung behind the chair. I studied the face for a resemblance to my hostess and her son, but it was the oval of a classic beauty. Only the coldness in the blue eyes made me think of Darraugh.

"My mother. It was a great disappointment to her that I inherited my father's looks: she was considered the most beautiful woman in Chicago when she was young." With her deliberate motions, Geraldine Graham moved the binoculars and glasses onto the books, then placed coasters for our mugs. Settling herself in her chair, she told me I might bring over one of those by the fireplace for myself. Her fluting voice started while I was still around the corner in the main part of the room.

"I probably shouldn't have bought a unit facing the house. My daughter warned me I would find it hard to see strangers in the place, but of course I haven't, except for the few months that they could afford the payments. A computer baron who melted like snow in last year's business upheavals. So humiliating for the children, I always think, when their horses are sold. But since they left, I haven't seen anyone until these last few days. Nights. I see nothing out of the ordinary during the day. Although my son hasn't said so, he seems to think I have Alzheimer's. At least, I assume he does, since he actually drove out to visit me Thursday evening, which is a rare occurrence. I am not demented, however: I know what I'm seeing. I saw you there this afternoon, after all."

I ignored the end of her statement. "Larchmont Hall was your home? Darraugh didn't tell me that."

"I was born in that house. I grew up in it. But neither of my children wanted the burden of looking after such a property, not even to hold in trust for their own children. Of course my daughter doesn't live here, she's in New York with her husband; they have his family's property in Rhinebeck, but I thought Darraugh might want his son to have the chance to live in Larchmont. He was adamant, however, and when Darraugh has made up his mind he is as hard as any diamond."

Why hadn't Darraugh told me he grew up here? Anger at feeling blindsided distracted me from what she was saying. What else had he concealed? Still, I could see that looking after Larchmont Hall would be a full-time job, not something a widower wedded to his business would take on willingly. I pictured Darraugh in a Daphne du Maurier childhood, learning to ride, to hunt, to play hide-and-seek in the stables. Perhaps it's only blue-collar kids like me who imagine that you'd feel nostalgia for such a childhood and find it hard to give up.

"So you watch the place to see how it's faring without you, and you've noticed someone hanging around there?"

"Not exactly." She swallowed noisily and set the mug down on her coaster with a jolt that sprayed drops onto the wood. "When you're old, you don't sleep long hours at a time. I wake in the night, I go to the bathroom, I read a little and doze in my chair here. Perhaps a week ago," she stopped to count backward on her fingers, "last Tuesday, it would be, I was up around one. I saw a light glow and go out. At first I assumed it was a car on Coverdale Lane. You can't see the lane from here, but you can see the reflection of the headlights along the façades."

Reflection along the façades. Her precise speech made her sound even more formidable than her commanding manner. I stood at the window and cupped my hands around my eyes to peer through the wintry twilight. Across Powell Road, I could just make out the hedge that shielded New Solway from the vulgar. Larchmont Hall lay on the far side, in a direct line from where I was standing. It was back far enough from the road that even in the dusk I could make out the whole house.

"Take the binoculars, young woman: they allow one to see in the dark, even an old woman like me."

The binoculars were a lovely set of Rigel compact optics, with a nightvision feature usually used by hunters. "Did you buy these so you could see in the dark, ma'am?"

"I didn't buy them originally to spy on my old home, if that's what you're asking: my grandson MacKenzie gave them to me when I still managed Larchmont. He thought they would be helpful to me since my vision was deteriorating, and he was correct."

The glasses brought the dormers of the attic into sharp relief. I couldn't make out great detail in the dark, but enough to see the skylight cut into the steep roof. The small windows underneath the eaves were uncurtained. The main entrance, where the local cop and I had both parked, was to the left, at right angles to the side facing Anodyne Park. Anyone coming onto the property from the road would be easy to spot from here, if you were looking, but if someone approached from the meadows at the rear, they would be shielded from view by the stable and greenhouse.

"I found empty bottles and so on when I was walking around," I said, still scanning the house for any signs of light or life. "People are clearly coming onto the property now that it's vacant. Do you think that's who you're seeing?"

"Oh, I suppose working people feel a certain triumph in having sex on the old Drummond grounds," she said dismissively, "but I have seen lights flicker in the attic late at night. The skylight is revealing of what's inside as well as what's out. It was the servants' common room when my mother managed Larchmont. As a child, I used to go up there and watch the maids play poker. She didn't know about their card games, but children and servants are natural allies.

"After Mother died, I shut up the attic and moved the remaining staff to the third floor. I wasn't entertaining on a grand scale, I didn't use those bedrooms. Or all those servants Mother thought essential for running Larchmont as if it were Blenheim Palace.

"It's been most odd to see those lights, as if my mother's servants had returned to play poker up there. My son assured me you were a competent investigator. I do expect you to take my complaint seriously, unlike our local police force. After all, my son is paying you."

I turned back to her, laying the binoculars on the piecrust table. "Did you or Darraugh report this business to the titleholder, or the estate agents? They'd be the ones most concerned."

"Julius Arnoff. He's courteous, but he doesn't quite believe me. I realize that I no longer own the house," she said. "But I still feel a keen interest in its well-being. I told Darraugh when the police were so unhelpful that I would prefer my own investigator, who would owe me the necessity of reports. Which reminds me: I don't believe you told me your name, young woman. Darraugh did, but I've forgotten it."

"Warshawski. V. I. Warshawski."

"Oh, these Polish names. They're like eels sliding around the tongue. What did my son tell me he calls you? Vic? I will call you Victoria. Will you write your phone number on this pad? In large numbers; I don't want to have to use a magnifying glass if I need to summon you in a hurry."

Horrifying visions of Ms. Graham feeling free to call me at three in the morning when she had insomnia, or at odd moments during the day when loneliness overtook her, made me give her only my office number. My answering service would deflect her most of the time.

"I hope Darraugh hasn't exaggerated your abilities. I will watch for you tonight."

I shook my head. "I can't stay out here tonight. But I'll be back tomorrow."

That didn't please her at all: if her son was employing me it was my duty to work the hours that they set.

"And if someone else hires me tomorrow, should I drop my work for Darraugh to respond to that client's demands?" I said.

The heavy lines around her nose deepened. She tried to demand what obligation could possibly take precedence over her needs, but I wasn't about to tell her. To her credit, she didn't waste a long time on argument when she saw I wasn't giving in.

"But you will tell me personally what you find out. I don't want to have to get reports from Darraugh: there are times when I wish he was more like his father."

Her tone didn't make that sound like a compliment. When I stood to leave, she asked me—ordered, really—to take the cups back to the kitchen. I turned them over before putting them in the sink: Coalport bone china. Mugs, indeed.

I spent the drive to Chicago going over her surprising remarks. I wondered why Darraugh hated Larchmont so much. I found myself constructing Gothic scenarios. Darraugh was a widower. Perhaps his beloved wife had died there, while his wastrel father absconded with Darraugh's wife's diamonds and his own secretary. Or perhaps Darraugh suspected Geraldine of drowning his wife—or even his father—in the ornamental pond and had vowed never to set foot on Drummond land again.

As I returned to the small bungalows of Chicago's West Side, I realized the situation was probably something far less dramatic. Darraugh and his mother no doubt merely had the usual frictions of any family.

Whatever their history, Ms. Graham resented her son's fail-ure to visit her as often as she wanted. I wondered if phantom lights in the upper windows were a way of forcing Darraugh to pay attention to her. I foresaw the possibility of getting squeezed between these two strong personalities. At least it beat fretting about Morrell.

3

Hands Across the Water

It was the thought of Geraldine Graham's binoculars that determined me to slide through the grounds around Larchmont Hall Sunday night without showing a light or making the kind of ruckus I'd set up if I tripped and broke an ankle. She had called once already during the day to make sure I was coming out. I asked if she'd seen her flickering lights the night before; she hadn't, she said, but she didn't spend the whole night looking for them as I would. Just as I was stiffening at being treated like a hired hand, she disarmed me, saying, "Even ten years ago, I was still strong enough to spend the night looking for intruders. I can't now."

I wore my night-prowler's costume: black jeans, dark windbreaker over a sweater, black cap pulling my hair flat against my head, charcoal on my cheeks to keep the moonlight from reflecting off my skin. Ms. Graham's eyes would have to be good to find me even with her Rigel optics.

For tonight's trip, I parked on one of the residential streets on the northeast corner of the New Solway township. I walked the two miles south along Dirksen, the road that divided New Solway from a golf course on its eastern boundary.

Dirksen Road didn't have any sidewalks, the idea of people on foot apparently being beyond New Solway's budget, or maybe their imagination. I kept having to duck into a ditch to get out of the way of traffic. When I finally reached the entrance to Coverdale Lane, I was out of breath, and peevish. I leaned against one of the pervasive stone pillars to pick burrs out of my jeans.

Once I left Dirksen Road, I was enveloped in night. The lights of the suburbs—the houses, the streetlamps, the relentless traffic—faded. Coverdale Lane was far enough from the hedge that guarded New Solway to block out both the streetlamps and the traffic beyond.

The dark silence made me feel untethered from the world. The moon provided some light, but clouds shrouded it, making it hard to stay on the asphalt. I kept veering into the weeds growing alongside the road. I'd measured the distance from Dirksen Road to the mansion in my car yesterday morning: two-thirds of a mile. About twelve hundred paces for me, but I lost count after six hundred something, and the dark distorted my sense of distance. The night creatures, moving about on their own errands, began to loom large in my mind.

I froze at a rustling in the underbrush. It stopped when I stopped, but started again after a few minutes. My palms grew wet on the flashlight as the rustling came closer. I gripped the stock so I could use it as a weapon and switched the beam on at its narrowest focus. A raccoon halted at the light, stared at me for a full minute, then sauntered back into the bushes with what seemed an insolent shrug of furry shoulders.

A few paces later, Larchmont Hall suddenly appeared, its pale brick making it loom like a ghostly galleon in the moonlight. I used my own night-vision binoculars now, but didn't see anyone in front of me. I circled the outbuildings cautiously, disturbing more raccoons and a fox, but didn't see any people.

I picked my way to the edge of the garden, where I could get a bit of a vantage point for the back of the house. The attic windows were dark. I perched on a bench to wait.

I'd been curious enough about Darraugh's family history to do a little research, spending the afternoon in the Chicago Historical Society's library, where I pored over old society columns and news stories. It felt soothing to be in a library, handling actual pieces of paper with people around me, instead of perching alone in front of a blinking cursor. I'd learned a lot of local history, but I wasn't sure how much of it illuminated Darraugh's life.

Geraldine Graham's grandfather had started a paper mill on the Illinois River in 1877, which he'd turned into a fortune before the century ended. The Drummond mills in Georgia and South Carolina once employed nine thousand people. They'd shut most of those plants in the downturn of the last decade, but still had one major mill going in Georgia. In fact, I had once done some work down there for Darraugh, but he hadn't mentioned its ties to his mother's family. Drummond Paper had merged with Continental Industries in 1940; the Drummond name remained only on the paper division.

Geraldine's father had built Larchmont for his wife in 1903; Geraldine, her brother Stuart, and a sister who died young had been born there. The *Chicago American* had reported on the gala around the housewarming, where the Taverners, the McCormicks, Armors and other Chicago luminaries spent a festive evening. The whole story was like one of those period pieces on public television.

Your roving correspondent had to rove with a vengeance to get to the opening of Larchmont Hall, riding the tram to the train and the train to its farthest reaches, where a chara-banc obligingly scooped her up along with the men deliver-ing plants, lobsters and all manner else of delightful edibles to adorn the fête. She arrived perforce in advance of the more regal guests and had plenty of time to scope the grounds, where tables and chairs were set up for taking tea alfresco. Dinner, of course, was served in the grand dining room, whose carved walnut table seats thirty.

The tessellated entrance floor took the Italian workers eight months to complete, but it is worth the effort, the green and sienna and palest ecru of the tiles forming a rich yet un-

obtrusive foretaste of the splendors within. Your correspon-
dent peeped into Mr. Drummond's study, a most masculine
sanctum, redolent of leather, with deep red curtains drawn
across the mullioned windows so that the great man isn't
tempted by the beauties of nature to abandon his important
tasks.

Of course, the greatest beauty of all is within. Mrs.
Matthew Drummond, née Miss Laura Taverner, was the
cynosure of all eyes when she appeared in her embroidered
tulle over pale cornflower satin, the gold chiffon tunic edged
with rhinestones (from Worth's own hands, my dears, as
Mrs. Drummond's maid whispered, arrived last week from
Paris), with a display of ostrich plumes and diamonds that
were the envy of every other lady. Mrs. Michael Taverner,
Mrs. Drummond's sister-in-law, seemed almost to faint with
misery when she saw how commonplace her rose charmeuse
appeared. Of course, Mrs. Edwards Bayard has a mind
above dress, as everyone who has seen that mauve bom-
bazine a thousand times or so could testify—or perhaps her
husband's extra-domestic activities are funded from her
clothes budget!

The coy correspondent recounted with a wealth of description the thirteen bedrooms, the billiard room, the music room
where Mrs. Drummond's spectacular performance on the piano
held dinner guests spellbound, the ornamental pool lined with
blue clay and the three motorcars which Mr. Drummond had in-
stalled in the new "garage, as we hear the English are calling the
structure for housing these modern conveyances."

How very modern of old Matthew Drummond. The garage,
which loomed to my right, could hold six modern motorcars
with room for a machine shop to repair them. Then, as now,
vast wealth needed flaunting. How else did others know you
had it?

After reading about Larchmont's wonders, I'd searched various indices, looking for news of Geraldine. I wanted actually

to see who Darraugh's father had been, or what had happened
to engender the contempt in Geraldine's voice when she mentioned him. It was more than idle curiosity: I wanted to know
what currents lay beneath my client's surface so I could avoid
falling in them and getting swept away.

I found Geraldine's birth in 1912—a "happy event," as the
language of a century ago put it, a baby sister to keep little Stuart Drummond company. The next report was of her coming-
out party in 1929 with other girls from the Vina Fields
Academy. Her Poiret tulle gown was described in detail, including the diamond chips bordering the front drapery. Apparently the crash in the market hadn't kept the family from
pulling out all the stops. After all, some people did make
money from the disaster—maybe Matthew Drummond had
been among them.

The next family news was a clip welcoming Geraldine home
from Switzerland in the spring of 1931, this time in a white Ba-
lenciaga suit, "looking interestingly thin after her recent illness." I raised my brows at this: was it TB, or had Laura
Taverner Drummond hustled her daughter to Europe to deal
with an unwelcome pregnancy?

There'd been a major depression on in the thirties, but you
wouldn't know that from the society pages. Descriptions of
gowns costing five or even ten thousand dollars dotted the gos-
sip columns. Money like that would have supported my father's
family in comfort for a year. He'd been nine in 1931, deliver-
ing coal in the mornings before school to help the family eke
out a living after his father got laid off. I'd never met my grandfather, whose health deteriorated under the strain of not being
able to support his family. He'd died in 1946, right after my
parents were married.

No considerations like that marred Geraldine Drummond's
1940 wedding to MacKenzie Graham. The ceremony was a no-
holds-barred affair at Fourth Presbyterian Church on North
Michigan Avenue—eight attendants, two young ring bearers,
followed by a reception at the Larchmont estate so lavish that I

was surprised the mansion hadn't collapsed from the weight of the caviar. The happy couple left for two months in South America—the European war precluded a French destination.

Reading between the lines, it sounded as though Geraldine had been force-fed to the son of some business crony of her father's. Her one brother, Stuart, had died in a car wreck without leaving any children, so Geraldine was presumably the heir to all the Drummond enterprises. Maybe Matthew and Laura Drummond chose a son-in-law they thought could manage the family holdings. Or maybe Laura had chosen someone she could control herself—in the wedding photos, the bridegroom looked hunted and unhappy.

MacKenzie Graham stayed at Larchmont Hall until his death in 1957. Tidy obituaries in all the papers, death at home of natural causes. Which could mean anything from cancer to bleeding to death from a shooting accident. Maybe that was what had turned Darraugh against Larchmont, seeing his father die here.

Cold was seeping through my layers of jacket and sweatshirt. Despite the unsettling mildness of the weather—here it was, early March, with no snow, and no hard freeze all winter—it was still too cold to sit for long. I got up from the bench and backed up to the meadow so I could see the upper windows. Nothing.

I made another circuit of the building, stubbing my toe on the same loose brick I'd hit the previous two times. Cursing, I sat on a step by the pool and listened to the night around me. For a time, I heard only the skittering of night creatures in the underbrush along Larchmont's perimeter. Every now and then, a car would drive down Coverdale Lane, but no one stopped. A deer tiptoed across the lawn. When it saw me move in the moonlight, it bolted back across the meadow.

Suddenly, over the wind, I heard a louder crashing in the undergrowth beyond the garage. That wasn't a fox or raccoon. Adrenaline rushed through my body. I jumped to my feet. The crashing stopped. Had the newcomer seen me? I tried to melt into the shrubbery lining the ornamental garden, tried not to breathe. After a moment, I heard the whicking of feet on brick: the newcomer had moved from dead leaves to walkway. Two feet, not four. A person who knew his way, coming purposefully forward.

I dropped to my belly and slithered around the pool toward the house, sticking to the paths so I wouldn't announce myself on dead leaves. When I reached the shelter of a great beech, I cautiously lifted my head, straining at the shadows of the trees and bushes. All at once, a darker shadow appeared, ectoplasmic limbs floating and wavering in the moonlight. A slight figure, with a backpack making a hump in the silhouette, moving with the ease of youth.

I put my face back down in the turf so that moonlight wouldn't glint from the white of my nose. The figure passed a couple of yards from my head, but didn't pause. When I heard him at the north wall of the house, I got up and tiptoed after him. He must have seen the movement reflected in the French doors, because he whirled on his heel. Before he could bolt, I was running full tilt, tackling him around the knees. He cried out and fell underneath my weight.

It wasn't a youth at all but a girl, with a pale narrow face and dark hair pulled back into a long braid. Her skin gave off the sour sweat of fear. I rolled away from her, but kept a strong grip on her shoulder. When she tried to break away, I tightened my hold.

"What are you doing here?" I demanded.

"What are *you* doing here?" she hissed, terrified but fierce. Our breath made little white puffs in the night air.

"I'm a detective. I'm following up a report of housebreakers."

"Oh, I see: you work for the pigs." Fear muted her scorn.

"That insult was old when I was your age. Are you Patty Hearst, stealing from your fellow robber barons to give to the terrorists, or Joan of Arc, rescuing the nation?"

The moon was riding high in the sky now; its cold light

shone on the girl, turning her soft young face to marble. She scowled at my mockery but didn't rise to the bait.

"I'm minding my own business. Why don't you mind yours?"

"Are you the person who's flashing a light in this house in the middle of the night?"

It's hard to read expressions in the moonlight, but I thought she looked startled, even afraid, and she said quickly, "I came here on a dare. The other kids thought I was too chicken to go through this big deserted place at night."

"And they're lurking on the perimeter to see you make good on your word. Try another story."

"You don't have any right to question me. I'm not breaking any law."

"That's true, not yet, anyway, although it looked as though breaking and entering was going to be your next step. Is this where you and your boyfriend come to make out?"

Her eyes squinched shut in disgust. "Are you with the sex police? If I want to fuck my boyfriend, I'll do it in comfort at home, not squirreling around in some abandoned attic."

"So you know that the light is coming from the attic. That's interesting."

She gasped but rallied. "*You* said it was the attic."

"No. I said the house. But you and I both know you know what's going on in here, so let's not dance that dance."

Her soft mouth puckered into a scowl. "I'm not breaking any laws, so let me go. Then I won't sue you for assaulting me."

"You're too young to sue me yourself, but I suppose your parents will do it for you. Since you came on foot, you're probably from one of these mansions. I suppose you're like all the other rich kids I've ever met, so overindulged you never have to take responsibility for anything you do."

That did rouse her. "I am responsible!" she shouted.

She wriggled out of my slackened grasp and rolled over. I grabbed at her arm, but only got her backpack. A furry wad came loose in my hands as she wrenched herself free. She sprinted through the opening to the gardens. I jumped up after her, stuffing the furry thing into my jeans as I ran.

As I crashed through the garden, she disappeared around the pond, heading for the woods behind the outbuildings. I charged up the path and tripped again on the loose brick. I was going too fast to catch my balance. I flapped my arms desperately, trying to keep upright, but tumbled sideways into the water. Weeds and leaves clogged the surface. The water was only five feet deep, but I panicked, terrified that I wouldn't be able to push my head through the tangled roots. When I finally broke through the rotting mass, I was several yards from the edge. I was freezing, my clothes so heavy with the brackish water that they pinned me like an iron shroud. My feet slipped on the clay bottom and I grabbed at the plants to stay upright. Instead my numb fingers closed around clammy flesh. One of the dead carp. I backed away in disgust so fast I fell over again. As I righted myself, I realized it wasn't a fish I'd seized but a human hand.

4

Once More unto the Pokey,
Dear Friends

I worked my way around to the head. It was a man, weighted down by his clothes, kept on the surface only by the tangle of weeds underneath him. I thrust my arm under his armpits and started dragging him, holding his head out of the water in case he wasn't really dead. My feet kept slipping on the clay bottom. Pulling his waterlogged weight through that muck made my heart hammer. After some enormity of time, I managed to haul him to the pool's edge. The water was half a foot below the pool's perimeter. I took a deep breath, squatted in the rank plants, and did a dead lift to get him out.

My arm and leg muscles burned with fatigue. My own legs weighed about a ton each now. I lay my torso across the marble tiles surrounding the pool and managed to swing my legs over the side. My teeth were chattering so violently that my whole body shook. I lay on the sharp stone for a minute, but I couldn't afford to stay here. I was remote from help; I'd die of cold if I didn't move.

I got to my hands and knees and crawled to the man. I rolled him onto his back and cleaned the weeds out of his mouth and undid his tie and pushed on his chest and blew cold trembly gusts into his mouth, and, after five minutes, he was still as dead as he'd been when I'd clutched his hand in the water.

By now I was so cold I felt as though someone was slicing my skull with knives. I pried the zipper of my windbreaker open and dug my cell phone out of one of the pockets. I couldn't believe my luck: the little screen blinked its green lights at me and I was able to connect to the emergency network.

The dispatcher had trouble understanding me, my teeth were chattering so loudly. Larchmont Hall, could I identify that? The first house you came to off the Dirksen Road entrance to Coverdale Lane? Could I turn on my car lights or the house lights so the emergency crew could find me? I'd come on foot? Just what was I doing there?

"Just tell the New Solway cops to come to Larchmont Hall," I croaked. "They'll find it."

I severed the connection and looked wistfully at the house behind me. Maybe the dot-com millionaires had forgotten a bathrobe, or even a kitchen towel, when they left. I was halfway to the house when I realized that this would be my one chance alone with the dead man. Larchmont Hall was sealed like Fortress America. Without tools, with my hands frozen, I'd be lucky to have a door open before the cops arrived, but I'd have enough time to look for some ID on the body.

I found my flashlight near the French doors where I'd wrestled with the girl. I took it back with me to the dead man.

Was this my teenager's boyfriend? Despite her smart remark about the sex police, were they meeting in the abandoned house—somehow bypassing the security system? Maybe he hadn't made tonight's rendezvous because he'd tripped over the same brick I'd stumbled on, fallen into the pond and hadn't been able to fight free of the weeds. He hadn't tried to take off his shoes or his clothes: I'd undone his tie and unbuttoned his shirt to give him CPR, but he had on a suit; belt, fly button and zipper were all tidily done up. The suit looked as though it had been a good one, a brown wool basket weave. He'd been wearing wing tips, not an outfit for the woods at night.

I moved my flashlight along the length of his body. He was about six feet tall, lean, not particularly athletic looking. His skin was a nut-brown, his hair African, which might explain the need for secret meetings in an abandoned house. Or maybe it was his age—he looked to be in his thirties. I could picture the girl attracted to an affair with an African-American: the need to do something dramatic, something daring, was clearly strong in her.

Who was he? Who would meet his end in such a remote and dreadful way? I dug gingerly into the pockets. Like my own, they had clammed shut from the weight of the water. I had a hard job of it, as cold as I was, and I wasn't rewarded with much when I finished. There was nothing in his jacket or his front trouser pockets but a handful of change. I gritted my teeth and stuck my hand under his buttocks. The back pockets were empty, too, except for a pencil and a matchbook.

No one in the modern age goes out in a suit and tie without a wallet, or at least a driver's license. But where was his car? Had he done like me? Parked two miles away and come on foot for a secret rendezvous?

My head was aching so with cold I couldn't think clearly, but I'd have been bewildered even if I were warm and dry. I know people drown in their baths in panic, and I myself had had a moment's terror when I couldn't get my head through those weeds, but why had he left all his papers at home? Had he come here on purpose to die? Was this some dramatic event planned for my teenager? Come out in the open about me or I'll kill myself? He looked in repose like a steady man, not the person for such dramatic actions. It was hard to picture him as Romeo to my young heroine's Juliet.

When the emergency crew arrived, I was still holding his matchbook and pencil. I stuck them into my own jacket pocket so I wouldn't be caught in the act of stripping the body.

Besides a fire department ambulance, the dispatcher had sent both the New Solway cops and the DuPage County sheriff's police. The body had turned up in unincorporated New Solway.

That technically meant it belonged to the DuPage County sheriff, but the dispatcher had also notified the New Solway police. Even in my frozen state, I could understand why. The houses along Coverdale Lane were a who's who of greater Chicago Big Money: New Solway cops would want an inside track on who to blame if the local barons—or baronesses—got testy.

The two groups jockeyed for dominance in inspecting the body. They wanted to know who I was and what I was doing there. Through my chattering teeth I told them my name, but said I couldn't talk until I was some place warm.

The two forces bickered for another long minute while I shivered uncontrollably, then compromised by letting the New Solway police ride along while the sheriff's deputies took me to Wheaton.

"My God, you stink," the sheriff's deputy said when I climbed into his squad car.

"That's just the rotting vegetation," I muttered. "I'm clean inside."

He wanted to open the windows to air out the smell, but I told him if I ended up with pneumonia I'd see he footed the medical bills. "You have a blanket or an old jacket or something in the trunk?" I added. "I'm wet and freezing and your pals waiting for the shift change so they wouldn't have to take the call didn't help any: it's been over forty minutes since I phoned."

"Yeah, bastards," he said, then cut off the rest of the sentence, annoyed with me for voicing his grievance. He stomped around to the trunk and fished out an old towel. It couldn't be any dirtier than I was: I draped it around my head and was asleep before the car left the yard.

When we got to the sheriff's headquarters in Wheaton, I was so far gone I didn't wake up until some strong young deputy yanked me out of the backseat and braced me on my feet. I stumbled into the building, joints stiff in my clammy clothes.

"Wake up, Sleeping Beauty," the deputy snapped. "You need to tell us what you were doing on private property out here."

"Not until I'm clean and dry," I mumbled through cracked

and swollen lips. "You must have some clothes out here I can borrow."

The deputy who'd brought me in said that was highly irregular, they didn't treat housebreakers like hotel guests in DuPage County. I sat on a bench and began undoing the zipper on my windbreaker. A chunk of some dead plant had worked its way around the pull. My fingers were thick with cold, and I worked slowly while the deputy stood over me wanting to know what in hell I thought I was doing. The zipper took all my attention. When I finally had the jacket undone, I pulled off the wet sweater underneath. I was starting to take off my bottom layer, a T-shirt, when he grabbed my shoulder and yanked me back to my feet.

"What are you doing?"

"What it looks like. Taking off my wet clothes."

"You can't do that out here. You produce some ID and some reason for being on private property in the middle of the night."

By now, a number of other officers, including a couple of women, had joined him. I looked past him and said to them, "Darraugh Graham asked me to check on Larchmont Hall. You know, the old Drummond estate where his mother lived until the year before last. It's been standing empty and she thought she was seeing housebreakers. I found a dead man in the pool behind the house and got thoroughly soaked pulling him out. And that's all I can say until I get clean and dry."

"And how you planning on proving that story?" my deputy sneered.

One of the women gave him a sour look. "Be your age, Barney. You never heard of Darraugh Graham? Come along," she added to me.

My eyes were swelling with the onset of a head cold. I squinted at her badge. S. Protheroe.

Protheroe led me to the women's locker room, where I toweled myself dry. She even dug up an old set of uniform trousers and a sweatshirt, a size or two too big on me but clean. "We keep spares out here for officers who've been through the

wringer. You can sign for 'em on your way out and get 'em back
to us in the next week. You want to tell me your name and what
you were really doing out here?"

I pulled on clean socks and looked with disgust at my shoes.
The tiled floor was cold, but my shoes would have been worse.
I sat on the locker room bench and told her my name, my relationship to Darraugh, his mother's belief that there were intruders in her old home, my fruitless surveillance—and the body I'd
stumbled on. I don't know why I didn't feed her my young
Juliet. Native caution, maybe, or maybe because I like ardent
young women. I dug my wallet out of my windbreaker and
showed her my PI license, fortunately walled in laminate.

Protheroe handed it back to me without comment, except to
say the state's attorney would want some formal statement
about finding the dead man. When she saw me rolling my foul
clothes into a bundle, she even found a plastic bag in a supply
cupboard.

Protheroe took me to a room on the second floor and called
someone on her cell phone. "Lieutenant Schorr will be along in
a minute. You do much work out here? No? Well, I know the
Cook County sheriff's office is a cesspool of Democratic patronage and favors. Out here it's different. Out here it's a
cesspool of Republican patronage. So don't mind the boys,
they're not all real well trained."

Lieutenant Schorr arrived with a couple of male sidekicks
and a woman who announced she was Vanna Landau, the assistant state's attorney. One of the New Solway police officers had
stayed for the meeting, as well. A fifth man came hurrying in a
minute later, straightening the knot in his tie. He was introduced
as Larry Yosano, a member of the law firm that had handled
Larchmont's sale—apparently a very junior member.

"Thanks, Stephanie," Schorr dismissed my guide. She gave
me a discreet thumbs-up and left.

I was used to Chicago police interrogation rooms, with their
scarred tables and peeling paint, and where strong disinfectants
don't quite cover the traces of vomit. Stephanie Protheroe had

brought me to something like a modern boardroom, with a television and camcorder ruling over blond furniture. Behind the modern façade, though, the smell of disinfectant and stale fear rose to greet me like an unwelcome neighbor.

Vanna Landau, the ASA, was a small woman who leaned across the table as if trying to make herself bigger by taking up as much room as possible. "Now just what were you doing on the land?"

In between coughs and sneezes, I explained in as mild a voice as I could summon.

"Spying on Larchmont Hall in the middle of the night?" Landau said. "That is trespassing, at a minimum."

I pinched the skin between my eyebrows in an effort to stay awake. "Would it have been better if I'd done it in daylight? Geraldine Graham was worried when she saw intruders around the house late at night. At her son's request, I went over to take a look."

Larry Yosano, the young lawyer, was trying to rub sleep out of his own eyes. "Technically, of course, it's trespass, but if you've ever dealt with Mrs. Graham, you'd know that she's never really acknowledged that she no longer owns Larchmont. She's a strong personality, difficult to say no to."

He turned to me. "Lyons Trust is the titleholder. They're the ones you should call if Mrs. Graham sees a problem with the property."

I didn't say anything except to ask for a Kleenex. One of the deputies found some paper napkins in a drawer and tossed them across the table at me.

"Or the police," Lieutenant Schorr said. "Did that ever occur to you, Ms. Private Eye?"

"Ms. Graham called the New Solway police several times. They thought she was a crazy old woman making stuff up."

The New Solway cop, whose name I hadn't heard, bristled. "We went out there three times and saw nothing. Yesterday, when someone really was on the property, we responded to the alarm within fifteen minutes. Her own son even says she could be making stuff up because she wants attention."

I sat up at that. "I met with Ms. Graham yesterday afternoon. She didn't strike me as delusional at all. I know she's old, but if she says she's seeing lights in that house she is. What about the man in the pool? If nothing else, him being there proves someone was using that abandoned estate for something."

"I don't think Mrs. Graham makes things up," Yosano agreed, "but she doesn't listen to advice. We, for instance, advised her to move away from New Solway when she sold, but her ties to the community are very deep, of course."

I had a picture of the hapless dot-com millionaire, fending off Geraldine Graham's efforts to help him run Larchmont the way her mother had done.

The young state's attorney seemed to feel the interview was slipping away; she demanded to know my relationship to the dead man.

"We kissed once, very deeply . . ." I waited until one of the deputies had eagerly written this down before adding, ". . . when I was doing CPR on him. His mouth was full of the crud in the pool and I had to clean that out first . . . Did you get that? Need me to spell any of the words?"

"So you don't admit to knowing him?" Vanna Landau said.

"The verb 'admit' makes it sound like you think knowing him is a crime." I sneezed again. "Does that mean you know who he is? Some DuPage County career criminal whom it would be dangerous to admit knowing?"

"Black guy on the land, what else was he but a criminal?" one of the deputies snickered to his fellow.

I reached across the table and ripped a sheet from the state's attorney's legal pad. "Let me just write this last comment down word for word to make sure I have the quote exactly right when I call the *Herald-Star* tomorrow. 'Black guy on the land, what else was he but a criminal.' Right?"

"Barney, why don't you and Teddy go get us some coffee while we wrap this up," Schorr said to his deputies. When they had left, he pulled the paper away from me and balled it up. "It's late, we're all pretty tired and not using our best minds on this problem. Let's just go over a few last questions and let you get back to Chicago where you belong. Do you, or do you not, know who the dead man is?"

"I never saw him until tonight. I can't add anything to this discussion. You have any preliminary report from the ME?" I could feel a sore throat rising up my tonsils.

Schorr and the ASA exchanged looks. She pursed her lips but picked up the phone at her end of the table. She had a brisk conversation with one of the ME techs and shook her head. Even under the cold light of the DuPage County morgue, no one had found any clues I'd overlooked.

"You'll run a photo in the papers and on the news, right?" I said to the ASA. "And a full autopsy, including dental impressions?"

"We know our job out here," she said stiffly.

"Just asking. I wouldn't want to think that because he was a black man, you wouldn't put your best effort into cause of death and so on."

"You don't need to worry about that," Schorr said, the fake good humor in his voice not masking the anger in his face. "You go on home and leave this investigation to us."

When I told him where I'd left my car, he gave an exaggerated sigh and said he supposed one of the deputies could drive me, but I'd have to wait in the front hall.

My hamstrings had stiffened while we sat. I stumbled on my way out of the room. Larry Yosano, the young lawyer, caught my arm to keep me from falling. When I thanked him, I wondered why he'd joined our happy band tonight.

He yawned. "I'm the junior on call for difficult problems this week. We handle affairs for most of the estates in New Solway; we have keys, so if the lieutenant had wanted to get into the house I could have let him in. In fact, when they called me, I drove over to Larchmont, but your group had already left for here. I took some time to check the alarm; it hadn't been set off, and it's still functioning. I had a quick look around the ground floor, but there wasn't any sign of an intruder."

He yawned more widely. "I wish Lyons Trust—they're the titleholders—would find a buyer. It's not good to have a place like that standing empty. We advised hiring a caretaker, but the bank didn't want to spend the money."

Deputy Protheroe, the woman who'd given me my dry clothes, appeared: she'd been elected to drive me. Yosano walked out with us. Before climbing into his BMW, he gave me a card. I squinted at it through my swollen eyes: he was an associate with Lebold, Arnoff, offices in Oak Brook and LaSalle Street. I'd never heard of them, but I don't often have to deal with the property issues of the superrich.

"Give Geraldine Graham my number the next time she calls," Yosano said. "I'll try to talk her out of more private surveillance at Larchmont."

My cards were gummed together in my wallet. I wrote my office number on a scrap of paper for him.

"You awake enough to get that car of yours home?" Protheroe asked when we reached the Mustang. "I don't want to be called out in half an hour to scrape your body off the tollway. There's a Motel 6 up the road. Maybe you'd better check in for what's left of the night."

I knew I was tired enough to be at risk behind the wheel, but I was feeling so rotten that I wanted my own bed. I summoned a travesty of bravado, sketching a two-fingered salute and a smile. The dashboard clock read three-fifteen when I pointed my little Mustang toward the city.

5

Stochastic Excursion

I was in a cave, looking for Morrell. Someone had handed me a wailing infant; I was hunched over, trying to get out of the way of massive roots that pushed down through the rocks. The air was so bad I couldn't breathe; the rocks themselves were squeezing the air out of me. The infant howled more loudly. Next to me lay the body of a black man in a brown weave suit, dead from the bad air. A buzzing in the distance meant an air-raid warning. From far away I could hear planes whining overhead.

The howling of the planes, the wailing of the infant, finally forced me awake. The phone and downstairs doorbell were ringing simultaneously, but my head cold left me too groggy to bestir myself. I didn't even stick out a hand for the phone but rolled over onto my side, hoping to relieve the pressure in my sinuses.

I was startled to see the clock read two-forty: I'd slept the whole day away. I tried to raise a sense of urgency about the man I'd found last night, or about the girl I'd tackled, but I couldn't manage it.

I was just drifting back to sleep when someone pushed the buzzer right outside my third-floor door. Three insistent hoots, and then I heard a key in the lock. That meant one thing: Mr. Contreras, who has keys to my place, with strict orders to save them for emergencies—which he and I define very differently. I couldn't deal with him while flat on my back. By the time his heavy tread sounded in my hall, I'd pulled on a sweatshirt and the pants I'd borrowed from DuPage County last night.

He started talking before he got to the bedroom door. "Doll, you okay? Your car's out front and you ain't been out all day, but Mr. Graham, he just sent over a messenger with a letter for you. When you didn't even come to the door, I got kinda worried."

"Yeah, I'm okay." My voice sounded like Poe's raven after a night mainlining chloroform.

"You sick, doll? What happened to you? It was on the news, you being out in wherever diving into a pond after a dead guy. You have pneumonia or what?"

The dogs pelted down the hall and circled around me with delighted yips. All was forgiven in the three days since I'd last force-marched them down Lake Michigan to the Loop—they were ready for action. I fondled their ears.

"Just a cold. I didn't get home until four this morning—been sleeping. 'Scuse minute." I snuffled down to the bathroom, blenching at the sight of my face in the mirror. I looked worse than I sounded. My eyes were puffy. I had a bruise across my cheekbone and more on my arms and legs. I hadn't noticed banging myself up so badly when I was hefting bodies around the Larchmont estate last night.

I turned the hot water on in the shower and steamed myself for a few minutes. When I emerged, clean, and, thankfully, dressed in my own clothes, my neighbor had produced a large mug of tea with lemon and honey. Unlike Geraldine Graham's gilt eggshells, mine were real mugs, thick, clunky—and cheap.

"When I heard the news, them saying you'd been brought in to DuPage County for questioning about this dead man, I thought maybe you'd been arrested. You been fighting? You got some case that's gonna kill you and you ain't said nothing to me?" His brown eyes were bright with hurt.

"Nothing like that."

When I'd croaked out enough explanation to satisfy him, he suddenly remembered Darraugh's letter. The blistering prose raised welts on my fingers. ·

*I have been trying to reach you all day to find out why you
sent the police to my mother without informing me first. Since
you aren't answering your phone or e-mail I am sending this
by hand. Call immediately on receipt of this message.*

How nice to be the man in charge and bulldoze your way
through people as if they were construction sites. I checked in
with my answering service. Christie Weddington, the operator
I've known longest, answered. "Is that really you, Vic? Just to be
safe I'd better do our security check. What was your mother's
maiden name?" When I'd spelled "Sestieri" she added severely,
"When you're going to hole up, can you let us know? Now that
Mary Louise has left your company, you don't have any backup
person to call for emergencies. We got like eleven calls from
Darraugh Graham's office, and five from Murray Ryerson."

Darraugh, or his PA, Caroline, had started in at ten and kept it
up every half hour. Geraldine Graham had phoned four times
herself, the first time at a quarter of ten. So the DuPage sheriff
had been to see her by nine. At least they were taking it seriously.
Murray had called early, before eight, presumably when he'd
looked at the morning wires. I got back to him first, in case he
knew something that would help me in my conversation with
Darraugh. Murray was indignant that I hadn't called him when
the blood was fresh enough to lick.

"Have they ID'd the guy yet?" I croaked into his barrage of
questions.

"You sound like a frog in a cheese grater, Warshawski. So far
the DuPage sheriff is clueless. I gather they're running your John
Doe's prints through AFIS. And they've put his picture on the
wires."

"They have a cause of death?" I wheezed.

"He drowned. What were you doing, Warshawski, turning up
so pat minutes after the guy plunged to his watery death?"

"You should write for the *Enquirer,* with prose like that. You
drive out to Larchmont? No one could plunge to a watery death
in five feet of water. Either he did like me, tripped and fell, or—"

A coughing fit interrupted me. Mr. Contreras leaped up to pour me more tea, and to mutter that Murray was an inconsiderate jerk, keeping me talking when I was sick.

"—or he went in on purpose or he was put there," Murray finished for me. "What's your theory? Did it look as though he'd struggled?"

I shut my eyes, trying to remember the body as I'd found it. "I only had my flashlight to augment the moon, so I can't say whether he had unusual bruises or scratches. But his clothes were tidy—no undone buttons, and his tie was still neatly knotted. I undid it when I was trying CPR."

"Cross your heart, you never saw him before?" Murray demanded.

"Hope to die," I coughed.

"So you didn't go out there to meet him?"

"No!" I was getting impatient. "He's what Professor Wright used to call a 'stochastic excursion' in my physics class."

"Then what about the 'Warshawski excursion'?" Murray asked. "What were you doing in the land of hope and glory?"

"Catching the cold of a lifetime." I hung up as a cough started racking me again.

"You oughta go back to bed, cookie," Mr. Contreras fussed over me. "You can't talk, you won't have any voice at all you keep at it. That Ryerson, he just uses you."

"Street runs both ways," I choked. "I have to call Darraugh."

Darraugh interrupted a meeting on the fate of his Georgia paper division to take my call. "Mother had the police with her this morning."

"That must have pleased her," I said.

"Excuse me?" The frost in his voice turned the phone to dry ice against my ear.

"She likes people to attend to her. You don't visit her enough, the cops didn't respond when she told them about intruders in your boyhood home. Now she's gotten the attention she thinks is her due."

"You should have reported to me at once when you found a dead man at the house. I don't pay you to leave me in the dark."

"Darraugh, you're right." My words came out with annoying slowness, the way they do when you don't have a throat. "Hear how I sound? I got this way falling into your pool. After hauling out a dead man, futilely trying CPR, spending two hours with the sheriff's deputies in Wheaton, it was three-thirty. A.M. I could have called you at home then, but I went to bed instead. Where I regret that I slept through ringing phones, sirens, doorbells and atom bombs. I wish I weren't so human, but there you have it."

"Who was that man and what was he doing at the house?" Darraugh barked after a moment's silence—he wasn't going to agree that I had mitigating circumstances on my side, but he wasn't going to go for my jugular any more right now, either—from him a concession.

I repeated what little information Murray had given me, then said, "Why didn't you tell me Larchmont was your boyhood home?"

Darraugh paused another moment, before saying abruptly he was in an important meeting, but he wanted me to report to him at once if I learned who had died in the pool, and why he'd been there.

"You want me to investigate?" I asked.

"Give it a few hours. Not until your voice is better: no one's going to take you seriously when you sound like this."

"Thanks, Darraugh: chicken soup for the PI's soul," I said, but he'd already hung up. Just as well. He has plenty of options among the big security companies that handle most of his heavy-muscle jobs. He stays with me not because he likes to support small businesses, but because he knows there will be no leaks out of my tiny operation—I get the jobs that he wants total confidentiality for, but, if he got fed up enough, he'd take the work elsewhere.

When Mr. Contreras finally left with the dogs, I lay down on the couch. I didn't go back to sleep—I actually felt better after being on my feet for a bit. I put on an old LP of Leontyne Price singing Mozart and watched the shadows change on the ceiling.

I had one little bit of information that no one else did: the teenage girl. It wasn't only a wish to keep a hole card, although of course I wanted one, but that her spunk and ardor reminded me of my own youth; I felt protective of her the way you do of your childhood. I wanted to find her on my own before deciding whether the cops or reporters ought to have a crack at her.

I assumed she lived in one of the Coverdale Lane estates. I tried to imagine a strategy for going door-to-door looking for her. I was her scoutmaster coming to collect her Girl Scout cookie sales money. I was looking for my lost Borzoi. I'd found emerald earrings when I was jogging and wanted to restore them to the owner.

Perhaps I could check the area high school, although who knows where people in mansions like those in New Solway send their children. Not only that, I'd only seen the girl briefly, by moonlight. I wasn't sure I'd recognize her again, let alone be able to describe her.

I shut my eyes and tried to conjure her face, but all I remembered was her long braid and the soft cheeks of youth, the planes or lines that might show character not yet formed. Had she said anything that might lead me to her? I was a pig, she'd bet with some of the other kids, she knew someone was in the attic. What had I said that got her so mad she'd run away? Something about not taking responsibility for—

And then I remembered the little thing that had come loose in my hand when she jerked free. I had stuffed it into my jeans pocket. And my jeans were in the garbage bag the sheriff's deputy had given me.

I'd dumped the bag in the front hall when I came in this morning. With a gingerly hand, I fished out the damp, mud-caked pants. Rotted leaves and threads of plant roots fell away when I shook them out. I had a feeling I was lucky be too congested to smell them. I had to pry the pocket flap open and pull the whole pocket inside out to get the thing I'd torn from my teenager's backpack. It was black with mud.

When I ran it under the kitchen tap for a few minutes, the mud washed off to show an ancient teddy bear. The last few years it's become kind of a fetish with kids, putting the toys of early childhood on their backpacks or binders. A high school senior had told me that the coolest kids use ratty crib toys; wannabes buy them new. So my girl was cool, or aspired to be: this little guy was missing both his eyes, and even without a night in my muddy pocket his fur had been pretty forlorn, worn down to the nub in places.

The distinguishing feature of the bear was a tiny green sweatshirt with gold letters on it. At first I thought it was a Green Bay Packers shirt, which would only narrow my search to the million Packer fans in the Chicago-Milwaukee corridor, but then I saw the tiny *V* and *F* monogrammed around a minuscule stick. The Vina Fields Academy.

Vina Fields Academy used to be a girls' school when Geraldine Graham had gone there, where they'd learned French, dancing and flirting. Since turning coed in the seventies, it's not only become the most expensive private school in the city but an important academic one. The stick on the teddy bear's little shirt was supposed to be the candle or lighthouse or whatever the school uses to illustrate that it's a beacon of light.

I only know all this because I see a life-sized version of the sweatshirt every time I go into La Llorona on Milwaukee Avenue. The owner, Mrs. Aguilar, wasn't noticeably proud of her daughter, Celine, getting a scholarship to attend Vina Fields: she only had one entire wall papered with her yearbook photos from sixth grade on, along with pictures of Celine with the school field hockey team, Celine accepting the top prize in mathematics for her class three years running, and the sweatshirt.

I hadn't eaten for almost twenty-four hours. I might as well drive down there for some of Mrs. Aguilar's chicken soup with tortillas.

Neighborhood Joint

Back when I signed a seven-year lease for my part of a warehouse at the south end of Bucktown, the surrounding neighborhood was chiefly Hispanic, with a handful of starving artists who needed cheap rent. Two *taquerias* within half a block of my front door served fresh tortillas past midnight and I had my choice of palm readers.

This evening as I drove south and west toward my office, all I could see was old six-flats like mine coming down and new town houses going up. Strip malls with identical arrays of Starbucks, wireless companies and home renovation chains were replacing factories and storefronts, as if the affluent were afraid to take chances on neighborhood places. The *taquerias* are a memory. Now I have to walk almost a mile farther south for the nearest good tostada. Of course, tenants like me are one reason the neighborhood is changing, but that doesn't make me any happier about it. Especially when I figure what my next round of lease negotiations will look like.

I drove past my office without stopping, although I could see lights in the tall windows on the north side; my lease partner, Tessa Reynolds, was working late on a sculpture.

A few blocks south of our building, Milwaukee Avenue narrows to Model T width, making for congestion at all hours of the day. I parked at the first meter I came to and walked the last two blocks to La Llorona, threading my way through the kinds of crowds that I knew from my South Side childhood. Worn-out women with litters of children straggling around them were stopping in the markets for dinner, or fingering clothes on the racks set out on the sidewalk. Boys darted in and out of the noisy narrow bars and I saw a girl of about eight slip a hair clip off a table and into her pocket.

When I got to La Llorona, some six or seven women were talking to Mrs. Aguilar while she packed up their families' dinner. Celine was at the cash register, her red-brown hair swept up in a ponytail. She was working math problems in between ringing up purchases.

"*Buenos dias, Señora Aguilar,*" I croaked when Mrs. Aguilar glanced over at me.

"*Buenos dias, Señora Victoria,*" she called back. "You're sick, no? What you need? A bowl of soup? Celine, *chica,* bring soup, okay?"

Celine sighed in the manner of all beleaguered teenagers, but she ducked smartly under the counter to fill a big bowl for me. While I waited, I glanced at her book: *Differential Equations for Math SAT Students.* A snappy title.

I sat at one of three high-topped tables that were stuck in the far corner of the storefront, drinking the soup slowly. When the shop was empty of other customers, I listened to Mrs. Aguilar's endless fret about her bad back and her rotten landlord, who was raising her rent but refused to fix the leaking pipe that had shut her store down for two days last week.

"He want to make it so I go away, then he take down the building and make condos or something."

She was probably right, so I didn't do anything but commiserate. I finally managed to steer the conversation to Mrs. Aguilar's third-favorite topic, Celine's education. I asked if she had a current yearbook for Vina Fields. Mrs. Aguilar came around in front of the counter and pulled it out from the drawer underneath the cash register.

"Field hockey, I don't understand this game, but at this

school it is important, and Celine is the best." Celine squirmed and moved with her equations to one of the high tables. When another handful of customers came in I took the yearbook with me to my table, asking for a refill on the soup.

"Don't get no food on that, Victoria," Mrs. Aguilar admonished me, as she ducked underneath the countertop and returned to her skillets.

I started going through the class pictures, seniors first. So many fresh-faced, self-confident girls, so many with long dark hair and arrogant poise. I stopped at each such face, trying to match it to last night's phantom. I didn't think it had been Alex Dewhurst, favorite sport, showing horses, favorite singers, 'NSYNC, or Rebecca Caudwell, who loved figure skating and wanted to become an attorney, although both were possible.

"What are you looking for?"

I'd been so absorbed I didn't notice Celine shutting down the till and coming to stand next to me. Señora Aguilar was scrubbing down her counters. Time to pack up.

"I ran into one of your classmates when I was on a job last night. She dropped something valuable, but I don't know her name."

"What does she look like?"

"Long dark braid, kind of narrow face."

Celine offered to take the found item with her to school and post a notice on their in-house WebBoard, but I told her the girl probably wouldn't want the circumstances of her loss publicized. When I finished the seniors and moved on to the juniors, I saw my Juliet almost at once. Her eyes were serious despite the half smile the photographer had coaxed from her, and tendrils from her French braid were spiraling around her soft cheeks, as if she'd been too impatient to comb her hair just for a picture. Catherine Bayard, who loved Sarah McLachlan's music, whose favorite sport was lacrosse and who hoped to be a journalist when she grew up. She probably would be: Bayard and publishing, the two words go together in Chicago like Capone and crime.

I didn't linger on Catherine's face—I didn't want Celine alerting her at school the next day. Instead, I shrugged as if giving up the search as a bad job. Celine eyed me narrowly. Girls who work advanced calculus problems find adults like me tiresomely easy to solve. She knew I'd spotted someone, but maybe she couldn't tell who it was.

Before giving the book back, I looked at the faculty section. The director was a woman named Wendy Milford, who had the strong expression principals put on to make you think their young charges don't terrify them. I asked Celine to point out her field hockey coach, and memorized the names of a math and history teacher. You never know.

I closed the book and handed it to her with money for my soup. Three dollars for two bowls—you wouldn't find that in 923 or Mauve, or whatever trendy name you'd see on whatever bistro ultimately muscled La Llorona out of business.

I stopped in my office on my way home. Tessa had left for the day and the building was dark. It was also dankly cold. Tessa mainly wrestles large pieces of steel into towering constructions, work which makes her sweat enough to keep the furnace at sixty. I turned up my thermostat and sat bundled in my coat while I brought my system up.

Calvin Bayard, one of the heroes of my youth. I'd developed a huge crush on him when he addressed my Con Law class at the University of Chicago. With his magnetic smile, his easy command of First Amendment issues, his ready wit in answering hostile questions, he'd seemed in a different world than my professors.

After his lecture, I'd gone to the library to read his testimony before the House Committee on Un-American Activities, which had made me glow with pride. Illinois's own Congressman Walker Bushnell, who'd been a leading member of the House Un-American Activities committee, had hounded Bayard for most of 1954 and 1955. But Bayard's testimony made Bushnell sound like a small-minded voyeur. He had walked away from the hearings without ratting out his friends, and